Therapeutic Gastrointestinal Endoscopy

Therapeutic Gastrointestinal Endoscopy
A problem-oriented approach

Edited by

David Westaby MA FRCP
Consultant Physician and Gastroenterologist,
Chelsea and Westminster Hospital, London

and

Martin Lombard MD MSc FRCPI FRCP(Lond)
Consultant Gastroenterologist and Senior Lecturer,
The Royal Liverpool University Hospitals,
Liverpool

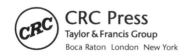

CRC Press
Taylor & Francis Group
Boca Raton London New York

CRC Press is an imprint of the
Taylor & Francis Group, an **informa** business

First published 2002 by Martin Dunitz Ltd

Published 2019 by CRC Press
Taylor & Francis Group
6000 Broken Sound Parkway NW, Suite 300
Boca Raton, FL 33487-2742

First issued in paperback 2019

No claim to original U.S. Government works

ISBN-13: 978-0-367-45508-8 (pbk)
ISBN-13: 978-1-899066-95-7 (hbk)

Visit the Taylor & Francis Web site at
http://www.taylorandfrancis.com

and the CRC Press Web site at
http://www.crcpress.com

British Library Cataloguing in Publication Data
A catalogue record for this title is available from the British Library.

Westaby, D (David), Lombard M (Martin)
Therapeutic Endoscopy
David Westaby, Martin Lombard (eds)

Always refer to the manufacturer's Prescribing
Information before prescribing drugs cited in this book.

Typesetting and image reproduction
Colour Gallery, Malaysia

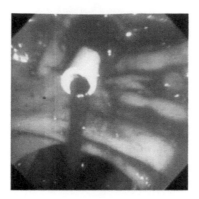

CONTENTS

Professor Hugh Barr MD ChM FRCS FRCSE
Professor and Consultant Surgeon, Cranfield Postgraduate Medical School, Gloucestershire Royal Hospital, Great Western Road, Gloucester GL1 3NN

Professor Stephen G. Bown MD FRCP
Professor of Laser Medicine and Surgery, Director, National Medical Laser Centre, Charles Bell House, 67–73 Riding House Street, London W1P 7PN

Dr Jane Collier
Senior Registrar, Addenbrooke's NHS Trust, Hills Road, Cambridge CB2 2QQ

Dr Peter D. Fairclough MD FRCP
Consultant Gastroenterologist, Barts and The London NHS Trust; Senior Lecturer in Medicine, West Smithfield London EC1A 7BE

Dr Alexander E. S. Gimson FRCP
Consultant Physician and Hepatologist, Medical Services, Box 210, Addenbrooke's NHS Trust, Hills Road, Cambridge CB2 2QQ

Dr Adrian Hatfield
Consultant Physician, Department of Gastroenterology, UCH Middlesex Hospital, Mortimer Street, London W1N 8AA

Prof Neville Krasner MD FRCP(Glas) FRCP
Consultant Gastroenterologist, Gastrointestinal Unit, University Hospital Aintree, Lower Lane, Liverpool L9 7AL

Mr Mark Lamah MB FRCS
Specialist Registrar, Egerton Road, Royal Surrey County Hospital, Guildford, Surrey GU2 5XX

Mr Roger Leicester OBE FRCS
Consultant Colorectal Surgeon, St George's Hospital, Blackshaw Road, Tooting, London SW17 0QT and Endoscopy Tutor, Department of Education, Royal College of Surgeons of England

Dr Martin Lombard MD MSc FRCPI FRCP(Lond)
Consultant Gastroenterologist and Senior Lecturer, The Royal Liverpool University Hospitals, Prescot Street, Liverpool L7 8XP

Dr Anthony I. Morris MSc MD FRCP
Consultant Physician and Gastroenterologist, Clinical Director of Gastroenterology, The Royal Liverpool University Hospitals, Prescot Street, Liverpool L7 8XP

Professor John P. Neoptolemos MA MD FRCS
Professor of Surgery/Head of Department of Surgery, Royal Liverpool University Hospitals, 5th Floor UCD, Daulby Street, Liverpool L69 3GA

Dr Paul A. O'Toole MRCP
Consultant Physician, Gastroenterology Unit, University Hospital Aintree, Lower Lane, Liverpool L9 7AL

Dr Kelvin R. Palmer MD FRCP(Ed)
Consultant Physician, Gastrointestinal Unit, Western General Hospital, Crewe Road, Edinburgh EH4 2XU

Dr Brian P. Saunders MD MRCP
Consultant Gastroenterologist, Wolfson Unit for Endoscopy, St Mark's Hospital, Watford Road, Harrow, Middlesex HA1 3UJ

Mr John Slavin MB BS BSc FRCS(Gen) MS
Senior Lecturer of Surgery, The Royal Liverpool University Hospitals, Daulby Street, Liverpool L69 3GA

Dr David Westaby MA FRCP
Consultant Physician and Gastroenterologist, Gastrointestinal Unit, Chelsea and Westminster Hospital, 369 Fulham Road, London SW10 9NH

Dr Mark L. Wilkinson BSc MD FRCP
Senior Lecturer and Consultant Physician, Department of Gastroenterology, Guy's King's and St. Thomas' School of Medicine, Guy's and St. Thomas' Hospital Trust, 4th floor, Thomas Guy House, London Bridge, London SE1 9RT

Dr Christopher B. Williams MA BM FRCP FRCS
Consultant Physician – Endoscopy, Wolfson Unit for Endoscopy, St. Mark's Hospital, Watford Road, London HA1 3UJ

Dr Simon G.J. Williams MA MD MRCP FRCS
Consultant Physician and Gastroenterologist, The Ipswich Hospital NHS Trust, Heath Road, Ipswich, Suffolk IP4 5PD

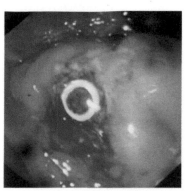

Endoscopy and its applications are now widely available, and the indications for its use continue to expand. It is an exciting and practical field in which to become involved, but developing skills, competence and expertise to undertake endoscopy can be technically demanding. This is even more true when the endoscopist begins to undertake therapeutic procedures. The skills required can only be acquired by practice and application. The trainee rightly has to focus on these skills and there are several 'how-to-do-it' books to help. In clinical practice, the questions of 'why do it, where to do it, and when to do it (or not!)' are often more pressing and we hope to address these questions in this book, in addition to practical advice on technique. The book therefore should be useful to endoscopists during the course of training but our co-authors have also included challenging areas which will interest even the established endoscopist. We have also included two chapters on screening as this ought not to be undertaken unless realistic therapeutic options are intended.

We are profoundly grateful to our friends who have contributed to this book. They bring a wealth of personal experience in the field, which has been acquired over many years. We hope that the concentration of that experience into this text will help you to make the right decisions for your patients. Inevitably, in a multiauthor tome, there will be repetition. We took editorial licence in moving some text between chapters among different authors for the purpose of integrating the material. We therefore acknowledge that some authors made contributions to several chapters.

Martin Lombard, *Royal Liverpool University Hospitals*
David Westaby, *Chelsea & Westminster Hospital London*

Introduction

1

M. Lombard and D. Westaby

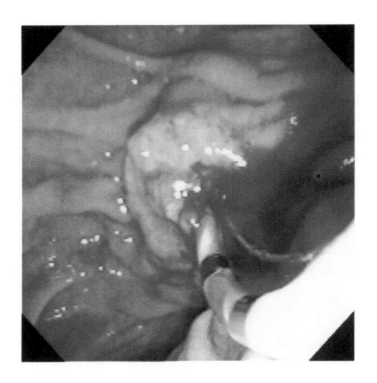

While many of the authors in this book were pioneers in endoscopic techniques and had to '*boldly go where no endoscopist had gone before*', it is now inconceivable that anyone would undertake advanced therapeutic procedures without personal tuition and training by an expert. We have had to assume in this book that basic endoscopic training has been completed, and there are many excellent texts which address this aspect. Nonetheless, there are some important points of preparation which we wish to emphasize before endoscopic therapeutic procedures are undertaken.

Patient preparation

It is vital that the patient understands what is entailed in therapeutic endoscopy. The general public have a reasonable appreciation that surgical operations carry an element of risk. However, many patients have come to be aware that endoscopy is a routine procedure, and frequently do not appreciate that there are risks associated with sedation and diagnostic upper or lower endoscopy. When therapeutic procedures are involved, it may be necessary to appraise the patient that this is a *surgical operation* undertaken through the endoscope, particularly where they are undertaken as 'day-case' procedures.

Consent

The question of informing the patient is increasingly important. The more open and honest approach adopted in recent years is certainly a great step forwards, in general. It requires, however, an increased level of skill, compared with the bland reassurances which were sometimes given in the past, for it to work well. Relatives and friends may try to collude with clinical staff, for example to shield the patient with cancer from 'distress', which may be merely their way of coping, or a genuine appreciation of the likely effect of bad news. Certainly a crude, early disclosure may be catastrophic. Patients must be given bad news in boluses which they can digest. The speed of first-rate, modern management can work against this process of gradual disclosure, understanding and acceptance. The judgement of the clinical team is crucial here. It is no longer appropriate, however – if it ever was – to commit a patient to dangerous, painful and unpleasant treatments without their being in possession of an appropriate understanding of what is going on. The legal background, with its emphasis on 'informed consent', has produced added challenges. Nevertheless, it remains a cruel and callous disregard of our patient care to provide a list of all the possible complications of a procedure without regard to the psychological effects this may have, not least on the ability of the patient to relax and cooperate through what can be a harrowing procedure. We need to temper our wish to tell all and avoid possible litigation with some common sense and compassion. Consent must be informed, but need not be omniscient.

Fasting and fluids

Traditionally, patients have been asked to fast for 8–12 hours prior to endoscopic procedures. In practical terms this usually means fasting from midnight before an elective procedure and, with increasing workload, the procedure may not take place until the late afternoon or evening. This can cause unnecessary discomfort to patients and for some can be dangerous. Recent work has indicated that fluids can be taken up to 4–6 hours before endoscopy without adverse consequence. It may be the case that small (thirst-quenching) sips can be taken right up to the time of endoscopy. The difficulties of allowing different limits for different patients in a busy service is more likely to require adherence to the '6 hour rule'.

For certain procedures fasting for longer may be necessary. For any patient – particularly for elderly patients – fasting for longer than 6 hours we feel an intravenous infusion of colloid is essential. This is particularly important for patients undergoing a therapeutic procedure as sedation is nearly always required and frequently the patient will have to fast for a variable period after the procedure until it is clear that there are no adverse consequences.

Jaundiced patients may have to fast for several procedures over several days, for example ultrasound scan, computed tomography (CT) scan and endoscopic retrograde cholangiopancreatography (ERCP). The elderly in this situation are particularly susceptible to dehydration and hepatorenal complications, and intravenous fluids can be vital for those patients.

Diabetic patients should be managed with a glucose infusion and a sliding scale of insulin. It may not always be possible to ensure that these patients are treated on a morning list. In this case, where it will not interfere with the specific planned procedure, a light breakfast can be given.

Bowel preparation

It is beyond the scope of this book to compare different means of bowel preparation. Suffice to say that large-bowel endoscopy, with its attendant risk of perforation, is generally not worthwhile without adequate preparation.

Undoubtedly, large-volume orthograde lavage solutions (e.g. polyethylene glycol solutions) give the best results, though they pose difficulty for some patients because of the volume required to be taken, and in the elderly can occasionally produce fluid and electrolyte imbalance. Lower-volume solutions with phosphate may be as effective for most patients. Occasionally, patients will require a combination of means with a fluid only diet for several days. It is important to discontinue iron supplements during the process of bowel preparation.

Purgation with phosphate enemas as proprietary preparations is often sufficient for left-sided colonoscopy.

Anticoagulation

For elective procedures, it is best to stop oral anticoagulants and use a heparin regimen which can be controlled and reversed if necessary, around a therapeutic procedure. For more acute procedures, a full therapeutic manoeuvre may not be possible, but valuable diagnostic information (e.g. source of bleeding) may still be obtained.

For patients with jaundice, a single intravenous dose of vitamin K is usually sufficient to correct the coagulopathy. There is no evidence to indicate that undertaking procedures with fresh-frozen plasma or with platelet transfusions will reduce the potential for complications in patients with an underlying coagulopathy.

Antibiotics

For most therapeutic procedures, antibiotics are unnecessary. They should be used for procedures in which there is a significant risk of perforation, where a normally sterile site will be breached or instrumented (e.g. the biliary tree or at gastrostomy), or where a patient is at risk for other reasons (e.g. valvular heart disease, cystic fibrosis, post-splenectomy).

Broad-spectrum antibiotics should be used and specific cover for coliforms is essential. Often, prophylaxis can be given orally on the morning of the procedure and orally again once the patient recovers.

PROCEDURES

Intravenous sedation, oxygen supplementation and monitoring

Many *diagnostic* endoscopic procedures can be undertaken with adequate explanation to the patient and without sedation. Topical pharyngeal anaesthesia with lignocaine 2% when used for gastroscopy has been shown to improve patient tolerance. Most comparative studies of upper endoscopy also indicate that, even where sedation is used, tolerance is further improved by the addition of topical oropharyngeal anaesthesia.

Most *therapeutic* procedures are undertaken with sedation, often in combination with analgesia and occasionally with a general anaesthetic.

Our preference is to use short-acting benzodiazepine such as midazolam. This has sedative, tranquillizing and amnesic properties. Heretofore, there has been a tendency to use midazolam in doses of 5–10 mg or diazepam in doses of 10–20 mg. Recent work and our own experience has shown that much lower starting doses (30 µg/kg; average 2–4 mg) with sequential increments if necessary during long procedures are effective. Thus in a personal series of over 1000 patients undergoing therapeutic ERCP, the average dose used was less than 5 mg midazolam and doses over 10 mg were used in only 2% of patients. Adverse excessive sedation can be reversed with flumazenil 250–500 µg intravenously (iv). In some units this has been used as routine reversal to shorten recovery. In our experience this is unpredictable, as flumazenil has an even shorter half-life than the agonist benzodiazepines and it can produce a false sense of security, particularly in elderly patients. It is also expensive. This practice is unnecessary with lower doses of midazolam.

Opiates are usually used in addition, e.g. pethidine 25–50 mg or fentanyl 50–100 µg. Adverse effects or hypotension can be reversed with naloxone 400 µg iv or intramuscularly (im).

Concern is occasionally expressed at the potential synergist effects of using opioids and benzodiazepines together. Clearly, the dosages used are important here. A safe practice is to give opiate first, followed by buscopan or atropine if required. Once the pulse begins to quicken (anticholinergic effect), the benzodiazepine is given in small boluses of 2–3 mg. as required, titrated to the anxiolytic response in the patient.

Systemic hypoxia can occur as a result of sedation, endoscopic intubation, the position of the patient for some procedures, or because of the patient's own underlying cardiorespiratory status. Published series indicate that severe hypoxia (saturation <90%) occurs in 10% to 70% of patients depending on those factors. Giving supplemental oxygen during the procedure can prevent this and pre-oxygenation may be particularly important in patients at risk as the greatest oxygen desaturation seems to occur immediately following intubation. Both nasal cannula and oral oxygen delivery systems seem equally effective.

It is clearly important that monitoring of vital signs is undertaken throughout the procedure. Electrical pulse oximetry and automatic blood pressure monitoring are useful adjuncts to personal nursing care, though there is no published data to indicate that they reduce complications.

Nursing and endoscopy assistants

Endoscopy nurses must be trained and highly skilled as they form an integral part of the clinical management team. It is not possible to undertake a number of the procedures described in this book without skilled technical assistance.

We recommend that all of our trainees spend time assisting these techniques, as it is the only way they gain an understanding of what they can expect from their assistants when they are performing the procedure themselves. It is also an excellent opportunity to become familiar with the equipment.

In addition to technical expert assistance, the importance of *nursing* the patient through the procedure cannot be overstated. Because of the amnesic properties of drugs used to achieve conscious sedation, patients need repeated reassurances during the procedures.

The moving patient

It can be tempting to equate the moving patient with a moving target where difficult therapeutic procedures demanding of patience and calm are concerned. However,

a major advantage of 'conscious sedation' over general anaesthesia is that some biological feedback is retained when potentially traumatic therapeutic procedures are undertaken, i.e. if the patient is in discomfort, they can usually signal this. This should not be interpreted by the endoscopist that more sedation is required. In our experience, patients who move during endoscopy do so for one of three reasons: (i) too much air is insufflated causing gaseous distention of a viscus (a common occurrence with the novice endoscopist); (ii) the patient is paradoxically stimulated by the hypnotic (common with a history of alcohol excess or longstanding use of anxiolytics); and (iii) a visceral perforation has occurred (rarely, it is hoped).

With expert nursing, the conscious sedated patient will remain quiet and relaxed throughout the procedure. Incremental sedation should be used for signs of wakeful distress or anxiety, not if the patient is trying to warn of an impending problem.

Recovery and postoperative care

As most procedures are undertaken with sedation, they will require a period of recovery in a sedated state. Thus, fasting is usually continued for 2–3 hours following a procedure and fluid replacement may be required for certain patients. The patient should continue to be monitored with nursing observations of pulse and blood pressure. By this time, if serious complications have occurred (e.g. perforation or haemorrhage), they should have become clinically apparent.

Feeding should always commence with clear fluids and any untoward effects or pain should be investigated at once. The particular investigation pathway will obviously depend on which procedure was undertaken. Thus, a patient with chest pain following oesophageal procedures will require a chest X-ray, electrocardiogram (ECG) and possibly a water-soluble contrast fluoroscopic examination.

For certain procedures, antibiotics may be continued afterwards, particularly if complications are suspected.

Patients can often seem wide awake and coherent following a procedure but remember nothing of the explanation or results given to them because of the amnesic properties of sedation. A copy of a written result or an explanation to an accompanying person is often useful in this regard.

Complications

These must be recognized early for optimum management.

It is essential that the endoscopist is aware of what may go wrong and anticipate early warning signs. Complication rates are dependent on the procedure itself, the nature of the pathology, the sedation used, the age and morbidity of the patient and the expertise of the endoscopist. It is essential that, in comparing complications between different procedures, individuals or institutions, these are defined in a uniform way. A complication has been variously defined as an incident occurring as a result of a procedure which represents a deviation from the normal or ideal course, i.e. a negative outcome. The severity of complications has been defined in terms of symptoms and their duration, the intervention required to alleviate it, the length of hospital stay and the functional incapacity at a specified time. Because endoscopic procedures are so often compared to surgical procedures, the 30-day complication

Table 1.1. Complication rates published for a range of procedures

Procedure	Morbidity (%)	Causes	Mortality (/1000)	Causes	Comments
Sedation	0.2–0.5	Cardiorespiratory	0.3–0.5	Cardiorespiratory	
Diagnostic gastroscopy	5	Bacteraemia	0.5		Significant if predisposed
	0.03	Perforation	0.01		Usually associated pathology
Upper gastrointestinal procedures	40	Bacteraemia			Peptic and achalasia
	6–7	Pain, perforation, fistula	10	Perforation	Malignant
Oesophageal dilatation	0.5	Perforation	1	Lower rates for benign strictures,	
	10	stricture	30	× 10 for malignant	
Variceal injection	10	Strictures	20	Various	
	20	Ulceration			
	20	Bacteraemia			
	40	Rebleeding	300	Underlying pathology	
Variceal banding	3	Strictures			
	25	Rebleeding			
PEG tubes	30	Infection, leakage, migration	150	Infection, premorbid condition	
Diagnostic colonoscopy	0.1	Increases with polypectomy and age	0.2	Perforation	
Polypectomy	1	Bleeding, increased % with larger polyps			
ERCP-diagnosis	5	Pancreatitis	1	Pancreatitis, haemorrhage	range 0–40%
	50	Hyperamylasaemia			
	10	Cholangitis			
Endoprosthesis	25	Stent occlusion @ 3/12	10	Sepsis Pancreatitis, perforation, myocardial infarction, premorbidity	
Sphincterotomy	2	Haemorrhage	0.2	Haemorrhage	
	10	Late sepsis (10 yrs)			

rate has been widely accepted to be a reasonable comparison of outcome. Some endoscopists have difficulty with this concept and try to make a judgement about direct relationship – for statistical comparison it is important to adhere to principles of 'intention to treat'.

Some complications are covered in more detail in the individual chapters. A table of published complications is given here for guidance but the 'ballpark' figures given are not directly comparable and the reader is referred to the extensive reference list on this subject. It is vital that any endoscopist undertaking these procedures is aware of the potential for complications – this is not a comprehensive list.

FURTHER READING

Arrowsmith J, Gerstman B, *et al.* Results from the American Society for Gastrointestinal Endoscopy/US Food & Drugs Administration collaborative study on complication rates and drug use during gastrointestinal endoscopy. *Gastrointest Endosc* 1991; 37: 421–427.

Clavien PA, Sanabria JR, *et al.* Proposed classification of complications of surgery with examples of utility in cholecystectomy. *Surgery* 1992; 111: 518–526.

Cotton PB. Complications, comparisons and confusion. In: Cotton PB, Tytgat GNJ, Williams CB, Bowling TE (eds), *Annual of Gastrointestinal Endoscopy*, 10th edn, London: Rapid Science, 1997, pp. 7–9.

Cotton PB. Outcomes of endoscopic procedures: struggling towards definitions. *Gastrointest Endosc* 1994; 40: 514–518.

Fleischer DE. Better definitions of endoscopic complications and other negative outcomes. *Gastrointest Endosc* 1994; 40: 511–513.

McCloy R. *Towards Safer Sedation Endoscopy*. Meditext Ltd, London, 1991.

Quine MA, Bell GD, *et al.* Prospective audit of upper gastrointestinal endoscopy in two regions of England: safety, staffing and sedation methods. *Gut* 1995; 36: 462–467.

Vallera R, Baillie J. Complications of endoscopy. *Endoscopy* 1996; 28: 187–204.

Zuckerman GR (ed.) *Complications of Gastrointestinal Endoscopy*. Gastrointestinal Endoscopy Clinics of North America. WB Saunders, Philadelphia, 1996.

2 *Benign oesophageal obstruction*

P. D. Fairclough

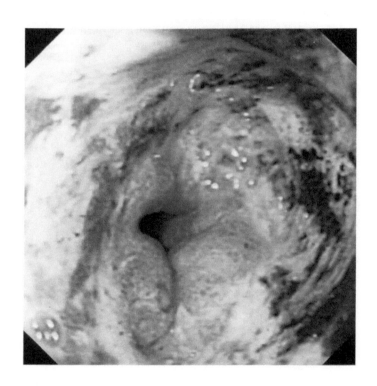

INTRODUCTION

Dysphagia is a common symptom, the cause of which can be clinically diagnosed in most cases. The difficulties of determining the incidence and prevalence of this symptom have been well reviewed [1]. There is little good information about the incidence and prevalence of dysphagia, but among hospitalized patients in Maryland, USA the most common causes were not primarily oesophageal: indeed, circulatory conditions, thought usually to be strokes, respiratory disease and 'symptoms, signs and ill-defined conditions' were the most common coded diagnoses. Digestive diseases and neoplasms accounted for only 15% of coded primary diagnoses associated with dysphagia. The limitations of these data are obvious.

Oesophageal dysphagia is characterized by a sensation of hindrance to the passage of food or fluid within 10 seconds or so of leaving the mouth – the maximum time normally taken for oesophageal transit. Clinicians recognize oropharyngeal dysphagia by the description of difficulty in transfer of food from the mouth to the oesophagus, associated with other symptoms such as regurgitation through the nose, nasal speech and coughing during swallowing. This is neuromuscular in origin, not generally amenable to endoscopic therapy, and will not be further discussed.

Table 2.1. Causes of oesophageal dysphagia

Neuromuscular	
Primary	Achalasia
	Diffuse oesophageal spasm
	Nutcracker oesophagus
	Hypertensive lower oesophagus
	Non-specific
Secondary	Scleroderma
	Collagen disorders
	Chagas' disease
Mechanical	
Intrinsic	Peptic stricture
	Schatzki ring (most common)
	Cancer
	Webs
	Diverticula
	Benign tumours
	Foreign bodies
	Injury, e.g. medication: drugs or poisons
Extrinsic	Goitre
	Vascular compression
	Mediastinal abnormality
	Osteoarthritis of the neck

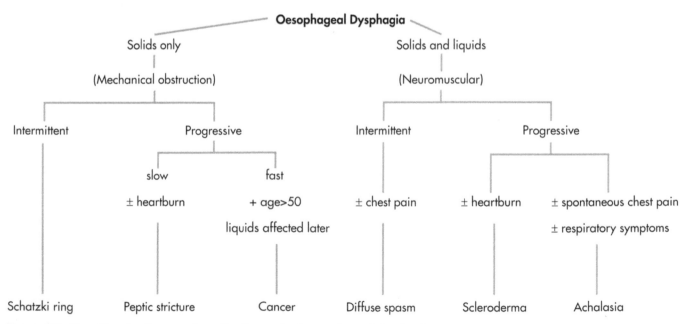

Figure 2.1. Algorithm for the symptomatic diagnosis of oesophageal dysphagia.

PRESENTATION

A simplified symptomatic analysis of the common symptom patterns is shown in the algorithm (Fig. 2.1). There are many other causes of dysphagia (Table 2.1).

In clinical assessment, the most important questions are:

- Are the symptoms induced by liquids or solids, or both?
- Did dysphagia for solids occur before dysphagia for liquids (indicating mechanical obstruction), or was the onset more or less simultaneous (indicating neuromuscular disorder)?
- Is the dysphagia intermittent or progressive?
- Is there heartburn?

CLINICAL SYNDROMES

Peptic strictures (Fig. 2.2)

These are characterized by intermittent dysphagia for solids at first, progressing over months or years to dysphagia for solids with each meal, despite the changes that the patient almost always makes toward softer foods and more liquids with meals. Most patients with peptic strictures have a history of heartburn. Episodes of bolus obstruction may occur, particularly with meat or bread.

Postoperative, sclerotherapy and radiotherapy-induced strictures

These occur after a variable period and have similar historical features to peptic strictures.

Schatzki rings (Fig. 2.3)

These usually present with intermittent, unpredictable episodes of complete bolus obstruction during which nothing can be swallowed. The episodes usually occur with meat or bread and are acutely embarrassing, often stopping the patient from eating away from home. When the obstructing bolus passes or is removed, swallowing usually returns immediately to normal, until the next episode. Symptoms are said to only occur when the diameter of the ring is less than 13 mm.

Neuromuscular disorders

When there is a history of difficulty in swallowing both solids and liquids from the start of the symptoms, the cause

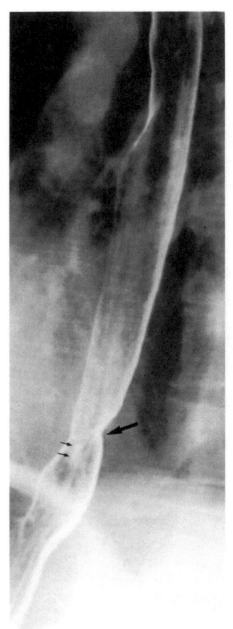

Figure 2.2. Barium demonstration of peptic stricture.

is usually neuromuscular. Diffuse spasm (Fig. 2.4) may be associated with spontaneous cardiac-type chest pain, but chest pain and respiratory symptoms are more common in achalasia, and the dysphagia tends to be more constant and progressive. Most patients with achalasia (Fig. 2.5) present between 20 and 40 years of age. Regurgitation of unchanged or putrid food occurs particularly at night, when it may cause aspiration and nocturnal cough. The symptoms often extend over a number of years, with gradually increasing severity and frequency of dysphagia.

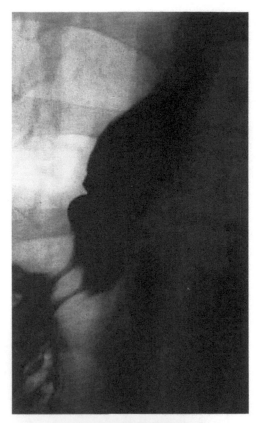

Figure 2.3. X-ray of Schatzki ring.

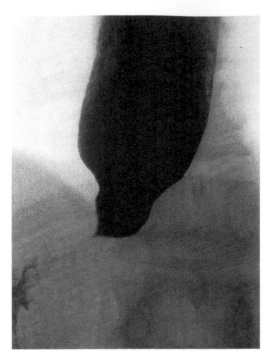

Figure 2.5. Barium demonstration of achalasia. Dilated body of oesophagus with 'bird's beak' appearance at lower end.

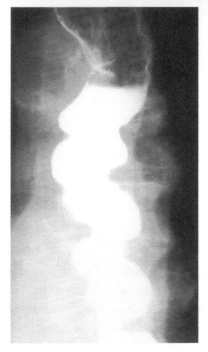

Figure 2.4. 'Corkscrew' oesophagus caused by spasm.

Scleroderma

If neuromuscular-type dysphagia is also associated with heartburn, scleroderma should be suspected and associated clinical findings should be sought.

Pharyngeal pouch and oesophageal diverticula

A large pharyngeal (Zenker's) diverticulum is classically associated with the symptoms of persistent cough, fullness and gurgling in the neck, postprandial regurgitation and aspiration. Traction diverticula (Fig. 2.6) in the oesophagus also can produce dysphagia.

Malignant dysphagia

Patients with malignant dysphagia (see Fig. 3.1) usually have a relatively short history of weeks of increasing dysphagia for solids, progressing rapidly to dysphagia for liquids, a feature almost never seen in peptic strictures.

DIAGNOSIS

Clinical diagnosis of dysphagia is surprisingly accurate, though it may take time and skill to elicit the salient features of the history. It is important to know that:

- the level at which the patient indicates obstruction is rarely of much value, most patients feeling the obstruction in the suprasternal area regardless of the level of the physical obstruction.
- Weight loss is of limited diagnostic help; it may occur with any cause of dysphagia.

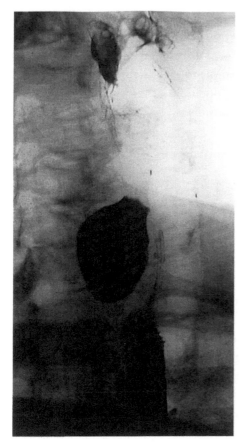

Figure 2.6. Oesophageal diverticula as seen on barium swallow.

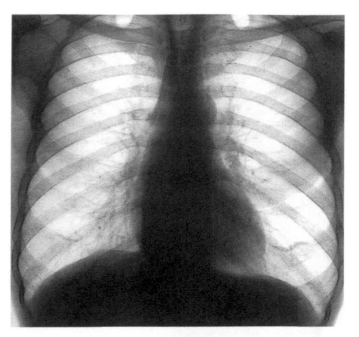

Figure 2.7. Chest X-ray demonstrating characteristic features of achalasia: dilated oesophagus behind the heart with absent gastric air bubble.

- Physical signs are uncommon. Supraclavicular or other lymphadenopathy may occur in association with advanced malignancy, or there may be signs of scleroderma. Occasionally, a mass in the neck indicates a goitre or a large Zenker's diverticulum.

INVESTIGATION OF DYSPHAGIA

Blood tests

These are rarely of help, except in general assessment and assessment of fitness for procedures, and in the finding of confirmatory antibodies in scleroderma. Mild anaemia is sometimes present with severe oesophagitis.

Radiology

Chest X-ray
Occasionally, this will show a dilated oesophagus in late achalasia (Fig. 2.7), classically associated with an absent gastric air bubble, due to the water-filled trap effect of retained fluid and food in the oesophagus. A fluid

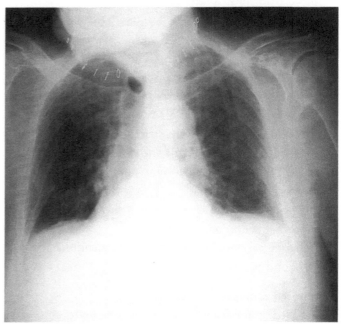

Figure 2.8. Chest X-ray. Fluid levels are seen behind the heart shadow in a hiatus hernia (note clips from recent thyroidectomy).

level may be seen behind the heart in an hiatus hernia (Fig. 2.8). In other forms of benign obstruction, it is usually normal.

Barium swallow
Many endoscopists use endoscopy as the first investigation

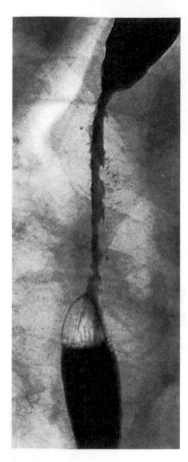

Figure 2.9. Barium examination showing tortuous tight stricture.

should be based on the history and clinical findings, and on the availability and expertise of radiologist and endoscopist. Given appropriate expertise, endoscopy is a very satisfactory first investigation for the more common causes of dysphagia, with the potential advantages of biopsy and therapy in the same session.

Endoscopic appearances

Benign strictures

Strictures in patients with reflux oesophagitis must be examined carefully to differentiate benign from malign lesions. Biopsy and brush cytology should be readily undertaken, both from the proximal and distal aspects of the stricture. Repeated endoscopy for biopsy may be necessary to show malignancy, and is mandatory in cases of clinical doubt. It is not advisable to attempt to dilate tight strictures with the endoscope; the more gradual dilatation achieved by dilators is generally accepted to be safer. Benign peptic strictures appear endoscopically as a concentric narrowing covered with exudate at least at the narrowest point, and are usually associated with signs of reflux oesophagitis above the stricture. However, early use of proton pump inhibitors (PPIs) has complicated the endoscopic picture. Signs of oesophagitis above and exudate within the stricture may be reduced or absent within weeks of starting PPIs, leaving a smooth benign-looking stricture, usually with reduction in the dysphagia. Strictures offer a variable resistance to passage of an endoscope, depending on the degree of narrowing and the size of the endoscope. Smooth strictures without accompanying reflux damage can be missed endoscopically if a small-diameter endoscope is used.

Endoscopic ultrasound (EUS) can be useful when the nature of a stricture is unclear (Fig. 2.10), particularly in differentiating intrinsic oesophageal lesions from extrinsic compression, and in the demonstration of malignant nodes. EUS is not histology, however, and findings of apparent malignancy must be followed by biopsy proof, either endoscopically or by transmucosal EUS-guided aspiration biopsy.

Scleroderma

Up to 60% of patients with scleroderma have erosive oesophagitis, and the frequency of stricture in these patients is high. The disease may be further complicated by

in patients with dysphagia. Barium study is particularly useful in patients suspected of:

- proximal, tortuous or tight strictures (Fig. 2.9), where endoscopy may be difficult and potentially more hazardous without a 'road-map', particularly in inexperienced hands;
- neuromuscular disorders in which there may be few abnormal endoscopic findings;
- a pharyngeal pouch which the unwary endoscopist may enter and perforate.

Computed tomography scan

Computed tomography (CT) or magnetic resonance scanning is useful for ruling out 'pseudo-achalasia' (see below) and distant metastases, and in the detection and local staging of tumours.

ENDOSCOPIC INVESTIGATION

Endoscopy or barium?

The choice of barium or endoscopy as the first investigation

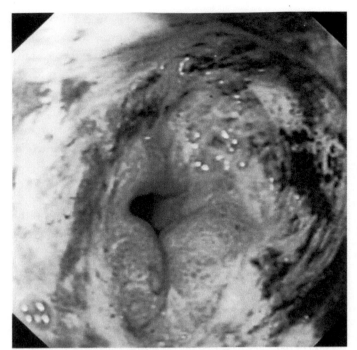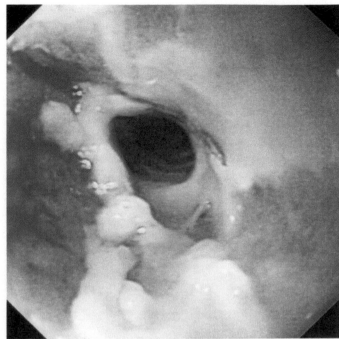

Figure 2.10. Endoscopic appearances of severe ulcerating oesophagitis (a) before and (b) after treatment with PPIs. A fibrotic stricture is developing at (b).

gastric metaplasia in the distal oesophagus, and mucosal candidiasis in up to 40% of cases.

Achalasia

The major purpose of diagnostic endoscopy in achalasia is the exclusion of malignancy causing a 'pseudo-achalasia', or squamous tumours complicating longstanding disease. The endoscopic appearances depend on the stage of the disease. The mucosa often appears normal, particularly in the early stages. In the later stages, when the oesophagus is dilated, surprising amounts of putrid food and secretions may be present, and a liquid diet followed by lavage with a large-bore tube to remove retained food is advisable before endoscopy. The oesophagus dilates as the disease advances, looks increasingly like sigmoid colon, and may be difficult to negotiate. Stasis may cause whitish mucosal plaques, erosions and ulceration. Passage through the gastro-oesophageal junction is usually easy. Significant resistance should prompt a particularly thorough search for extraluminal pathology or gastric cardiac tumours causing 'pseudo-achalasia'.

Malignant lesions

Endoscopy has a major role in diagnosis, staging and therapy of oesophagogastric malignancy (see Chapter 3).

Early squamous lesions can be most readily detected using Lugol's iodine spray: the normal oesophagus stains brown, dysplasia does not stain. Not all unstained areas are dysplastic, but lack of staining acts as a guide for targeted biopsy [2]. More advanced lesions are usually easily recognized. Biopsy and cytology combined give a positive diagnosis in almost 100% of cases. Adenocarcinoma is the second most common malignant tumour of the oesophagus, and may be the most common in some geographic areas. It usually arises in the distal oesophagus affected by intestinal metaplasia in association with reflux (Barrett's oesophagus), but may arise from oesophageal mucous glands. Gastric fundal adenocarcinoma may involve the hiatus. It may be difficult to determine the precise site of origin of a tumour affecting the distal oesophagus.

Endoscopic ultrasound

This new imaging modality is becoming more available in specialist centres. It is useful for establishing the precise local extent of a tumour, and for clarifying involvement of local lymph nodes [3]. Early cancers are often associated with minor symptoms, which should not be ignored as the prognosis for endoscopic or surgical treatment of early lesions is relatively good. In benign disorders, CT and EUS are of limited value, except where there is a suspicion of tumour (see Chapter 3).

Manometry and pH studies

These investigations are useful in neuromuscular disorders, for assessment of the results of antireflux therapy, for confirmation of achalasia when barium studies are equivocal, and for definition of less well-defined conditions. Peptic stricture and reflux oesophagitis are *prima facie* evidence of reflux, so neither pH nor manometry are required for diagnosis. Manometry is useful in achalasia for confirmation of the diagnosis, and for assessment of the results of treatment.

MANAGEMENT AND EVIDENCE

The aims of management of benign conditions causing dysphagia are:
- improvement of symptoms;
- avoidance of complications of disease and therapy

Benign peptic stricture

Conservative management
Medical therapy can significantly alleviate dysphagia by reducing inflammation, resulting in significant improvement in dysphagia scores. By the time a peptic stricture has formed, powerful antacid drugs are usually required. PPIs are effective; H_2 receptor blockers are usually much less so. The usual antireflux lifestyle measures (weight loss, antacids, postural change, small meals, stopping smoking, avoiding precipitating drugs, fat, caffeine and alcohol) may be of overall benefit to the patient, but do little for the stricture.

Dilatation
Combined with dilatation, PPIs are more effective treatment for reflux strictures than dilatation alone [4]. Dilatation is appropriate where dysphagia has not responded to drug therapy alone, or when conservative treatment is obviously going to be inadequate. Dilatations may need to be repeated for prolonged benefit. Weight loss and absence of heartburn may predict a need for frequent dilatation [5].

Endoscopic dilatation is applicable to all types of stricture in all ages. Relative contraindications include bleeding disorders, severe respiratory insufficiency, recent myocardial infarction, recent oesophageal surgery, gross thoracic aortic aneurysm, extrinsic oesophageal compression and unstable cervical spine disease, but all may be overridden if the clinical situation demands. General anaesthesia may be needed for occasional patients who cannot cooperate under sedation. Despite a multiplicity of available dilators and studies of dilatation, there are few randomized controlled trials on which to base recommendations.

Stenting
Insertion of an endoprosthesis for benign strictures is rarely required, and can only be justified if the benefits outweigh the costs, both medical and financial. For example, a stent might be justified in a patient with recurrent stricture formation which is resistant to maximal medical therapy and dilatation, and in whom surgery would be an unacceptable risk. Recurrence of dysphagia can occur due to epithelial hyperplasia. [6].

Surgery
Strictures which fail medical treatment and dilatation should be considered for surgical management. This is especially true for young patients in whom the likelihood of recurrent dilatation and prolonged PPI therapy is unacceptable [7]. Dilatations may be necessary in the initial phase after surgery, but if an effective antireflux procedure has been performed they should not be needed long term.

Achalasia

Conservative management
Medical therapy for achalasia is occasionally useful, mostly as a temporizing measure. Nitrates and calcium channel blockers are the principal agents, but rarely relieve the dysphagia adequately.

Dilatation
Dilatation has for years been the mainstay of treatment, though neither the technique nor the dilator are standardized [8] and the series are therefore difficult to compare. Fixed-diameter polyethylene balloons have now largely superseded earlier dilators. The Rigiflex over-the-wire (OTW) dilator which requires screening, and the scope-mounted Witzel dilator which does not require screening, seem to be the most widely used (Fig. 2.11).

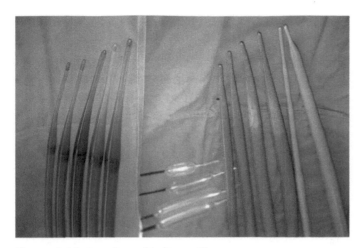

Figure 2.11. Bougie and balloon dilators.

Either dilator is available in 30, 35 and 40 mm models. The larger balloons should be reserved for those who fail two dilatations with the 30-mm balloon. Dilatation produces good symptomatic relief in 60–80% of patients in the short term, but the 5-year response to single dilatations is only around 25%, with at least 50% of patients requiring one or more further dilatation in this time [9,10]. In a study assessing favourable factors, best results were obtained in patients over 45 years of age with symptoms for at least 5 years, and without gross oesophageal dilatation [11].

Injection therapy

Injection of botulinum toxin (BoTox) into the lower oesophageal sphincter (LOS) has been shown in a double-blind, placebo-controlled trial to produce symptomatic and manometric improvement in achalasia [12]. Of 31 patients reported by Pasricha *et al* [13] 28 improved initially, but the response was sustained for longer than 3 months in only 20 cases. Older patients (aged >50 years) and those with vigorous achalasia responded best. The duration of the symptomatic response ranged from 5 months to 2.4 years. It has been suggested that failures of dilatation are due to failure to rupture oblique muscle fibres in the LOS, so that BoTox may be more effective because the orientation of muscle fibres is irrelevant.

Ethanolamine oleate has been injected into the LOS for treatment of achalasia, with apparent success [14]. Although promising, this therapy was accompanied by stricture formation, particularly in the early part of the series, and remains experimental.

There are no fully published studies randomly comparing dilatation with BoTox, but preliminary data comparing Witzel dilatation with BoTox indicated that 50% of BoTox patients failed to respond initially, or had recurrent symptoms in a mean of 12.5 months, compared with a 7% initial failure rate with Witzel dilatation, followed for a mean of 10.5 months [8]. It would seem that the safety of BoTox might favour its use as the first manoeuvre, particularly in those at risk for surgery or dilatation. If it is effective, further injections can be given when symptoms recur. Dilatation could perhaps be reserved for failures of BoTox.

Surgery

Endoscopists generally reserve open surgery for those who fail endoscopic therapy, because open surgery is a much more major procedure, and it is widely known that there is a higher incidence of reflux problems [15].

However, the results of surgery are impressive. In the comparative study by Csendes *et al* [10], 95% of 42 patients treated by surgery had good or excellent results at 5 years, compared with only 65% of 39 dilated patients. On the other hand, there was a 28% incidence of reflux after surgery – measured by pH monitoring, and mostly asymptomatic – compared with only 8% after dilatation [10].

Laparoscopic myotomy with a Dor antireflux procedure seems comparable in effectiveness with the more traditional thoracoscopic approach, with 86–90% patients having no dysphagia or dysphagia less than once a week, and a very low incidence of reflux [16].

Scleroderma

Management is directed at control of reflux, usually with H_2-receptor blockers or PPIs, with endoscopic dilatation for management of strictures. Long-term acid-suppressant medication is usually needed to control symptoms and to try to prevent recurrent stricture formation. Antireflux surgery is rarely indicated, partly because the associated motility disturbance confers a high risk of postoperative dysphagia.

Diffuse spasm

There are few controlled data available to guide therapy. The aims of treatment are to relieve symptoms and improve quality of life. Reassurance that a positive diagnosis has been made, and that heart disease and cancer excluded, are important. Drug therapy with nitrates or calcium channel blockers may be helpful. Bougienage may afford temporary relief. Balloon dilatation of the LOS should be reserved for refractory symptoms – for example, one study reported marked improvement of symptoms in eight of nine patients followed for up to 3 years, but there was no change in the pattern of oesophageal motility [17]. Use of BoTox has been reported in a limited number of patients with motility disorders, with hopeful results in one-third [18]. Surgical longitudinal myotomy is a last resort.

Schatzki rings

Reassurance is important here, and treatment of reflux oesophagitis may resolve the symptoms.

Patients should eat more slowly, chew their food well, and avoid large boli of meat or bread. Glucagon injection during bolus obstruction may allow the bolus to pass, avoiding an endoscopic disimpaction procedure. Although there are few convincing data, bougienage with a single large dilator is believed to achieve the best results. Balloon dilatation is rarely necessary, and carries a higher risk of perforation than bougienage.

PRACTICALITIES

General principles

The nature of the stricture should be established before the dilation procedure by radiology, endoscopy, biopsy and cytology. A pre-procedure chest X-ray is generally not necessary for reflux strictures which can be traversed by the endoscope, but is recommended for all others. X-ray screening is not necessary for straightforward procedures when a standard 10-mm endoscope can be passed into the stomach, but is necessary if it cannot, and for all balloon dilatations.

The patient should fast for at least 4 hours for benign strictures, and for 24 hours before dilatation of achalasia, where lavage with a large-bore oro-oesophageal tube may be necessary before the procedure.

Equipment

Mechanical dilatation is an ancient procedure: the urethras of

Egyptians at the time of the Pharaohs were dilated with reeds, and bougies have been used for oesophageal dilatation since the 16th century [19]. Balloon dilators are a relatively recent development. The physics of oesophageal dilatation has been well reviewed [20], and the characteristics required of the ideal dilator are listed in Table 2.2. Sadly, but not surprisingly, no dilator fulfils all these aspirations.

Bougies, dilators and balloons

Bougies and balloons are available with different characteristics, and some of these are shown in Table 2.3. Important factors influencing their suitability for different purposes are:
- the minimum diameter of the tip;
- the length of the dilating segment;
- the maximum diameter; and
- the slope or angle of incidence of the dilating segment of the bougie with the stricture.

Bougies convert axial force into radial dilating force, in a ratio depending on the slope of the dilating segment. There is always a component of axial force stretching the oesophagus longitudinally. Short dilating segments are useful after gastrectomy. High angles of incidence provide greater tactile feedback but more abrupt dilatation; low angles of incidence provide smoother, gentler dilatation, but require a longer segment of gut distal to the stricture.

Balloons are theoretically safer because they exert radial force alone, but this has not proved to be so in practice, and balloons seem to be less effective than bougies, except in

Table 2.2. Characteristics of the ideal dilator

Passes easily through the oropharynx and stricture of any diameter
Allows the operator to 'feel' the stricture
Produces a long-lasting functional passage for food and fluid (> 16 mm) *with a single introduction*
Carries no risk of perforation
Is radio-opaque, to allow use of X-ray when necessary
Is suitable for use after partial or total gastrectomy, or in difficult hiatus hernias
Is useable in children
Is quick and easy to use

Table 2.3. Specification of common bougies and balloons

Dilator	Diameter[a] Min : max (mm)	Leader[b] (mm)	Angle of incidence[c] (degrees)	Passages[d]	X-ray?
Rigiflex balloon	2.8 : 20	80	–	1	+
Rigiflex TTS balloon	1.8 : 20	80	–	1	±
Celestin	3.7 : 18	160	6	2	–
Eder-Puestow	3.7 : 19.3	21	49	M	–
KeyMed 'Advanced'	3 : 17.3	82	12	3	–
Savary	5 : 20	177	6	M	–

a   tip diameter : maximum diameter
b   start of dilator to point of maximum diameter
c   angle at the start of the dilating segment
d   number of passages normally needed to achieve maximum dilatation; M = multiple
X-ray?   need for x-ray screening

achalasia, although a realistic comparison is not possible because a 30-mm bougie would not pass safely through the pharynx. Initial dilatation of very tight strictures can be easiest with a wire-guided through-the-scope (TTS) balloon.

Balloon dilators are used in achalasia to stretch the LOS forcefully, usually to a set diameter of 30 mm, and occasionally to 35 or 40 mm. The danger of rupture precludes the use of balloons of this size in benign strictures. The Rider–Moeller waisted dilating bag which was mounted on a flexible metal shaft has largely been superseded by the Rigiflex achalasia dilator (Microvasive, Boston Scientific). This is made of modified polyethylene (Polytuss 150), mounted on a flexible polyethylene shaft, with a relatively soft, tapered, radio-opaque Percuflex tip. It maintains its size and shape on inflation, and is designed to rupture in a safe longitudinal tear, rather than a potentially damaging blow-out. The Witzel and other similar endoscope-mounted dilators (Sakai, Troidl, Frimberger) are mounted on the shaft of a forward-viewing endoscope, and introduced into the sphincter under radiological or endoscopic control.

Choice of technique

The choices are often dictated by availability of equipment and local expertise. Based on evidence or experience, the following can be recommended:
- Bougies are preferable to balloons for organic stenoses of the oesophagus, because bougie dilatation is probably more effective in dysphagia relief [21].
- Endoscopic and/or wire-guided methods under radiological control are usually needed for long, tight

or tortuous strictures, and those associated with large hiatus herniae or fistulae.
- Anastomotic strictures are often best dilated with a balloon, because of the short segment of catheter ahead of the dilator.
- For achalasia, BoTox injection therapy is probably the first choice in the elderly or infirm, because of its safety. For dilatation, a 30-mm diameter × 50-mm long balloon (Rigiflex or similar) is the first choice, because it is predictable and relatively safe.
- Though there is continuing debate about the merits of surgery for achalasia [22], endoscopists should keep in mind that it is very effective.

Techniques

Guidewires

A small-diameter endoscope is preferable so that a larger proportion of strictures can be dilated without screening. The endoscope should be introduced under direct vision. A guidewire is passed via the biopsy channel of the endoscope and placed across the stenosis, with its tip in the gastric antrum. X-ray screening after endoscopic injection of contrast may be helpful for difficult strictures. Too much guidewire in the stomach predisposes to kinking or knotting of the wire in the stomach. The position of the guidewire in the stomach can be confirmed radiologically during and after removal of the endoscope. Stiff 'piano wire' guidewires offer the most support to the dilator, but more flexible biliary-type wires may be needed to traverse complex strictures. J-tip wires introduced into the top end of the stricture within an endoscopic retrograde cholangiopancreatography (ERCP) Teflon guiding catheter are atraumatic, effective, available and cheap. Hydrophilic wires can also be useful, but are less available and more expensive.

The dilator is passed over the guidewire, and its progress monitored radiologically. The guidewire is maintained in position relative to a fixed point outside the patient (usually the edge of the endoscopy trolley worktop), with the tip in the gastric antrum, and by reference to the X-ray and to marks on the wire itself.

Bougienage (Fig. 2.12)

Lubricating jelly is applied to the tapered segment of the bougies. Dilatation is achieved by the successive passage of progressively larger dilators through the stricture. For very tight strictures, it is advisable not to attempt full dilatation in a single session. Benign strictures which can be traversed by a 10-mm endoscope can normally be safely dilated to 18 mm in a single session.

Balloon dilatation

'Over-the-wire' balloons (Fig. 2.13)

The procedure is similar to bougienage except that a balloon is positioned in the stricture over-the-wire (OTW). Preliminary submucosal injection of 0.2–0.5 ml of lipiodol contrast, which is more accurate than external radio-opaque markers, is of use in this situation for accurate positioning of the balloon. The diameter and length of the balloon to be used depends on the dimensions of the stricture. The guidewire is introduced via the endoscope (or under radiological guidance alone), and the endoscope is withdrawn. Over the naked guidewire, and under entirely radiological control, the balloon is inflated within the stricture, using an inflation device with a pressure gauge to avoid rupturing the balloons (which are expensive!). The maximum pressure recommended by the manufacturer is often required for adequate dilatation. I prefer to use dilute water-soluble contrast to monitor inflation, as liquids are less compressible than air and it is easier to see the loss of the waist in the balloon, which indicates that full dilatation has been achieved. The balloon is normally inflated for 1 min, though there are few data to validate this practice. Unlike bougies, resistance is difficult to judge with balloon dilatation.

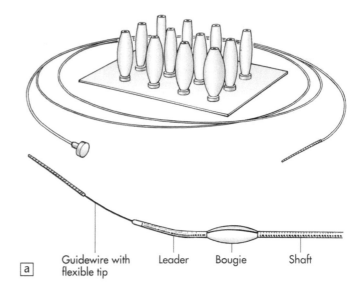

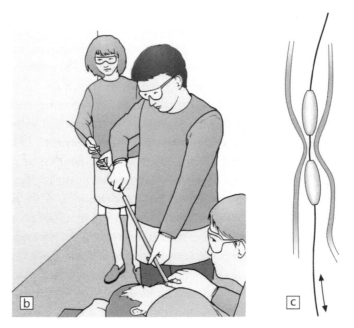

Figure 2.12. Illustration of Eder-Puestow dilator being 'railroaded' along a wire. The olives come in graduated sizes and are serially mounted on a pushing device over guidewire (a), the device is 'railroaded' over a preinserted guidewire (b) and passed through the stricture (c).

'Through-the-scope' balloons

Through-the-scope (TTS) balloons have the advantage that the endoscope does not need to be removed, dilatation takes place under direct vision, and fluoroscopy is usually not required. The completely deflated balloon, after being lubricated with silicone oil and mounted on a guidewire, is passed through the biopsy channel of the endoscope. The

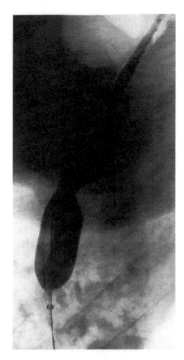

Figure 2.13. X-ray of waisted balloon across a stricture.

guidewire is advanced ahead of the balloon under direct vision and X-ray control, and the balloon positioned within the stricture. Alternatively, the guidewire can be passed alone, followed by the balloon when the wire has traversed the stricture. The deflated balloon can also be passed without a guidewire, as is commonly done for colonic strictures. There is a risk that the relatively rigid leading segment of the balloon will perforate the side wall of the oesophagus, but this is small if the stricture is known to be short and uncomplicated.

Postoperative management

Post-dilatation endoscopy may be performed if further biopsies are needed, or to examine the stomach and duodenum if previously inaccessible.

Post-procedure observations of pulse, temperature, respiration, chest pain and subcutaneous emphysema should be routine to provide early evidence of possible perforation. Their frequency and duration depends on the difficulty of the dilatation, which gives a rough guide to the likelihood of perforation. During the observation period, the patient should be kept nil-by-mouth. Post-procedure chest X-ray is generally not necessary if the patient has neither chest pain nor clinical signs of perforation 4 hours after the dilatation.

In the absence of clinical signs, a post-procedure X-ray study with water-soluble contrast is unnecessary (though this is routine in some centres).

Patients can normally drink water when sufficiently recovered from sedation, provided that there are no signs of perforation. This is an ideal time for the endoscopist to review the patient, and to observe them drink water. Food may normally be taken the following day.

The patient should be discharged with any necessary medication and a follow-up plan and dietary advice provided if indicated.

Protocols of management

Dilatation can be repeated within a few days in severe cases, and every few weeks if necessary until swallowing is normal. Half of the patients with benign strictures do not need dilatation within a year, even without PPI therapy [23].

Severity, as reflected in the need for further dilatation, is dependent on the diameter of the original stricture, but more importantly on whether there is peri-oesophageal fibrosis – as in caustic strictures, or after a perforation – which tend to recur and need frequent dilatation. The need for dilatation is judged by the amount of dysphagia. If the major symptom is not dysphagia – nocturnal cough for example – deciding when to redilate may be more difficult, and measurement of stricture size with wax-impregnated balls may be helpful [24]. If the stricture measures 12 mm or more, patients are unlikely to benefit from dilatation.

The 'rule of three'

It was said that the amount of dilatation in one session should not exceed three increases (2–3 F) in dilator size once the operator feels significant resistance. This is still a good principle for the inexperienced. Unless a peptic stricture is of pin-hole size, or is particularly fibrotic and difficult to dilate, we normally dilate to 18 mm in the first session. Endoscopists need to develop a personal sense of what is safe.

SPECIAL CASES

Achalasia

Botulinum toxin injection

This is performed as follows:

- The oesophagus is emptied by lavage and endoscopic suction.
- Using a varices injector with a 5-mm needle, BoTox is injected into the sphincter rosette, typically just at the

squamocolumnar junction. It is important to note that the available preparations are not equipotent. Pasricha *et al.* recommend 80 units of a US preparation (Oculinum; Allergan Inc., Irvine, CA) injected in four 1-ml aliquots of 20 U each into each quadrant of the LOS. After initial failures using a smaller dose, we now use a total of 400 units of the preparation available in the UK (DysPort Speywood BoTox), diluted in 10 ml of saline, injected in four 2-ml aliquots. This appears to be effective in a small personal experience.

- Relief of dysphagia can be expected the following day.
- If dysphagia is not relieved despite an apparently adequately sited injection, dilatation or surgery can proceed immediately.

Balloon dilatation (Fig. 2.13)

The steps are:

- The OTW technique is used, normally with a 30-mm diameter Rigiflex balloon designed for the purpose. The guidewire is placed in the gastric antrum. During withdrawal, the approximate position of the LOS in relation to the diaphragm is determined by screening the tip of the endoscope positioned at the LOS.
- The balloon is placed at the oesophagogastric junction (OGJ) under radiological control, and partly inflated with dilute water-soluble contrast. The position of the catheter is adjusted so that the waist of the partly inflated balloon caused by the LOS is at the mid-point of the balloon. (Dilatation can be performed, under endoscopic control alone, but I prefer to screen because perfect placement and dilatation can be confirmed and documented by taking X-rays.)
- Maintaining the balloon catheter in position by fixation against the bite guard, the balloon is fully inflated with dilute water-soluble contrast.
- Full inflation is confirmed by the loss of the waist at the mid-point of the balloon. This is often accompanied by pain or restlessness. Inflation is maintained for 1–3 minutes. There are no comparative data to define the correct duration of inflation. In my hands, a single dilatation of 1 min seems adequate, though others suggest three 1-min dilatations, or a single dilatation of 3 min duration. Pressure gauges are recommended by the manufacturer, but in my experience, true achalasia dilates at a low pressure easily achievable by hand at well below the burst pressure of the Rigiflex balloon, so I never use a gauge for this indication. If the stricture does not dilate easily, I am very suspicious that achalasia is not the cause. Successful dilatation is usually accompanied by minor bleeding due to mucosal tearing, with blood on the balloon on withdrawal.

- A water-soluble contrast examination immediately after the dilatation to look for perforation is sometimes recommended. We order a contrast examination only if there is clinical suspicion of perforation.
- A second dilatation with a 30-mm balloon can be performed as soon as one week later, and if this is not successful, further pairs of dilatations with progressively larger balloons (35 and 40 mm) can be undertaken. If these are not successful, an alternative injection or surgical technique should be used.

Alternative techniques using other dilators are essentially similar. The important points are that the dilator be of fixed size, and that it be precisely placed in the LOS. With the Witzel dilator, this can be ensured by X-ray screening if desired, or by retroverting the endoscope in the stomach to view the position of the dilating balloon from below.

Anastomotic strictures

Strictures at the oesophagogastric anastomosis after total gastrectomy are most easy to dilate using a balloon, because there is insufficient space into which to advance the tapered end of a bougie. Care must be taken to exclude malignancy, but adequate biopsies may not be possible until after dilatation.

Children

Balloon dilators would seem an obvious choice in children, but there are no controlled data to compare balloon and bougie dilatation, and the X-ray exposure should be avoided if possible.

Food impaction

Food boli can be disrupted with forceps, or removed with a basket or grasping forceps through an overtube to prevent aspiration, but the best method is often to dilate the stricture. The guidewire is passed beside the obstructing bolus into the stomach, and the stricture dilated as usual, allowing the bolus to pass.

Radiotherapy strictures

The tissues are often friable, making the oesophagus liable to perforation. Care should be taken to avoid excessive dilatation; gentle dilatation with Savary–Gilliard dilators in more than one session seems safest. In one recent study, relief of dysphagia was adequate in 66% of 103 patients, with persistent pain in seven patients, unexplained fever in two, perforation in two, and tracheo-oesophageal fistula in one patient. It has been suggested that perforation may be no more common in radiation-treated oesophagus, but that the complications may be more severe [25].

Sclerotherapy strictures

These are similar to peptic strictures, and can be dilated with bougies or balloons.

COMPLICATIONS

Complications of dilation of benign oesophageal obstructions are relatively uncommon [24,25], though probably more common in achalasia than was thought [26,27]. They include:

- *Transient chest pain.* This is common during the dilatation of tight strictures. Persistent pain or fever usually indicates a complication of dilatation.
- *Perforation of the oesophagus.* This is the major hazard. In the ASGE 1974 survey of all techniques and disorders, the incidence of perforation was 1 in 500 [28]. The most common site is the cervical oesophagus, and at or just proximal to the stricture. Faulty technique and over-enthusiastic dilatation is probably the major cause. The mortality rate of endoscopic perforation ranges from 6% to 25%, because the population at risk is elderly. There are insufficient data to indicate that any single commercial dilator is particularly hazardous in peptic strictures. Perforation is most likely to occur in malignant, caustic and post-radiation strictures. In malignant strictures, perforation rates of around 10% are reported, particularly when prosthesis placement is attempted at the procedure. This rate is probably significantly less with use of expanding metal stents which require little or no instrumental dilatation. Caustic strictures which tend to be longer, tighter and associated with more mucosal damage may be more at risk for perforation. In the long term, more than 15% of patients with caustic strictures were perforated – about three times the rate in a comparison group of peptic strictures [29].
- *Aspiration pneumonia.* This probably occurs more frequently than is recognized, because symptoms are treated by general practitioners after discharge from hospital, and are never reported.
- *Bacteraemia and pyaemic infection.* Bacteraemia occurs during many endoscopic procedures, but so it does during tooth brushing. Thus, it is perhaps not surprising that so few infective complications occur. Reported rates of bacteraemia after oesophageal dilatation are up to 50% – ten times more often than after upper endoscopy alone [30]. Bacteraemia is related to the degree of dilatation damage, involves oropharyngeal organisms and those from the dilator surface, and does not occur when dilators are passed in volunteers without strictures [31,32]. Metastatic abscesses and bacterial meningitis have been described. On general grounds, immunosuppressed patients should be considered for antibiotic prophylaxis, and guidelines for patients at risk for infective endocarditis must be followed. Disinfection of endoscopic equipment must be thorough, though the major source is probably endogenous bacteria from the pharynx and nose.
- *Haemorrhage.* It is common for benign stricture and achalasia to bleed slightly after dilatation, but significant bleeding needing transfusion is uncommon.
- *Rare complications.* Knotting of the guidewire requires surgery for removal. Rupture of the spleen, atrio-oesophageal fistula and pneumothorax are described.

REFERENCES

1. Kuhlmeier KV. Epidemiology and dysphagia. *Dysphagia* 1994; 9: 209–217.

2. Fagundes RB, de Barros SGS, Putten ACK *et al.* Occult dysplasia is disclosed by Lugol chromoscopy in alcoholics at high risk for squamous cell carcinoma of the esophagus. *Endoscopy* 1999; 31: 281–285.

3. Hiele M, DeLeyn P, Schurmans P *et al.* Relation between endoscopic ultrasound findings and outcome of patients with

tumours of the esophagus or gastro-esophageal junction. *Gastrointest Endosc* 1997; 45: 381–386.

4. Smith PM, Kerr GD, Cockel R *et al*. A comparison of omeprazole and ranitidine in the prevention of recurrence of benign esophageal stricture. *Gastroenterology* 1994; 107: 1312–1318.

5. Agnew SR, Pandya SP, Reynolds RP, Preiksatis HG. Predictors for frequent esophageal dilatations of benign peptic strictures. *Dig Dis Sci* 1996; 41: 931–936.

6. Tan BS, Kennedy C, Morgan R *et al*. Using uncovered metallic endoprostheses to treat recurrent benign oesophageal strictures. *Am J Roentgenol* 1997; 169: 1281–1284.

7. Wo JM, Waring JP. Medical therapy of gastroesophageal reflux and management of esophageal strictures. *Surg Clin North Am* 1997; 77: 1041–1062.

8. Koshy SS, Nostrand TT. Pathophysiology and endoscopic/balloon treatment of esophageal motility disorders. *Surg Clin North Am* 1997; 77: 971–992.

9. Eckhardt VF, Aignerr C, Bernhard G. Predictors of outcome in patients with achalasia with pneumostatic dilatation. *Gastroenterology* 1992; 103: 1732–1738.

10. Csendes A, Braghetto I, Henriquez A, Cortes C. Late results of a prospective randomised study comparing forceful dilatation and oesophago-myotomy in patients with achalasia. *Gut* 1989; 30: 299–304.

11. Vantrappen G, Hellemans J. Treatment of achalasia and related motor disorders. *Gastroenterology* 1980; 79: 144–154.

12. Pasricha PJ, Ravich WJ, Hendrix TR *et al*. Intrasphincteric botulinum toxin for the treatment of achalasia. *N Engl J Med* 1995; 332: 774–778.

13. Pasricha PJ, Rai R, Ravich WJ *et al*. Botulinum toxin for achalasia: long-term outcome and predictors of response. *Gastroenterology* 1996; 110: 1410–1415.

14. Moreto M, Ojembarrena E, Rodriguez ML. Endoscopic injection of ethanolamine as a treatment for achalasia: a first report. *Endoscopy* 1996; 28: 539–545.

15. Hunter JG, Richardson WS. Surgical management of achalasia. *Surg Clin North Am* 1997; 77: 993–1015.

16. Patti MG, Arcerito M, De Pinto M *et al*. Comparison of thoracoscopic and laparoscopic Heller myotomy for achalasia. *J Gastrointest Surg* 1998; 2: 561–566.

17. Ebert EC, Ouyang A, Wright SH *et al*. Pneumatic dilatation in patients with symptomatic diffuse esophageal spasm and lower esophageal sphincter dysfunction. *Dig Dis Sci* 1983; 28: 481–485.

18. Miller LS, Parkman HP, Schiano TD *et al*. Treatment of symptomatic non achalasia esophageal motor disorders with Botulinum toxin injection at the lower esophageal sphincter. *Dig Dis Sci* 1996; 41: 2025–2031.

19. Earlam R, Cunha-Melo JR. Benign oesophageal strictures: historical and technical aspects of dilatation. *Br J Surg* 1981; 68: 829–836.

20. Abele JE. The physics of oesophageal dilatation. *Hepato-Gastroenterology* 1992; 39: 486–489.

21. Cox JGC, Winter RK, Maslin SC *et al*. Balloon or bougie for dilatation of benign oesophageal stricture? *Dig Dis Sci* 1994; 39: 776–781.

22. Gadenstatter M, Nehra D. Achalasia: dilation or myotomy? A continuing enigma. *Am J Gastroenterol* 1997; 29: 1572–1573.

23. Patterson DJ, Graham DY, Smith JL *et al*. Natural history of benign oesophageal strictures treated by dilatation. *Gastroenterology* 1983; 85: 346–350.

24. Dyet JF, Bennett JR, Buckton G, Ashworth D. The radiological measurement of oesophageal stricture diameter. *Clin Radiol* 1983; 34: 647–649.

25. Clouse RE. Complications of endoscopic gastrointestinal dilation. *Gastrointest Endosc Clin North Am* 1996; 6: 323–341.

26. McBride MA, Ergun GA. The endoscopic management of esophageal stenosis. *Gastrointest Endosc Clin North Am* 1994; 4: 595–621.

27. Eckhardt VF, Kanzler G, Westermeier T. Complications and their impact after pneumatic dilation for achalasia: prospective long-term follow up study. *Gastrointest Endosc* 1997; 45: 349–353.

28. Khandelwal M, Ouyang A. Pneumatic dilation for achalasia: are all complications revealed? (Editorial). *Gastrointest Endosc* 1997; 45: 437–439.

29. Silvis SE, Nebel O, Rogers G, Sugawa C, Mandelstam P. Endoscopic complications. Results of the 1974 American Society for Gastrointestinal Endoscopy survey. *JAMA* 1976; 235; 928–930.

30. Broor SL, Kumar A, Chari ST *et al.* Corrosive esophageal strictures following acid ingestion: clinical profile and results of endoscopic dilatation. *J Gastroenterol Hepatol* 1989; 4: 55–61.

31. Newcomer MK, Brazer SR. Complications of upper gastrointestinal endoscopy and their management. *Gastrointest Endosc Clin North Am* 1994; 4: 551–570.

32. Stephenson PM, Dorrington L, Harris OD *et al.* Bacteraemia following oesophageal dilatation and oesophagogastroscopy. *Aust NZ J Med* 1977; 7: 32–35.

3 Malignant oesophageal obstruction and tracheo-oesophageal fistulae: endoscopic palliation

A.I. Morris

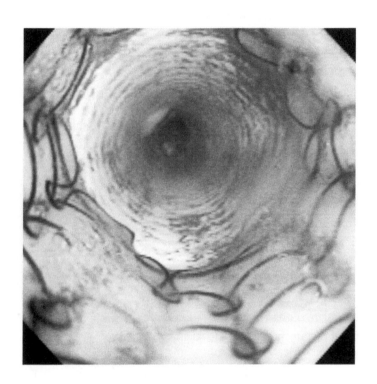

INTRODUCTION

Patients with dysphagia often ignore their symptoms and find ways of dealing with their difficulty, usually by changing their dietary habits. As discussed earlier in Chapter 2, there are many benign causes of dysphagia, but oesophageal malignant obstruction most commonly presents with this symptom. Frequently patients misinterpret the symptom and describe it as either vomiting or regurgitation of saliva. The classical story of progressive dysphagia with difficulty in swallowing solids initially, followed by difficulty in managing semi-solids and subsequently liquids, is present in only a minority of patients. Increasingly, patients are being referred with only dysphagia for solids, and it is of course important that all referring doctors always take the onset of dysphagia as a serious symptom.

PRESENTATION

There are no specific associated features that will help to differentiate benign from malignant causation (see Chapter 2). Although not all patients with dysphagia will have a malignancy, it must be assumed that this is the case until investigation has proven otherwise. Despite this widely promulgated dictum, at presentation only about 40% of patients with oesophageal malignancy will be suitable for surgery, either because of distant metastases, local spread or lack of fitness for surgery.

A less common, and widely missed, diagnosis on the basis of symptoms is the presence of a tracheo-oesophageal fistula (TOF). If the patient complains of coughing bouts precipitated by drinking fluids or swallowing, then it should be considered that there is either a TOF, a very high stricture in the oesophagus, or some neurological cause for the dysphagia. The presence of nasal regurgitation or dysphonia would favour a neurological cause.

Occasionally, patients may present with more generalized symptoms that do not focus one's attention on the oesophagus, such as anorexia, weight loss, a gastrointestinal bleed or less specific dyspeptic symptoms.

It is probably wise to pay little attention to the site at which patients say their food sticks as there is a poor correlation between the site of stricture – whether benign or malignant – and the level indicated by the patient. It is also important to ask the patient whether food sticks on the way down, as well as whether they can swallow properly. Many patients think the act of swallowing is limited to getting food out of their mouth.

DIAGNOSIS AND INVESTIGATION

The first role of investigation is to determine the cause for the patient's symptoms, and in particular whether there is a malignant obstruction or not. The initial diagnosis can be made by either endoscopy or barium studies, unless a TOF is suspected when a water-soluble contrast medium should be used. There are advantages and disadvantages to both techniques, and in some cases both will be required.

Barium studies

Although barium studies can demonstrate a stricture (Fig. 3.1), and features can be suggestive of malignancy, they

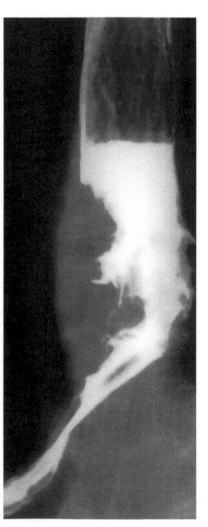

Figure 3.1. Barium swallow demonstrating features of malignant stricture.

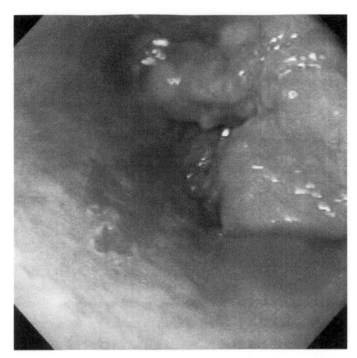

Figure 3.2. Endoscopic appearance of malignant oesophageal stricture.

cannot confirm the diagnosis histologically. In very tight tortuous strictures barium studies can give an accurate estimate of its length.

Some gastroenterologists still insist on a barium study before an endoscopy for dysphagia, but this is probably not needed unless access to barium studies is much quicker than to endoscopy. All patients with a provisional diagnosis of malignant stricture – or indeed any stricture seen at barium study – will require endoscopy both for histological diagnosis and for symptomatic relief until further assessment is made.

Endoscopy

An endoscopy will nearly always give an experienced endoscopist the diagnosis (Fig. 3.2), but occasionally negative biopsies will need to be repeated to confirm the endoscopic impression. The main problem with endoscopic diagnosis is when a tight stricture is found. Unless the patient and endoscopist are prepared to go on to a therapeutic procedure, then assessment of the length of the tumour will not be possible.

Patients with dysphagia should be treated as an urgency. In many units, patients with dysphagia are endoscoped within a week and are consented and prepared for a dilatation at the time of the diagnostic endoscopy. This saves a further procedure, is appropriate whether the stricture is benign or malignant, and – if undertaken with care and to not too large a diameter – is safe.

Further investigations

Radiology

Appearances of extrinsic compression by tumour either at endoscopy or on barium will mandate at least a chest X-ray, as well as a computed tomography (CT) scan in most centres. As with other tumours, an important part of the assessment is whether there has been local infiltration. It should also be apparent whether or not bony or pulmonary metastases are present.

Endoscopic ultrasonography (EUS)

In some patients with atypical achalasia, or a difficult benign stricture which will not respond to standard dilatation techniques, submucosal infiltration by cancer must be excluded. This is best done by EUS.

Blood tests

A routine blood test to exclude anaemia, abnormal liver function tests and urea and electrolyte disturbances are also appropriate. Abnormal liver enzymes may indicate metastatic disease, and under such circumstances a liver ultrasound should be considered.

MANAGEMENT

If a malignancy is confirmed or suspected on initial investigation, then the next part of the diagnosis is to determine the type of malignancy and then the extent of the tumour. It is important to treat the dysphagia as soon as possible to allow adequate nutrition while other investigations are being organized and a decision made about long-term management.

The main aims of management are:

- to provide symptomatic relief;
- to stage the cancer;
- to decide between potentially curative or palliative treatment;
- to arrange the necessary treatment;
- to provide salvage procedures as required; and
- to support the patient, their relatives and carers.

Symptomatic relief

Before a definitive plan for the patient's management is formulated, it is essential to provide some relief of their symptoms for both psychological and nutritional reasons.

Pain relief

Pain is an important consideration as, more than any other symptom, it drains the patients of any will to live. If the diagnosis of malignancy is confirmed there should be no limits to the strength or dose of analgesic used to obtain complete pain relief. Advice from a pain relief clinic, Macmillan nurse or palliative care team should be sought if there are problems. In the presence of severe dysphagia, alternative routes of administration may be appropriate until swallowing is improved. Sublingual, transcutaneous, rectal or parenteral preparations offer a wide choice in this difficult situation.

Relief of dysphagia

This is paramount in improving the life of these patients. It is my practice at the initial endoscopy to try and dilate the stricture at least to a slight degree. If the diagnosis is in doubt, then a dilatation either with a through-the-endoscope balloon (TTS) or with an over-the-wire (OTW) bougie-type dilator is appropriate. If the stricture can not be passed by the endoscope, then my preference is to use a balloon dilator of 12 mm inflated diameter (Fig. 3.3).

The advantage of such a balloon is that it has only a short leading tip, so that in the presence of a tortuous stricture it is unlikely to give rise to a false passage, as may occur with a guidewire unless passed under X-ray screening control. It is essential in a malignant stricture to dilate to

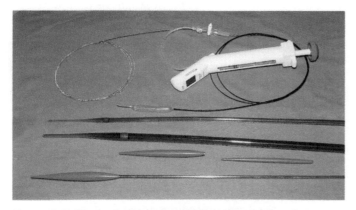

Figure 3.3. Through-the-scope (TTS) and over-the-wire (OTW) dilators.

Table 3.1. Factors against consideration of cure

Factors preventing curative treatment
Metastases
Local tumour spread
Biological age
Concomitant medical conditions

only a small degree at the first dilatation in order to avoid overstretching and splitting a tumour.

These initial dilatations are only designed to improve swallowing while staging and other decisions are made, and it must be accepted that the benefit that they produce will be of short duration, lasting a few days only. Repeated dilatations may be required, and simple dilatation alone is not an effective means of treating malignant dysphagia in the long run.

If it is apparent that the patient is not going to be suitable for curative therapy from the start (Table 3.1), then with appropriate explanation and preparation it may be possible to plan for definitive endoscopic treatment at the initial endoscopy, such as laser therapy (see Chapter 4) or stenting. In many cases, however, it is more sensible to temporize with a simple dilatation allowing more time for greater explanation to patients and relatives, staging to be completed, and patient choice to be allowed.

Staging the cancer

The purpose of staging is to prevent patients being subjected to attempted major surgical resection when there is evidence of either metastases or spread which would render the patient incurable. On the other hand, it is essential to ensure that all those patients who are potentially curable are referred to the appropriate specialist with minimal delay. If staging is carried out properly, there is great benefit both to the patient in avoiding falsely building up their hopes of cure, and also in health care costs in preventing, or reducing the number of 'open and close' operations.

Initial staging is achieved with relatively inexpensive, and widely available techniques with the aim of excluding distant metastases. Useful modalities include:
- standard chest X-ray
- liver function tests
- either an ultrasound or CT of the liver and upper abdomen.

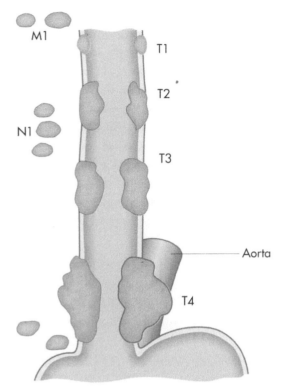

Figure 3.4. EUS staging of oesophageal tumours: 1> mucosa and submucosa; 2> through to muscularis propria; 3> through to adventitia; 4> into neighbouring structures.

Initial staging must be undertaken speedily so as to avoid unnecessary delay in definitive decision making and undue stress to the patient (Fig. 3.4). If these initial screening tests are negative and there are no contraindications to consideration of resection, patients should proceed to EUS (Figs 3.5, 3.6). This has been shown to be the best method

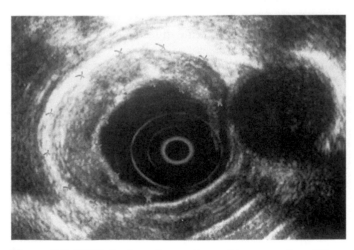

Figure 3.5. TNM staging of oesophageal tumours stage T2.

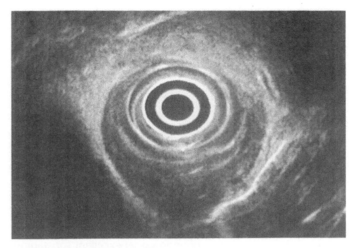

Figure 3.6. EUS image of TNM stage T3.

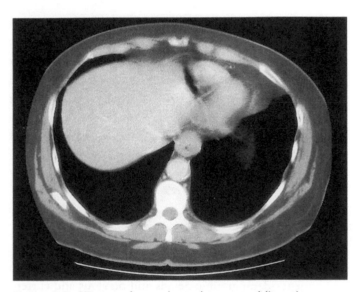

Figure 3.7. CT scan of oesophageal tumour obliterating lumen.

of T, N staging of the oesophagus in comparison with thoracic CT (Fig. 3.7).

In the absence of EUS, a thoracic CT would be appropriate, but is less sensitive at identifying local invasion, spread through the wall and small nodes. If the patient then clears this stage, referral to a skilled and preferably specialist oesophageal surgeon would be appropriate.

Many such surgeons will now undertake laparoscopy before carrying out a major resection, to exclude peritoneal deposits and local invasion. If the tumour is in the upper and mid oesophagus, many surgeons will also undertake a bronchoscopy to exclude tracheobronchial involvement or invasion. EUS, if available, would obviate

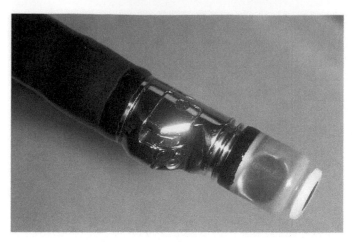

Figure 3.8. Radial array echoendoscope: excellent for staging oesophageal tumours but may not pass through all tumours.

the need for this. The disadvantage of EUS is the nature of the rather large endoscope (Fig. 3.8), which will fail to pass malignant strictures, without prior dilatation in about 25–40% of cases. The use of a blind wire-guided ultrasound probe of narrower diameter enables most strictures to be passed, and the use of the mini-probe through the biopsy channel will enable the vast majority of strictures to be examined by this means. However, all of these alternatives are very expensive.

Deciding on the type of therapy

Surgery

In most patients an experienced endoscopist armed with the patient's demographic details and previous and current medical history will be able to decide whether curative treatment is going to be possible. Even in those patients who have had what was thought to be a curative resection, the 5-year survival rate is only about 5–10%, or up to 15% in the best series.

Patients with severe pre-existing cardiovascular, respiratory or other coexistent disease which would adversely affect the outcome of surgery should not be subjected to resection. The presence of metastases would also indicate incurability and thus referral for surgery would be inappropriate. Most specialist surgeons would resect those tumours that are staged as T1, 2 or 3, although the presence of nodes – particularly in T3 lesions – would be enough for many surgeons to decline to operate. Palliative resections are probably no longer indicated, in view of less expensive, lower morbidity and mortality endoscopic palliative techniques.

Radiotherapy

Palliative radiotherapy alone has some success, but often results in deteriorating dysphagia scores at least initially, and in up to 30% of cases may result in subsequent fibrotic stricturing, even if tumour seems to have been abolished in the oesophagus. Radical radiotherapy aimed at cure does not have a significant role in adenocarcinoma, but some series of patients with squamous cell carcinoma have shown similar results to those obtained with surgical resection. Some radiotherapists believe that the use of brachytherapy significantly improves the results of external beam treatment, but this is still controversial.

Endoscopic therapy

The available choice of palliative endoscopic technique seems to be increasing as new techniques come on stream. However, the 'ideal' endoscopic technique does not exist (Table 3.2).

The choice of technique will depend upon the techniques available in the hospital, the experience of the endoscopist, and to some extent personal preference. There is no single technique or type of equipment that will meet every requirement, and so for good palliation a range of options must be available. This is the main reason why treatment for these patients should be concentrated in specialist centres.

The type of lesion to be palliated, and its site in the oesophagus, is the most important consideration. There are four types of malignant oesophageal obstruction:

1. Exophytic, predominantly intraluminal
2. Stenosing, predominantly intramural
3. Extrinsic compression
4. Tracheo-oesophageal fistulation

Table 3.2. The ideal endoscopic treatment for oesophageal malignancy

Characteristics
Simple *and* safe to use
Requires a single procedure
Produces instant and lasting complete relief from dysphagia
Is associated with a low morbidity and no mortality
Is inexpensive
Salvage techniques are available

Palliation of exophytic lesion

Injection methods

These lesions can be treated by most of the available palliative techniques. Injection with absolute alcohol or a sclerosant using a through-the-scope (TTS) flexible injection needle has been shown to be of benefit in this type of tumour; however, the effects are delayed and less predictable than with other tumour ablative methods. This technique has the advantage of being inexpensive, and requires limited training.

Thermal methods (Fig. 3.9)

Thermal ablation using either diathermy, heater probe, argon beam coagulation or laser produces more predictable damage, but as with all treatments of an ablative type may need to be repeated frequently (see Chapter 4). How much tumour is treated at any one session is a matter of debate and experience. Some authors attempt extensive tumour destruction in a single session, and then only repeat the therapy if dysphagia returns or deteriorates.

Dilatation

Simple dilatation is probably least effective with very exophytic tumours, and relief of dysphagia rarely lasts longer than a few days. However, it may be required as a prelude to the methods discussed above or in order to place an endoprosthesis (as discussed below) for stenosing lesions. Stents for exophytic tumours are likely only to be effective if there is a considerable bulk of tumour, and/or a degree of stenosis, because if the tumour is small and soft, with little stenosis, most stents migrate. Details of types of stent and their particular advantages and disadvantages are described below.

Chemotherapy/radiotherapy

There is no definite place for chemotherapeutic alleviation of dysphagia. Palliative radiotherapy can help patients with exophytic lesions.

Photodynamic therapy (PDT)

PDT has been used for palliation, but judging the dose of light exposure to produce enough tissue penetration is difficult, and overtreatment in a patient with transmural spread may produce a perforation. Because of the delay in tissue necrosis, the degree of palliation can be difficult to predict.

Palliation of stenosing lesions

Although repeated dilatation can produce effective improvement in dysphagia, the results – as have been

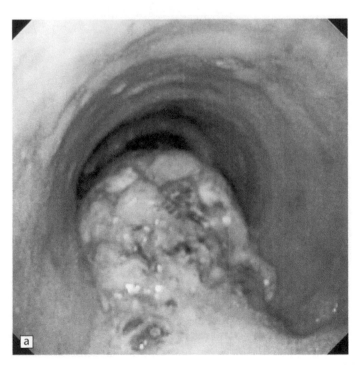 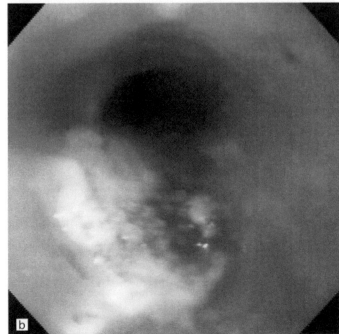

Figure 3.9. Exophytic tumour (a) before and (b) after thermal laser ablation.

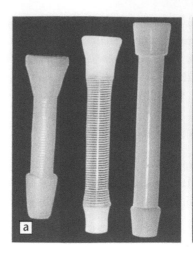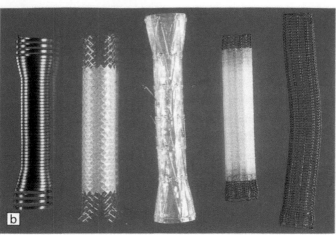

Figure 3.10. Examples (from left to right) of older rigid tubes (a) Atkinson, Celestin Cook and (b) more recent semi-flexible and covered endoprostheses Endocoil, covered wallstent, covered Gianturco, covered Ultraflex, uncovered Ultraflex.

mentioned – are short-lived. Thermal methods are not very effective and, if transmural tumour exists, these may give rise to perforation. This is also true for PDT. The longer the lesion, the more difficult and time consuming it can be to try and produce effective palliation of dysphagia with thermal or injection therapy, and the more suitable stent placement becomes.

Endoprostheses

The mainstay in the treatment of stenosing lesions is placement of stents or prosthetic tubes (Fig. 3.10a,b). Initially, these were put in under general anaesthetic by surgeons at open operation. A tapered rubber or plastic tube with a proximal flange or funnel to reduce distal migration was pulled through the tumour from below via a gastrotomy, the tapered narrowed end then being cut off and the distal end sutured to the gastric wall. The Mousseau–Barbin tube was the frequently used type, but was soon replaced by an endoscopically placed semi-rigid stent such as the Atkinson or Celestin (Fig. 3.11).

In this case, the stent was pushed through the tumour, over a guidewire and often under X-ray control, by a rammer tube. As a prerequisite for such a stent the stricture had to be dilated to 18 mm. Even in expert hands, a perforation rate of up to 10% is to be expected because of the need for the wide dilatation. Furthermore, as the lumen of the prosthetic tube was rarely more than 9 mm internal diameter, patients could rarely swallow normally and were usually confined to a puréed diet.

These semi-rigid stents (Fig. 3.10a) provided the mainstay of palliation until the development of expandable, flexible stents of which currently there are four main types. They are

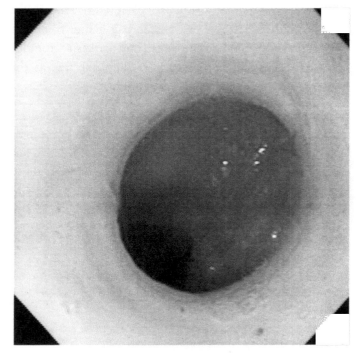

Figure 3.11. Endoscopic view through a rigid endoprosthesis within the oesophagus.

all introduced in a compressed form on a relatively slim introducer, so that it is not necessary to dilate the stricture to more than 12 mm diameter. As a result, the risk of perforation is greatly reduced. The characteristics of an ideal expandable stent are shown in Table 3.3 but, not surprisingly, none fully meets these demands as yet.

Several expandable stents are available (Fig. 3.10b). The following flexible stents are currently available in the UK:
- Ultraflex (Boston Scientific) (Fig. 3.12). Knitted nitinol wire. Available as coated and uncoated. Removable.

Slim introducer with easy deployment. Available as pre-selected proximal or distal release. Not redeployable. Shortens on deployment.

- Gianturco–Rosch (Wilson Cook). Stainless-steel wire. Coated. Not removable. Complex introducing system. Distal release, but partially redeployable. Does not shorten.

- Wallstent (Schneider) (Fig. 3.13). Stainless-steel wire. Coated or uncoated. Not removable.
- Slim introducer with easy deployment. Distal release, but partially redeployable. Shortens on deployment. Available in TTS and OTW forms.

Table 3.3. The ideal self-expanding stent

Characteristics
Easily introduced
Simple release mechanism not requiring dilatation
Should be radio-opaque
Should not shorten on deployment
Should be of narrow dimensions when compressed
Should be deployable from proximal or distal ends
Should be removable or partially redeployable
Should resist external compression, prevent tumour ingrowth and not migrate
Should be inexpensive

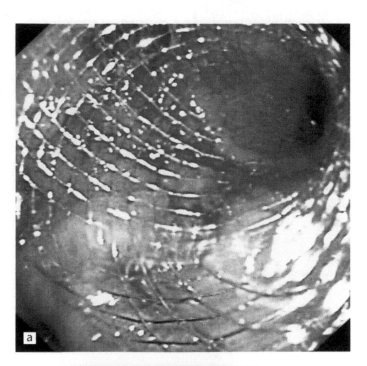

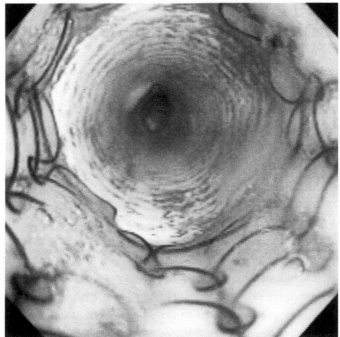

Figure 3.12. View through the covered Ultraflex stent overlaying a previously placed rigid stent.

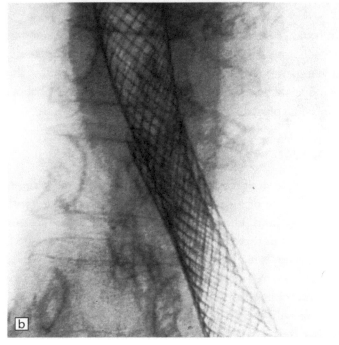

Figure 3.13. The Schneider Wallstent stent: endoscopic view (a) and X-ray appearance (b).

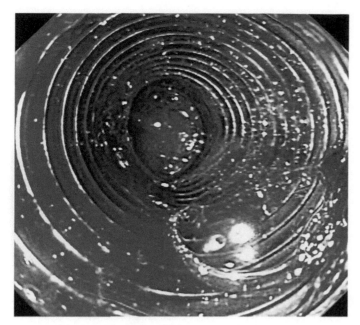

Figure 3.14. The Instent esophagocoil *in situ*.

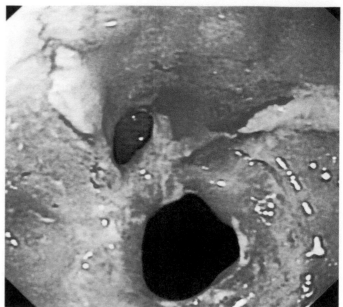

Figure 3.15. Tracheal fistula visible anterior to the oesophageal lumen: a covered flexible stent should prevent aspiration.

- Esophagocoil (Instent) (Fig. 3.14). Nitinol coil. Uncoated. Removable with difficulty. Simple release mechanism. Release from proximal, distal or middle selected *in situ*. Not redeployable. Shortens on deployment.

Extrinsic compression

In terms of management, this is dealt with in the same way as stenosing lesions. CT scan is probably the most useful investigation to clarify the nature of the lesion and, if this is inoperable, then the endoscopic methods described above can be employed to relieve symptoms.

Tracheobronchial fistulae

The palliation of tracheo-oesophageal fistulation can transform the life of a patient from that of abject misery with coughing and choking whenever food or fluids are swallowed to that of a symptom-free existence. Apart from being symptomatically unpleasant, few patients with a fistula live for more than 6 months, due to recurrent respiratory infections.

The only means of palliation is by covering the fistula with a covered stent (Fig. 3.15). As most of these patients also have a degree of dysphagia, the stent serves to treat both problems simultaneously. When placing the stent in this situation, it is preferable to mark the site of the fistula with either endoscopically placed clips or by suitable external markers, and aim to place the stent so that the fistula is sited at the mid-point of the stent, rather than simply placing the stent to bridge the tumour, as described below. This is to ensure that there is a considerable area of covered stent above the fistula which may not arise from the mid-point of the visible tumour. It is sensible to pick a stent with as large an upper expanded area as possible in order to get good occlusion around the top edge of the stent so that seepage of fluid around the outside of the stent into the fistula will be prevented.

Failure completely to seal such a fistula may require an additional stent being placed above and partially overlapping the original oesophageal one. This is possible if there is sufficient space above the stent in the oesophagus; if there is not sufficient space, a tracheobronchial stent may be placed to occlude the fistula from the other side.

Problems can occur after radical radiotherapy when exophytic tissue has been destroyed and the walls of the oesophagus and trachea or bronchus have been destroyed by extensive radionecrosis. This can lead to large fistulous openings, even sufficient to get a large-diameter endoscope through from the oesophagus into the respiratory tract, with little stricturing or exophytic growth remaining to hold the stent in place.

There is no simple solution to this problem except to try and use the largest diameter stent available. However, in some cases an attempt at heroic surgery to reconstruct the respiratory tract, or to bypass the oesophagus, may be worthwhile in those with no remaining tumour and otherwise good performance status.

Principles of stent selection

Although most stents can be used in most circumstances some are more suited than others at particular sites and in certain clinical conditions. A covered stent is ideal when trying to occlude a tracheo- or broncho-oesophageal fistula.

For very tight extrinsic compressive lesions an Esophacoil or Gianturco–Rosch stent provides the greatest radial force. High oesophageal lesions, within a few centimetres of the upper sphincter, are best treated by either the non-shortening Gianturco–Rosch, or the proximal release Ultraflex or the Endocoil, released proximally first. These stents permit more accurate placement to avoid the upper end of the stent protruding into the pharynx, and thus being uncomfortable or indeed intolerable to the patient.

PRACTICALITIES

Placement of stents

There are several important principles in the placement of stents, over and above the choice of which stent to use. The degree of pre stent placement dilatation is important, for if too great the stent will migrate caudally. Generally if a standard 9- to 10-mm endoscope (the 'P' series Olympus scopes) will pass through the stricture I would not dilate the stricture, but if the scope could not be introduced into the stomach then dilatation to 12 mm is all that is required. The stent should be selected so that it covers the malignancy and preferably 2–3 cm above and below the malignancy (Fig. 3.16).

Some compromise is necessary if attempting to stent very high upper-third lesions, to avoid the stent overriding into the pharynx and being felt by the patient. Very angulated tumours should be stented with a firmer stent to avoid kinking. Once the procedure is under way, with a guidewire placed into the antrum, it is important to mark the upper and lower limits of the tumour for correct stent placement (Fig. 3.17).

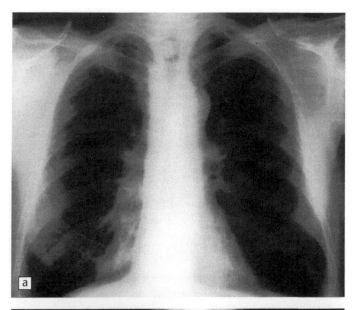

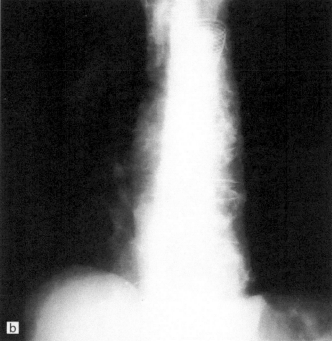

Figure 3.16. (a) The Schneider Wallstent and (b) Instent oesophagocoil in position across a malignant stricture.

Internal marking with intramucosal lipiodol injection, or mucosal metal clips, are probably the best way of defining the tumour extent for radiological screening purposes, although the latter are quite expensive. External radio-opaque markers such as paper clips stuck to the skin with adhesive tape can be adequate if the patient is well sedated and does not move significantly during the procedure, some endoscopists preferring the patient to lie prone during the procedure.

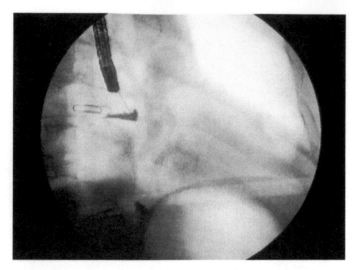

Figure 3.17. Marking the limits of stent placement by contrast injection (internal marking) and paper clip (external marking) at tumour margins.

After the stent has been released (Fig. 3.18) and the introducer withdrawn, it is sensible to check with an endoscope that the stent is in the correct position and has fully expanded. Although these expanding stents will continue to expand, sometimes taking up to 24–48 hours to get to their fully opened diameter, if there is less than 75% full deployment it is sensible to try and increase the degree of opening by balloon dilatation, either with a TTS or OTW balloon dilator. Care must be exercised not to apply longitudinal, shearing, forces to the partially opened stent as this might dislocate it from the ideal position; it is for this reason that balloon rather than bougie dilatation is employed. Similarly, when using a balloon dilator it is important to ensure that the leading end of the balloon has not been inserted through the mesh of the stent, as inflation will damage the structure and integrity of the stent, and may create a false passage.

Salvage procedures

Whatever technique is used to endoscopically treat oesophageal malignancy and tracheo-oesophageal fistulation, problems are likely to arise even in the most experienced hands. Most of the problems relate to specific

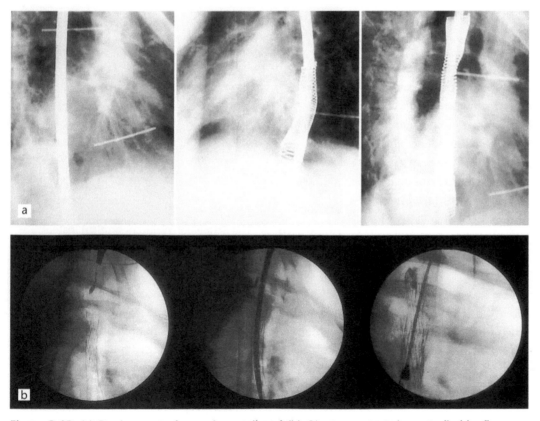

Figure 3.18. (a) Deployment of oesophagocoil and (b) Gianturco stents is controlled by fluoroscopy.

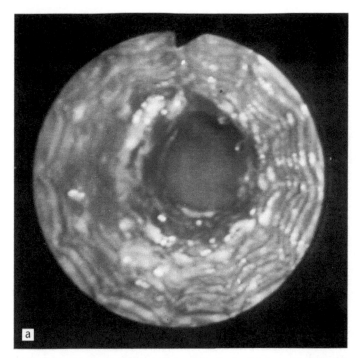
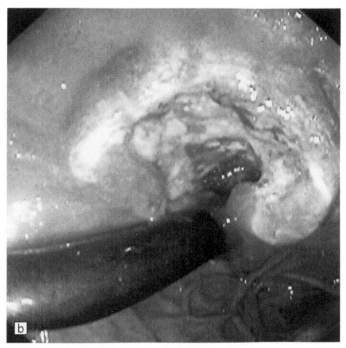

Figure 3.19. (a) Tumour overgrowth at the lower end of an Ultraflex stent and (b) retroverted endoscopic view showing extensive tumour growth below previously placed oesophageal stent.

complications of the procedures, and when such a complication arises, it needs to be diagnosed quickly and dealt with expeditiously. As with all aspects of therapeutic procedures careful and full pre-procedure explanation should have taken place with appropriate mention of major possible complications. Some common problems include the following.

Stent overgrowth (Fig. 3.19)

Whether at the top or bottom of the stent, this can be easily managed with any thermal method of tumour destruction. If there is a long bulk of tumour, placement of a second stent to override the overgrowth is another, albeit more expensive, option (Fig. 3.13b).

Stent ingrowth (Fig. 3.20)

The management of this complication is the same as that for stent overgrowth; however, repeated passage of a wide-diameter endoscope through the stent will often abrade sufficient tumour to improve dysphagia. Rarely food bolus obstruction can occur and the stent may require removal (Fig. 3.21).

Stent kinking (Fig. 3.22)

If a stent is placed in a very angulated tumour, particularly

if the tumour is very firm, then kinking may occur. This is especially the case with the softer, less rigid stents such as the Ultraflex. This problem may also arise from failure of

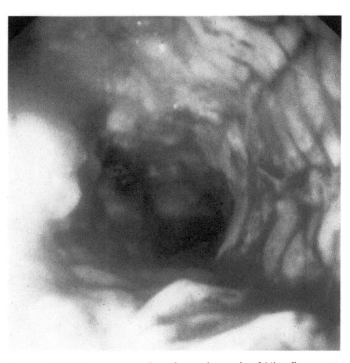

Figure 3.20. Tumour growing through mesh of Ultraflex stent.

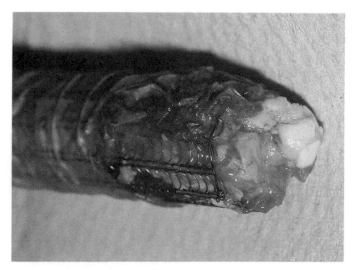

Figure 3.21. An extreme example of tumour ingrowth obstructed with food debris in an endoprosthesis removed by endoscopy.

full expansion of a stent. Initially, an attempt should be made to expand the stent fully by insertion of a balloon dilator, but if this does not work, or if the problem rapidly returns, then placement of a second stent through the original one should provide a solution to the problem.

Stent migration (Fig. 3.23)

If the stent is only partially migrated, then overlap stenting may be performed provided that there is enough room above the original stent (if appropriate). If the first stent has slipped right through the tumour, then restenting with a different and certainly wider stent would be reasonable. A stent that has migrated into the stomach can be left *in situ*, and may even pass down the gut. Attempts at removal should only be undertaken if the stent is causing symptoms, such as obstruction.

Bleeding from under the stent

There is little that can be done if the bleeding is occurring from under a covered stent. If it is not covered, or the bleeding is from tumour that is accessible endoscopically, then thermal methods – particularly argon beam coagulation – may reduce the rate of blood loss.

Perforation at dilatation

Providing this is recognized at the time, perforation is best managed by immediate stenting with a covered stent, intravenous fluids and feeding, and treatment with broad-spectrum antibiotics. If the perforation is recognized after the initial procedure has been completed, then a contrast study should be undertaken to assess the size of the

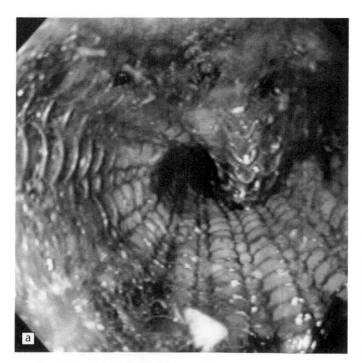
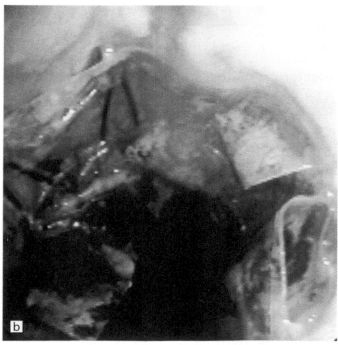

Figure 3.22. (a) Stents causing partial obstruction by kinking or (b) disuption of membrane covering stent.

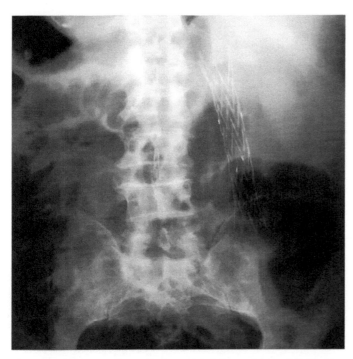

Figure 3.23. Oesophageal stent which has migrated through to stomach.

perforation. If small with minimal mediastinal infiltration, then conservative management with nil-by-mouth, parenteral feeding and intravenous antibiotics should suffice. If there is a large defect, then stenting would be appropriate. Detailed discussion with the patient and their relatives is essential. If the patient has been selected for palliation correctly then it should be rare to have to involve a surgeon, though most of these cases are best managed with a multidisciplinary team of endoscopists, radiologists, surgeons and oncologists.

Recurrent stricturing

This often occurs after radiotherapy or intensive laser therapy. Both of these modalities induce a fibrotic reaction, and some endoscopists believe that these strictures – which can be very firm – are prone to split. Either repeated dilatation, or in recurrent difficult cases stenting, may help. If dilatation is undertaken it should be in small gradually increasing steps in order to avoid splitting and perforation.

FURTHER READING

Tytgat GNJ. Endoscopic therapy of esophageal cancer: possibilities and limitations. *Endoscopy* 1990; 22: 263–267.

Loizou LA, Grigg D, Atkinson M *et al.* A prospective comparison of laser therapy and intubation in endoscopic palliation of malignant dysphagia. *Gastroenterology* 1991; 100: 1303–1310.

Sargeant IR, Lozou LA, Tobias JS *et al.* Radiation enhancement of laser palliation for malignant dysphagia: a pilot study. *Gut* 1992; 33: 1597–1601.

Knyrim K, Wagner H-J, Bethge N *et al.* A controlled trial of an expansile metal stent for the palliation of esophageal obstruction due to inoperable cancer. *N Eng J Med* 1993; 328: 1302–1307.

Krasner N. The use of laser in the upper gastrointestinal tract Ch 6 p 87–102. In; *Practice of Therapeutic Endoscopy* Eds Tytgat, GNJ and Classen M. Edinburgh: Churchill Livingstone, 1994.

Tytgat GNJ. Endoprosthesis palliation of esophagogastric malignancy Ch 5 p 67–86. In; *Practice of Therapeutic Endoscopy* Eds Tytgat, GNJ and Classen M. Edinburgh: Churchill Livingstone, 1994.

Lightdale CJ, Heier SK, Marcon NE *et al.* Photodynamic therapy with porfimer sodium versus thermal ablation with Nd-YAG laser for palliation of esophageal cancer: A multicenter randomized trial. *Gastrointest Endosc* 1995; 42: 507–512.

Mitty RD, Cave DR, Birkett D. One stage retrograde approach to Nd-YAG palliation of esophageal carcinoma. *Endoscopy* 1996; 28: 350–355.

Segalin A, Bonavina L, Carazzone A *et al.* Improving results of esophageal stenting: a study on 160 consecutive unselected patients. *Endoscopy* 1997; 29: 701–709.

Fleischer D. Four things to recall about esophageal cancer. *Endoscopy* 1998; 30: 311–312.

Lambert R. Endoscopic treatment of esophagogastric tumours. *Endoscopy* 1998; 30: 80–93.

Savary JF, Grosjean P, Monnier P *et al.* Photodynamic therapy of early squamous cell carcinomas of the esophagus: a review of 31 cases. *Endoscopy* 1998; 30: 258–265.

Inoue H, Tani M, Nagai K *et al.* Treatment of esophageal and gastric tumours. *Endoscopy* 1999; 31: 47–55.

Bartelsman JFW, Bruno MJ, Jensema AJ *et al.* Palliation of patients with oesophagogastric neoplasms by insertion of a covered expandable modified Gianturco-Z endoprosthesis: experiences in 153 patients. *Gastrointest Endosc* 2000; 51: 134–138.

Siersema PD, Hop WCJ, Blankenstein M-V, Dees J. A new design metal stent (Flamingo stent) for palliation of malignant dysphagia: a prospective study. *Gastrointest Endosc* 2000; 51: 139–145.

4 Upper gastrointestinal malignancy: palliation with thermal laser, photodynamic therapy and argon beamer

N. Krasner

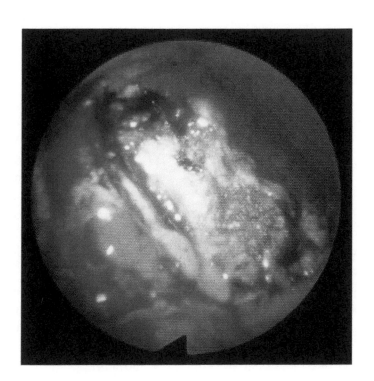

INTRODUCTION

The incidence of carcinoma of the oesophagus and gastric cardia is rising sharply in the Western world, including the UK [1], and the majority of patients are incurable at presentation [2]. For the purposes of this chapter, oesophageal cancer will include the gastric cardia.

PRESENTATION

Dysphagia

As indicated in the earlier chapters on this subject, dysphagia is the most common feature, being present in some 95% of patients. It is, however, remarkable that the initial accommodation to the swallowing problem allows patients to tolerate a symptom which should require rapid access to medical advice and timely investigation and treatment.

Weight loss

Weight loss and inanition are common terminal features of such tumours, the former being an obvious warning sign but – particularly in the older age groups – acceptance of a modified soft or even liquid diet may, for a time a least, allow the patient to maintain a reasonable calorie intake.

Pain

Pain in the chest or in the upper epigastrium is not an invariable feature, but discomfort on swallowing becomes increasingly common as the obstruction progresses. Initially, enhanced proximal peristalsis to overcome the block may be a source of chest pain, as may oesophageal spasm and disordered motility due to invasion of nerve supply and interference with the nerve conduction mechanism.

Bleeding and anaemia

Overt bleeding from the tumour is a relatively common initial presentation (Table 4.1), though anaemia from occult blood loss is more frequent. Once palliative treatment has been commenced, bleeding may occur from the treated cancer surface.

Table 4.1. Symptoms of oesophageal cancer

Symptoms of oesophageal cancer	
Common symptoms	Regurgitation and/or vomiting
	Progressive dysphagia
	Weight loss
	Chronic iron-deficiency anaemia
	Pain on swallowing (odynophagia)
Uncommon symptoms	Aspiration pneumonia
	Hoarseness of voice
	Severe gastrointestinal bleed
	Oesophago-tracheal/pleural fistula

DIAGNOSIS

Dysphagia may result from inflammatory conditions, neural or muscular disorders, and a variety of sources of mechanical block, as discussed in Chapter 2. As emphasized in Chapter 3, the possibility of a malignant origin must be considered at an early stage, even in relatively young subjects in their 30s and 40s, if there is to be any realistic hope of cure. A 'fast-track' protocol to identify the problem, together with education of the public and primary and secondary care staff, is essential to allow earlier diagnosis and improve the prospect of cure.

Surgery remains the only realistic hope of cure [3], and the value of early diagnosis has been demonstrated by the Japanese whose operative mortality rate for radical resection can be restricted to 4%, with a 5-year survival rate of 30% [4].

Early endoscopy with histological confirmation, with or without a barium swallow, will provide initial information on the tumour bulk, degree of obstruction and the possibility of extrinsic compression. A bleeding, friable tumour surface points to the source of anaemia. Forceps biopsy is most useful but, where obstruction proximally prevents direct vision of the malignancy, brush biopsy is also useful. Preliminary dilatation with balloon, Savary–Gilliard bougie type or KeyMed Advanced olive dilators, cautiously applied (see Chapter 3), should allow assessment of the full luminal extent of the tumour, as indicated in Table 4.2.

Careful staging is necessary to avoid inappropriate surgery, as discussed earlier. Endoluminal ultrasound provides the most accurate assessment of depth of tumour and local invasion [5], while standard or coiled computed

Table 4.2. Characteristics of oesophageal tumours influencing choice of treatment

Features
Position and length
Concentric or exophytic
In the oesophageal wall itself, intraluminal or extrinsic
Degree of obstruction (does not necessarily correlate with degree of dysphagia).

tomography (CT) or positron emission tomography (PET) scanning determine distant spread. Ideally, these imaging modalities should be used in tandem but, as yet, they are not routinely available in many centres.

MANAGEMENT AND EVIDENCE

Objectives

The ideal palliative treatment provides relief from symptoms by a simple, safe and easily reproducible and repeatable method with minimum disturbance to the patient, and an acceptable level of morbidity and mortality. The primary objectives for oesophageal carcinoma in the simplest form are shown in Figure 4.1.

There are five questions to be asked in this respect:

1. Is dysphagia adequately relieved, and for how long?
2. Is the gain worth the pain, i.e. does the patient tolerate the procedure?
3. Is the general quality of life improved?
4. Is the treatment cost effective (value for money)?
5. Does the treatment measure up in a cost–benefit analysis (value to the patient)?

Restoration of functional patency by relief of luminal narrowing or reduction in tumour bulk is the basis of

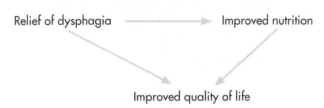

Figure 4.1. Integrated approach to management of oesophageal cancer.

treatment but, once achieved, attention must be given to the type and consistency of dietary intake which will maintain nutritional status and weight and, by so doing, improve general well-being.

Prevention of anaemia and reduction in transfusion requirements is another priority. Stenting or intubation may provide initial tamponade, but bleeding from under the stent/tube surface is not an uncommon complication and may be difficult to access. Thermal ablation by laser, argon plasma coagulator or bipolar electrode are all effective in cauterizing a bleeding tumour surface, although sloughing of the charred or coagulated surface may well result in further bleeding.

Choice of palliation

It is clear from the list of options available (Table 4.3) that the ideal form of palliation has not yet been achieved, and that different approaches may be more applicable in particular patients. For this reason, as emphasized in Chapter 3, patients should be referred early to specialist centres where

Table 4.3. Palliative modalities in oesophageal carcinoma

Modality	
Dilatation	Balloon, bougies
Intubation	Semi-rigid tubes
	Expandable metal stents (coiled, open mesh, membrane-covered)
Laser therapy	Thermal (Nd-YAG, diode)
	Photodynamic therapy (dye laser, diode)
Argon plasma coagulator	
Bipolar electrocoagulation	BICAP
Radiotherapy	External beam
	Brachytherapy
Chemotherapy	
Alcohol and sclerosant injection	
Percutaneous endoscopic gastrostomy (PEG) feeding	
Surgery	

BICAP = Bipolar coagulator
PEG = Percutaneous endoscopic gastrostomy

a multidisciplinary range of treatment options should be available. The most commonly applied techniques are placement of a prosthesis using a semi-rigid tube or a variety of the expanding metal mesh stent, and thermal ablation of the obstructing tumour using a laser or, more recently, the argon plasma coagulator. Photodynamic therapy (PDT) using a laser or non-laser light source is still largely a research technique that is available in only a few centres in the United Kingdom.

PRACTICALITIES

Equipment

Thermal ablation
Since the early 1980s the primary use of thermal lasers has been in the palliation of upper and lower gastrointestinal malignancies. It has become apparent however, that for selected patients with small, non-invasive cancers, the laser can be applied as primary therapy, particularly when surgery is hazardous because of the patient's general condition. Thermal laser treatment of oesophageal malignancy can be applied using the high-power neodymium–yttrium–aluminium–garnet (Nd-YAG) or gallium–aluminium–arsenide (GaAlAs) diode lasers which have been demonstrated to be effective, relatively safe and easy to apply with the patient under conscious intravenous (iv) sedation. The potassium–titanyl–phosphate (KTP) laser with an operative wavelength of 532 nm has a very superficial depth of penetration, and is useful only to coagulate or cauterize a bleeding surface, although it is used primarily as a cutting instrument and in conjunction with the Nd-YAG laser. The depth of penetration of the laser beam depends on absorption by water and relates to the wavelength of light used (Fig. 4.4).

Nd-YAG laser
This laser emits a light beam in the near infra-red range at 1064 nm (Fig. 4.2). Focused on to a 600-nm quartz fibre, and protected by a Teflon sheath, the laser delivery assembly is passed through the instrument channel of a standard end-viewing endoscope [6]. A twin-channel scope obviates the need for a separate venting tube to prevent unnecessary gaseous distension. A coaxial jet of CO_2 gas maintains the tip clear of debris and prevents destruction of the tip by overheating; alternatively a water-cooled system

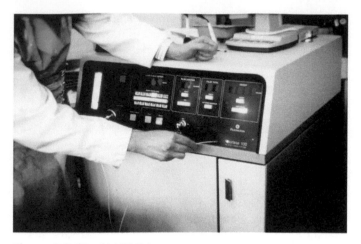

Figure 4.2. The Nd-YAG laser.

can be employed which reduces the production of smoke and abolishes the need for constant suction. If a video electronic system is employed, it is unnecessary to wear protective glasses or to fit a filter within the endoscope eyepiece.

Diode laser
An identical set-up is involved in the application of the GaAlAs diode laser (Fig. 4.3), which operates at 810 nm. At this wavelength, tissue penetration is enhanced, although with the lower power levels employed – 30–45 W as against 60–80 W with the Nd-YAG laser – depth of necrosis achieved is up to 3 mm with the diode system and up to 5 mm with the Nd-YAG. Duration of laser application is a variable feature, but my usual practice is to apply 1- to 2-second bursts with the Nd-YAG laser, but with the diode laser to use continuous application, 'painting' the target surface to achieve safe debulking. With both lasers, a very

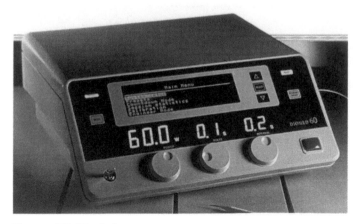

Figure 4.3. Diode laser.

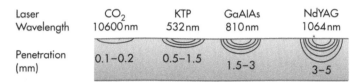

Laser Wavelength	CO$_2$ 10600 nm	KTP 532 nm	GaAlAs 810 nm	NdYAG 1064 nm
Penetration (mm)	0.1–0.2	0.5–1.5	1.5–3	3–5

Figure 4.4. Tissue penetration versus wavelength. Note: depth of penetration depends on absorption of laser light by water, e.g. CO$_2$ – strong; NdYAG – weak.

low-power aiming beam allows precise application. Ideally, non-contact laser probes should be held about 1 cm from the target tissue, and the laser is activated via a foot pedal.

A smoke extraction system removes unpleasant and theoretically hazardous fumes and particulate matter. Single-use fibres are generally employed and, although this appears to add to the cost of the procedure, there is a saving in the cost of sterilizing and repolishing the multi-use fibre. Sapphire-tipped contact probes are also available, the use of which reduces the energy required and reduces the smoke produced by tissue vaporization, but lengthens the duration of the laser procedure. A comparison of tissue penetration of these techniques is shown in Fig. 4.4.

Argon plasma coagulator (APC)

APC is a means of applying a monopolar electrosurgical current to tissue via an ionized argon gas stream (argon plasma) (Fig. 4.5). The argon gas remains ionized for 2–10 mm distal to the tip of the applicator where the energy delivery to the tissue is uniform, contact-free and penetrates to a maximum coagulation depth of about 3 mm. There are the additional benefits of better visualization because of the low volume of smoke produced, and the limited depth of penetration makes perforation of a hollow viscus less likely. The corollary is that there is less efficient debulking of large tumours. However, the limited effectiveness in destruction of tumours due to physical restrictions on the zone of thermal necrosis is largely offset by extending the duration of application sufficiently to induce tissue shrinkage by desiccation.

A main benefit of the APC is its ability to coagulate large surface areas, particularly a bleeding surface. The argon plasma beam not only acts in a straight line along the axis of application, but in seeking conductive bleeding targets, the beam can also 'bend' and thus treat lesions tucked behind mucosal folds or intestinal angles. The APC device consists of a flexible Teflon tube with a tungsten electrode contained in a ceramic nozzle at its distal end to prevent tissue adherence.

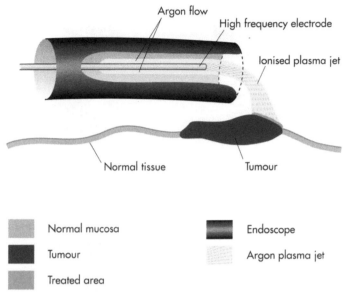

▨	Normal mucosa	▬	Endoscope
■	Tumour	▨	Argon plasma jet
▬	Treated area		

Figure 4.5. Argon beamer.

Techniques

Preliminaries

Following a minimum period of fasting of at least 5 hours to allow for complete gastric emptying, patients are sedated intravenously with midazolam (3–10 mg). In the occasional patient who has experienced chest discomfort from the heating effect of the laser, fentanyl 50–75 mg is added pre-procedure. A pulse oximeter should always be employed. Preliminary dilatation with a balloon dilator or Savary bougie to 12–15 mm may be required to allow luminal access to the tumour by a standard end-viewing gastroscope. Note that the wider the attempted dilatation, the more likely is an oesophageal tear or perforation to occur, which would preclude the use of the laser. This also applies to the other treatment modalities to be discussed.

Painting technique (thermal laser)

Ideally, treatment should be in a retrograde direction (Fig. 4.6), commencing at the distal end of the tumour since tissue oedema from the heating effect of the laser might otherwise limit access to the whole length of the lesion. Immediate, though incomplete, relief from dysphagia is anticipated if this technique is followed. Where luminal occlusion is so complete that a guidewire cannot be safely passed as a prelude to dilatation, the laser should be directed at the proximal surface of the tumour and ablation proceeds cautiously to try and open a swallowing channel (Fig. 4.7). In this situation, several laser sessions may be necessary,

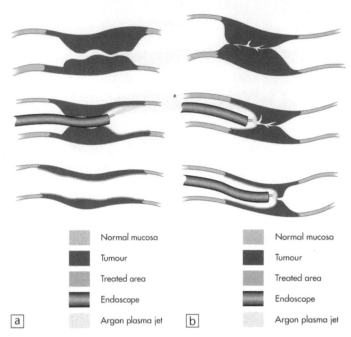

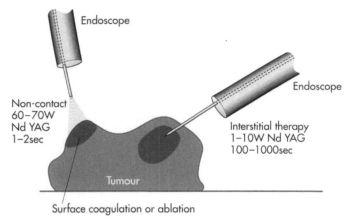

Figure 4.6. Approaches to tumour ablation. (a) Distal to proximal; (b) 'burning' a way through.

Figure 4.8. Thermal laser 'inserted' into exophytic tumour to induce necrosis by 'cooking'. Note: multiple fibres can be inserted interstitially via the percutaneous route to provide a larger volume of confluent necrosis.

ideally at intervals of 2–3 days. While single sessions can be conducted on an outpatient or overnight stay basis, if a series of treatments is required to achieve safe and useful swallowing, the in-patient period can be usefully employed to conduct a full nutritional assessment and plan the individual needs of the patient.

Tissue adherence to the probe is minimized by the instillation of water at droplet rate. Interstitial administration of the contact probe is useful for the treatment of large exophytic lesions where tissue necrosis is induced by 'cooking' the tumour at low power (2–5 W) at multiple sites for up to 10 seconds (Fig. 4.8). The hyperthermia induces a

combination of coagulation necrosis and vascular damage resulting in a reproducible volume of necrosis of about 2 ml per insertion. Once the lumen has been established, further laser treatments planned on a day-case basis every 4–6 weeks will maintain luminal patency at an acceptable level. A simple grading system will allow patient comfort and nutritional intake to be monitored [7].

Spraying technique (APC)

Application of the coagulator closely resembles that of laser treatment (Fig. 4.9). Preliminary oesophageal dilatation may be applied cautiously as necessary. The Teflon delivery tube is passed through the instrument channel of a standard end-viewing gastroscope. Settings of 40–60 W, but up to 100 W, are usual with pulses of 1–2 seconds for small lesions or continuous application for large surface areas, including bleeding tumours. The instillation of gas, if excessive, can lead to uncomfortable gaseous distension which requires frequent suction or a separate venting tube.

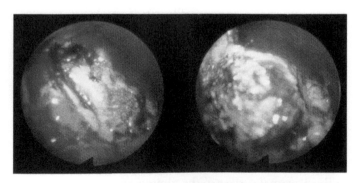

Figure 4.7. Painting technique used with thermal laser. Note: the laser has been applied across the whole surface of the tumour to achieve haemostasis and tumour shrinkage.

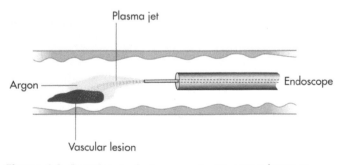

Figure 4.9. Spraying technique used with argon beamer.

Preliminary studies suggest that small or early tumours in the oesophagus can be as effectively palliated with APC as with Nd-YAG laser [8,9].

PHOTODYNAMIC THERAPY (PDT)

General principles

PDT involves the local destruction of tissue by light of a specific wavelength matched to the absorption of a previously systemically administered photosensitizer. The photosensitizer is retained with some selectivity in tumours and is activated by light to produce a local cytotoxic effect that is probably mediated by singlet oxygen species, though damage to vasculature is an additional source of tissue necrosis. Note that it should be borne in mind that PDT has the potential to damage normal tissue also, albeit this retains a lower concentration of the sensitizing drug than tumours.

Photosensitizing agents

A variety of photosensitizers is currently under study for use in PDT. Photofrin is most widely used clinically, although other agents such as 5-amino-laevulinic acid (5-ALA), chlorins and phthalocyanines are undergoing investigation and clinical trial (Table 4.4). The ideal sensitizer should be administered orally or topically, it should be stable chemically, non-toxic and rapidly metabolized to minimize photosensitivity; a favourable tumour to normal tissue concentration gradient would also be an asset. This ideal has not yet been achieved,

and is not at this stage on the near horizon. The second major problem area relates to the most effective light delivery system. Tissue penetration by light is limited to less than 5 mm, and to achieve an even light distribution in a solid or hollow organ requires individually adapted probes. Laser-induced PDT was introduced by Dougherty and colleagues in the mid 1970s [10] at virtually the same time as the introduction to gastroenterology of endoscopically delivered thermal lasers [11], but while the use of the latter is now an established technique in the palliation of oesophagogastric carcinoma, PDT for the management of this condition is of limited availability and still considered as largely a research procedure.

Light delivery system

Light of an appropriate wavelength is derived from an argon or KTP pumped dye laser, a copper vapour laser, a diode laser or, most recently, a non-laser light source, the Paterson lamp [12]. The patient is administered the photosensitizer, usually intravenously, at between 6 and 96 hours previously, depending on the predicted peak tissue levels of the individual photosensitizer. The light delivery system is deployed under endoscopic control, the probe usually being passed over a guidewire and the endoscope subsequently withdrawn. Light exposure varies from 2 to 8 min at each 2- to 3-cm segment of oesophageal tumour, and the energy density is usually restricted to 200 J/cm^2 with a power of 100–150 mW/cm^2 to prevent tissue damage by thermal effect. Unlike the effect of thermal lasers on tissue which is seen immediately as blanching, and is indicative of protein coagulation, tumour necrosis is seen within hours of laser

Table 4.4. Characteristics of photosensitizers used in PDT

Photosensitizer	Wavelength activation (nm)	Route of administration	Trial status
Haematoporphyrin derivative (HpD)	630	iv	Licensed
Photofrin II	630	iv	Licenced
Benzporphyrin derivative (BPD)	690	iv	Phase II
Aluminium sulphonated phthalocyanine (AlSPc)	675	iv	Phase II
5-Aminolaevulinic acid (5-ALA) (Protoporphyrin IX)	630	Oral, topical, iv	Phase III
Mesotetrahydroxphenyl chlorin (mTHPC)	652	iv	Phase III

treatment and, until mucosal regeneration has taken place, a sloughy-based ulcer is apparent.

Practicalities

As with thermal laser therapy, the procedure is performed under conscious iv sedation. Since most oesophageal cancers have extended into and beyond the muscularis propria at the time of diagnosis, laser light will only penetrate the superficial aspect of the tumour and, at best, even with the latest generation of photosensitizers, achieve a depth of penetration not exceeding 4–5 mm. This, however, offers considerable potential for the effective treatment of dysplasia or carcinoma *in situ* in Barrett's oesophagus [13]. The most comprehensive series to date of PDT for oesophageal cancer reports an overall 5-year survival of 25% but, when disease-specific survival was considered, this rose to 74% [14].

Safety considerations

The main advantage of PDT over thermal methods of palliation relates to the improved safety profile. Whereas with thermal treatment, healing of damaged areas takes place with scarring, the collagen and stroma is preserved in PDT and there is no reduction in mechanical strength of the organ and consequently a greatly reduced risk of perforation. This advantage, however, is offset by the duration of skin phototoxicity.

Note that careful advice must be given to patients warning of the avoidance of exposure to bright lights or sunlight for an appropriate period (up to 6 weeks in some cases). For the first few days, house lights should be dimmed and, if daytime exposure to light is necessary, dark glasses, a wide-brimmed hat and a long-sleeved garment should all be worn. During this time, standard proprietary high-level 'sun-block' creams will limit the possibility of phototoxicity which presents as a sunburn effect that varies from mild scorching of the skin to frank blistering and third-degree burns, depending on the duration of light exposure. Subsequently, graded exposure to light will help to 'photobleach' or degrade the photosensitizer and those reduce the potential period of phototoxicity. The advantage of using 5-ALA as a photosensitizer is that it is metabolized within 24 hours, which is therefore the limit of the sunburn period.

COMPLICATIONS

General considerations

One of the basic requirements of good palliation is that the therapy applied should be safe, or at least be associated with an acceptable level of complications. The advent of Atkinson and Wilson–Cook semi-rigid tubes represented a significant advance in the palliation of oesophageal cancer, but their insertion was associated with procedure-related mortality and morbidity rates of 3% to 12% and 5% to 15%, respectively [15]. Additionally, food bolus obstruction was a common problem, necessitating further endoscopy, and migration of the tube (early or late) occurred in up to 40% of cases [16]. In addition, overgrowth at the proximal or distal end of the tube required thermal laser treatment or alcohol injection to restore luminal patency. The more recent development of expanding metal mesh stents (MMS) has resulted in a lower perforation rate and better nutritional intake because of the wider diameter of the MMS. However, the open mesh stent is associated with tumour ingrowth, and covered or open stents can also be complicated by tumour overgrowth. Indeed, there is unlikely to be any prosthesis in the future where overgrowth might not be a problem, and the longer the tube or stent is *in situ*, the more likely is overgrowth to occur.

Thermal techniques

Thermal laser treatment or the use of APC is effective in elimination of the obstruction. While the Nd-YAG laser may melt the MMS in whatever form, the diode laser, APC and PDT [17] can all be used without damage to the open mesh stent, though the membrane-covered stents will be damaged by any thermal method if applied within the lumen of the stent [18].

A significant improvement in the overall quality of life has been achieved with Nd-YAG laser therapy in patients undergoing palliation of oesophageal carcinoma [7]. Perforation, which occurs in 4–6% of patients with the Nd-YAG laser, can often be managed conservatively with peripheral parenteral feeding and antibiotic cover as necessary. Accurate information on perforation rates for the diode laser and APC is sparse, but rates appear lower than for the Nd-YAG laser. In more than 50% of such perforations or tears, it appears that preliminary dilatation is

Table 4.5. Complications of laser and APC treatment

Minor	Nd-YAG/Diode laser	Photodynamic therapy	Argon plasma coagulation
Transient retrosternal pain	+	+	+
Transient pyrexia	+	+	+
Gaseous distension (benign pneumoperitoneum)	+	−	+
Pneumomediastinum	Uncommon	−	Not recorded
Photosensitivity	−	+	−
Major perforation	+	−	Not recorded
Tracheo-oesophageal fistula	+	+	Not recorded
Bleeding from tumour	Uncommon	Uncommon	Not due to therapy
Septicaemia	Rare	Not recorded	Not recorded
Chronic severe dysphagia	+	+	Not recorded
Oesophageal stenosis	+	+	Not recorded
Aspiration pneumonia	Uncommon	Uncommon	Uncommon

responsible rather than the treatment modality *per se*. As a consequence, it is suggested that dilatation to the smallest practical diameter to allow access to the target tissue should be practised. Large tears and tracheo-oesophageal fistulae require the placement of a membrane-covered MMS or 'cuffed' Wilson–Cook tube. Surgical intervention in this situation is inevitably accompanied by an increased mortality rate.

Complications associated with thermal laser therapy, PDT and APC are outlined in Table 4.5. By and large, PDT is a safe procedure and the most frequently encountered problems are oesophageal stenosis, particularly if circumferential treatment is given (though this is readily amenable to dilatation), and skin photosensitization. A recorded perforation rate of less than 2% (six in 325 treatment sessions throughout the gastrointestinal tract) suggests that APC is a safer procedure than thermal laser therapy, though there is evidence that it is less effective in reducing oesophageal tumour bulk [8]. As yet, experience with endoscopically applied APC is limited and it is difficult to make valid comparisons with alternative methods of palliation.

CHOICE OF TECHNIQUE

'To a man with a hammer, a lot of things look like a nail that needs pounding'.

Mark Twain

Any new treatment technique attracts enthusiasts who, because of their application, become expert in the use of their particular new therapy. It is important, therefore, to be able to step back, and subject the new method to critical appraisal and controlled trial, but also be aware that a combination of available methods may in fact be the best option for the individual patient. The list in Table 4.3 might suggest that treatment modalities are mutually exclusive – a philosophy which should be discounted. While laser or APC or PDT may be applied initially, the speed of tumour growth may ultimately require intubation, and this can be used to advantage in a complementary fashion [19]. Controlled trials have shown comparable outcomes in terms of quality of life and survival, though complications occur more frequently with the insertion of semi-rigid tubes [16]. Comparable data are not yet available for MMS.

Intubation and stenting are considered elsewhere in this book, but careful consideration should be given to the optimum timing when either is used in tandem with laser treatment or APC. Relative indications for palliation with laser therapy or stenting/intubation are shown in Table 4.6.

Radiotherapy

Palliative radiotherapy, either external beam or intracavitary (brachytherapy) used as single modality therapy is effective in selected groups, and may prolong survival in patients with relatively good swallowing. However, individuals

Table 4.6. Relative indications for laser therapy or intubation stenting

Laser (Nd-YAG or diode)	Insertion of prosthesis (metal mesh stent or semi-rigid tube)
Complete oesophageal obstruction	Stricture length > 5 cm
High cervical tumour	Tortuous stricture
Stricture <5 cm, exophytic type	Rapidly growing tumour
Haemorrhage from tumour	Sealing perforation/tear or tracheo-oesophageal fistula
Debulking tumour before:	Need for single treatment
Radiotherapy	
Chemotherapy	
Intubation	
Nutritional support before surgery	
Tumour overgrowth of prosthesis	

with severe obstruction and marked dysphagia respond less well [20]. Two studies from the National Medical Laser Centre, London, investigated the effects of preliminary Nd-YAG laser therapy followed by external beam radiotherapy [21] and brachytherapy [22]. The only significant benefit appears to be the prolongation of the initial dysphagia-free interval, although this may provide an acceptable option for those who are relatively fit and prefer a single, more lengthy admission to hospital for combination laser/radiotherapy therapy at the start of their treatment.

Injection methods

Injection of concentrated ethanol produces tumour necrosis [23], and is a useful starting point in any Unit which practices therapeutic endoscopy. This technique, however, has not been subjected to a controlled trial against laser therapy, and is likely to find its place in the therapeutic armamentarium as a holding technique to relieve dysphagia prior to more definitive treatment with laser therapy or APC. Controlled trials of chemotherapy in combination with other methods of palliation raise ethical questions, but on an anecdotal basis, laser therapy has proved more effective if tumour shrinkage with cytotoxic drugs has proved successful.

Thermal ablation

Laser therapy has an established place in the palliation of oesophageal carcinoma. However, as with all forms of therapeutic endoscopy, there is a learning curve and close supervision is necessary until proficiency is achieved. None-

theless, in the hands of an experienced practitioner, thermal lasers are an efficient, reproducibly effective and relatively safe method of clearing bulky, even totally obstructive tumour, throughout the length of the oesophagus. It is used ideally in the straighter middle two-thirds of the organ, and is probably the only practical method for tackling very high cervical lesions. Angulation at the cardia and gastro-oesophageal junction renders tumours technically difficult to treat, and every care must be exercised to avoid penetrating through to the lower thorax or upper peritoneal cavity. The bulky Nd-YAG laser, which requires a special water and electricity supply and is fixed in one location, is likely to give way progressively to the much smaller, mobile, simple plug-in diode laser which can be used more safely in a continuous mode of application.

The characteristics of the APC with the relatively superficial ablative or coagulative effect make it ideal for smaller, non-obstructive tumours. While exophytic tumours can usefully be treated – albeit more slowly than with the thermal laser – the APC offers an advantage in safety with a reduced perforation rate in the management of flat and intramural tumours. The efficacy in achieving surface haemostasis from bleeding tumours, even beyond mucosal folds and round bends, represents a definite asset. Further trials are required to establish more precisely the optimum indications for its use.

Photodynamic therapy

At this stage, PDT cannot be considered as a routine service tool in the palliation of oesophageal carcinoma. However, the technique holds definite promise as a primary treatment modality for the treatment of small, early, non-invasive tumours, carcinoma *in situ* and the management of dysplastic Barrett's mucosa when the problems of light delivery and most practical photosensitizer have been resolved. The role of PDT as a major tumour debulking technique is likely to be limited though there may be a use in tumour clearance from blocked MMS.

COST IMPLICATIONS

With stringent budgets and close scrutiny of the cost of delivery of health care to patients, clinical directors are required to justify to their Trusts the cost effectiveness of their approach to the management of individual conditions. Discounting the initial diagnosis of inoperable oesophageal carcinoma, palliation is relatively cost-intensive for the predicted median survival of about 5 months. A recent paper by Kay *et al.* [24] calculated that by using a metal stent, the mean overall cost of palliation was £2817, as against a variety of 'conventional' methods using alcohol injection, BICAP diathermy and Atkinson tubes, where the mean bill was £4566. If, as originally proposed, intubation or stenting were a single, virtually no follow-up procedure, the cost would be much reduced, although mesh stents cost £600–800. An Oxford group estimated that the current cost of palliation of an oesophageal cancer with a metal stent is equivalent to the cost of laser treatment at £315 per session or £1260 for a median of four treatments per patient [25]. (Atkinson tubes are 1/10th of the cost but are quickly being superseded.) However, 40% of patients develop complications and require further endoscopy, tube placement or clearance of tumour ingrowth or overgrowth. Hence, the overall cost of stenting probably approximates to the cost of thermal laser therapy, in spite of the need for repeated treatments with the latter.

The major consideration for many Units will be the initial capital outlay and subsequent running costs of thermal lasers, dye lasers or APC. A Nd-YAG laser costs £50 000 to £60 000 and a diode laser in excess of £45 000, though this is likely to drop significantly as diode technology rapidly advances. Dye lasers vary widely in price, between £45 000 to £70 000, and combined thermal/dye laser instruments are available at about £90 000. If these expensive instruments are placed in a central location and used in other specialties, e.g. thoracic medicine, urology, gynaecology and surgery, then the expense can more readily be justified. As photodynamic therapy establishes and extends its role in oesophageal cancer palliation, serious consideration should be given to the acquisition of one of the recently developed multi-wavelength capability non-laser light sources which are likely to be priced at about £10 000. Although styled as (readily) tunable, most dye lasers operate at a narrow band wavelength, whereas the non-laser instruments have the facility of rapid replacement of a filter to provide light wavelength for a wide range of photosensitizers.

Although more widely used in surgery, there is increasing application of endoscopic APC, the cost of which is just about £15 000. If subsequent trials show that results obtained are equivalent to or nearly match those obtained with thermal lasers, this would seem to be a worthwhile option, bearing in mind that the argon ion tube must be replaced from time to time. It is likely that the learning curve for its use is shorter and the potential hazards less serious. Full training is nonetheless required.

A major issue is the referral population and the numbers likely to be attracted. A small or peripheral unit may find it difficult to justify major expenditure, and be prepared to resort to expensive extra-contractual referrals as and when necessary, or even deny the patient referral to a tertiary unit because of financial restrictions.

It is a source of concern that long delays still occur in the diagnosis of cancer of the oesophagus and gastric cardia [26]. If survival rates and cure rates are to improve, health education and a mechanism for streamlining of investigations must be put in place if palliation is not to remain the mainstay of treatment for this unpleasant malignancy. There is a need for regional or sub-regional tertiary referral centres which have access to a fairly complete range of therapeutic options and clinical expertise and which will be able to help with the more difficult or unusual cases. Every moderate sized district general hospital should have access to this multidisciplinary expertise whether or not they have a modality for tumour ablation in addition to the facility of metal mesh stent insertion. The choice of instruments available is likely to be determined by either the pragmatic needs of service requirements, or the specialist or research interests of individual gastroenterologists, medical or surgical.

REFERENCES

1. Blot WJ, Devesa SS, Fraummeri JF. Continuing climb in rates of oesophageal adenocarcinoma: an update. *JAMA* 1993; 270: 1320.

2. Watson A. Surgery for carcinoma of the oesophagus. *Postgrad Med J* 1988; 64: 860–864.

3. Watson A. Carcinoma of the oesophagus. In: Misiewicz JJ, Pounder RE, Venables CW (eds). *Diseases of the Gut and Pancreas*. Blackwell Scientific Publications, Oxford, 1994; p. 182.

4. Isono K, Sato H, Nahayama K. Results of a nationwide study on the 3 field lymph node dissection of oesophageal cancer. *Oncology* 1991; 148: 411–420.

5. Tis TL, Colne PPLO, Schouwink MH, Tytgat GNJ. Esophagogastric carcinoma : pre-operative TNM classification with endosonography. *Radiology* 1989; 173: 411–417.

6. Krasner N, Barr H, Skidmore C, Morris AI. Palliative laser therapy for malignant dysphagia. *Gut* 1987; 28: 792–798.

7. Barr H, Krasner N. Prospective quality of life analysis after palliative photoablation for the treatment of malignant dysphagia. *Cancer* 1991; 68: 1660–1664.

8. Wahab PJ, Mulder CJJ, den Hartog G, Theis JG. Argon plasma coagulation in gastrointestinal endoscopy: pilot experiences. *Endoscopy* 1997; 29: 176–178.

9. Sessler MJ, Flesch BHD, Grund KE. Therapeutic effect of argon plasma coagulation on small malignant gastrointesinal tumours. *J Cancer Clin Oncol* 1995; 121: 235–238.

10. Chang CT, Dougherty TJ. Photo-radiation therapy: kinetics and thermal dynamics of porphyrin uptake and loss in normal and malignant cells in culture. *Radiat Res Sec* 1978, 74: 498–499.

11. Fruhmorgen P, Bodem F, Reidenbach HD *et al.* The first endoscopic laser in the human GI tract. *Endoscopy* 1976; 7: 156–157.

12. Whitehurst C, Byrne K, Moore JN. The development of an alternative light source to laser for PDT: 1. Comparative *invitro* dose response characteristics. *Lasers Med Sci* 1993; 8: 259–267.

13. Barr H, Shepherd NA, Dix A *et al.* Eradication of high grade dysplasia in columnar lined (Barrett's) oesophagus by photodynamic therapy with endogenously generated protophorphyrin IX. *Lancet* 1996; 438: 584–585.

14. Sibille A, Lambert R, Souquet JC *et al.* Long term survival after photodynamic therapy for oesophageal cancer. *Gastroenterology* 1995; 108: 337–344.

15. Buset M, des Marez B, Baize M *et al.* Palliative endoscopic management of obstructive esophago-gastric cancer: laser or prosthesis. *Gastrointestinal Endosc* 1987; 33: 357–361.

16. Barr H, Krasner N, Raouf A, Walker RJ. Prospective randomised trial of laser therapy only and laser therapy followed by endoscopic intubation for the palliation of malignant dysphagia. *Gut* 1990; 31: 252–258.

17. Tan WC, Sturgess RP, Watt P, Krasner N. Photodynamic therapy for dysphagia due to failure of metallic metal endoprosthesis. *Illustrated Case Reports in Gastroenterology* 1995; 2: 31–34.

18. Madhotra R, Raouf A, Sturgess R, Krasner N. Laser therapy in the maintenance of the patency of expandable metal stents. *Lasers Med Sci* 1999; 14: 20–23.

19. Bown SG. Palliation of malignant dysphagia: surgery, radiotherapy, laser, intubation alone or in combination. *Gut* 1991; 32: 841–844.

20. Caspers RJL, Wilvaart K, Verkes J *et al.* The effect of radiotherapy on dysphagia and survival in patients with oesophageal cancer. *Radiother Oncol* 1988; 12: 15–23.

21. Sargeant JR, Tobias JS, Blackman G *et al.* Radiotherapy enhances laser palliation of malignant dysphagia: a randomised study. *Gut* 1997; 40: 362–369.

22. Spencer G M, Thorpe SM, Sargeant IR *et al.* Laser and brachytherapy in the palliation of adenocarcinoma of the oesophagus and cardia. *Gut* 1996; 39: 726–731.

23. Nivokolo CN, Payne-James JJ, Silk DBA *et al.* Palliation of malignant dysphagia by ethanol induced tumour necrosis. *Gut* 1994; 35: 299–303.

24. Nicholson DA, Haycox A, Kay CL *et al.* The cost effectiveness of metal oesophageal stenting in malignant disease compared with conventional therapy. *Clin Radiol* 1999, 54: 212–215.

25. Savage AP, Baigine RJ, Cobb X *et al.* The palliation of malignant dysphagia by laser therapy. *Dis Esophagus* 1997; 10: 243–246.

26. Martin IG, Young S, Sue-Ling H, Johnston D. Delays in the diagnosis of oesophago-gastric carcinoma: a consecutive case series. *Br Med J* 1997; 314: 464–470.

5

Endoscopic screening for upper gastrointestinal malignancy

H. Barr

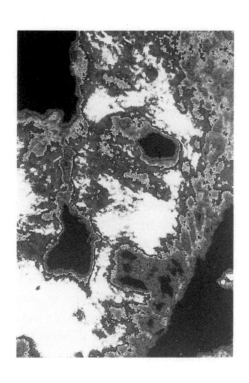

INTRODUCTION

Cancer of the upper gastrointestinal tract shows widespread variation and remains a significant health care problem. In Japan, gastric cancer attains almost epidemic proportions, with an incidence 70 per 100 000 males, and the cumulative risk of developing the disease by the age of 75 being 11%. Indeed, in Japan gastric cancer is said to be the 'national disease', and in 1960 accounted for nearly 52% of deaths from malignancy in men and 38% of such deaths in women. Other countries with a high incidence (>30 per 100 000 males) include Chile, Costa Rica, Hungary, Poland, Portugal, Iceland, Romania, Indonesia and Italy [1].

The Western world is currently facing an increasing problem of cancer arising at the gastro-oesophageal junction and related to gastro-oesophageal reflux disease and Barrett's oesophagus. Adenocarcinoma occurs 30 to 100 times more often in patients with Barrett's oesophagus than in a matched population. Currently, adenocarcinoma in Barrett's oesophagus has an incidence of 800 per 100 000, whereas the incidence of lung cancer in men over 65 is 500 per 100 000. Cancer incidence may be expressed as a percentage of a particular population developing cancer per year. For adults with Barrett's oesophagus, the annual rate is 0.8% [2]. The significance of the problem is emphasized by the current rate of rise which is outstripping any other cancer including melanoma, lymphoma and small-cell lung cancer [3].

A common feature in all these tumours is that they are mucosal cancers. They arise first on the surface and then penetrate deeper to become invasive and finally metastatic. Once these latter two events have occurred, the prognosis is extremely poor. Thus, there is a clear rationale for early detection. Endoscopic screening is highly appropriate since the first changes are surface abnormalities that may be seen at endoscopy. If found early, then dysplastic and superficial changes may be eradicated endoscopically, and the disease prevented from progressing to invasive cancer [4].

POPULATION SCREENING

Screening for oesophageal cancer

Consideration must be given to the current methods of screening so that lessons can be learned for endoscopic screening. In particular, consideration must be given to the remarkable experience in China. This has shown that squamous cell carcinoma is curable if detected early by screening when asymptomatic. The screening method used is based on cytology of cells from the oesophagus obtained by 'lawang'. A balloon covered with a fine mesh is swallowed, inflated and pulled up the oesophagus. Those found to have malignant cells have endoscopy and biopsy. The accuracy detection rate is 80%, and surgical cure was possible in 90% in patients with early asymptomatic cancer. A large series examined and followed up patients who were found to have early oesophageal squamous cancer and early adenocarcinomas but who refused all treatment. The period for the early carcinoma to progress to an advanced stage was 4–5 years. This clearly indicates that there may be a large window of opportunity to detect cancer endoscopically and eradicate it. In the United Kingdom and the USA there is the major problem of oesophageal adenocarcinoma arising in Barrett's oesophagus, and screening or surveillance is becoming a priority for these patients.

Screening for gastric cancer

Screening the asymptomatic population has been implemented in Japan, Chile and Venezuela where prevalence rates are high. In Europe, screening has focused on high-risk groups. Others advocate a low threshold for endoscopy in patients with dyspepsia using open-access endoscopy. In Japan, government-subsidized mass screening has been introduced for some years. The initial methods used are predominantly radiological, with photofluorographic radiology performed at designated centres, or by mobile units such that approximately 5 million people are screened per year. After 25 years of screening, deaths in men from gastric cancer have decreased from over 50% of all deaths caused by malignant disease to 33%. Similarly, deaths in women due to gastric cancer have been reduced from 38% to 28%. The incidence/detection of early gastric cancer had risen from under 2% in 1945 to 63% in some centres. The overall 5-year survival rate from gastric cancer had risen to greater than 50%. There are clear shortcomings in using survival rate in evaluating the effectiveness of screening. In particular, there is concern at the definition of early gastric cancer and its distinction from dysplasia, or 'worrying mucosal appearance'. Also most studies report 5-year survival and there may well be a lead time bias. Recently, a detailed follow-up has demonstrated that two-thirds of patients with screen-detected cancer in Osaka were cured of their disease 15 years after resection.

Screening of asymptomatic patients has not been considered feasible elsewhere. In Japan, 25% of cancers are identified by screening programmes. Despite the wider use of the flexible endoscope in the West, the detection of early stage I cancers has not increased. However, it is still recommended that patients with dyspepsia have access to early and prompt endoscopy as the only method for the detection of early and potentially curable gastric cancer.

In the West, screening of some high-risk groups has been feasible, and certain centres have introduced programmes to allow early endoscopy of dyspeptic patients over the age of 40, and serial endoscopy until healing of all patients with gastric ulcer. Patients with atrophic gastritis, dysplasia or adenomatous polyps are offered endoscopy on an annual basis. Of 2659 patients examined in this scheme, 57 cancers were identified; of these, 20% were early gastric cancers, but overall only 60% of all detected cancers were suitable for attempted curative surgery.

CONTROVERSIAL ISSUES AND QUALITY PROBLEMS

Endoscopic examination

The efforts of the Japanese to detect polyps and tumours at very early stages has highlighted some important aspects of the quality of endoscopic examination required in order to detect early cancer. It has become evident that the time spent by Japanese endoscopists in examining suspicious lesions with endoscopic staining techniques appears to be more meticulous than a standard United Kingdom open-access endoscopy for dyspepsia. In one study, despite open-access endoscopy the overall incidence of gastric cancer detected at an earlier stage remained low at 13% [5]. These authors concluded that the advantages of open-access endoscopy appeared to be compromised by delayed referral and failure of the endoscopist to recognize early disease.

Pathological issues

The excellence of the results of surgery for gastric cancer in Japan has fuelled debate as to whether the disease in that country differs from that in the West. In all countries, Stage I disease is associated with a relatively good prognosis, yet the overall 5-year survival rate in Europe for this stage of disease was reported as 70% compared with 98% in Japan, suggesting that there are differences in tumour biological behaviour. Clarification of this issue occurred with a detailed review of tumour classification. The British Society of Gastroenterology reviewed the histology of 319 patients from 41 hospitals with histopathological findings of dysplasia and early gastric cancer. There was good agreement between pathologists on the difference between dysplasia and cancer, but over one-third of patients thought to have early gastric cancer were found to have more advanced disease on reassessment. The true 5-year survival rate of the group redefined as having early gastric cancers was 90%, compared with 75% of the group initially defined as early gastric cancer. Thus, European survival rates for the disease approach those in the East if strict Japanese criteria are used. Unfortunately, the issue cannot yet be regarded as completely resolved. In Japan there is a higher incidence of better-prognosis tumours, and some tumours may behave differently in the East and West; however, when direct comparisons are made between like tumours, the results appear similar.

The pathological diagnosis of cancer remains a much-debated subject between Western and Eastern pathologists. The presence of invasion is the most important diagnostic criterion for most Western pathologists, but morphological and cytological features are pre-eminent to the Japanese [6]. Certainly in Japan gastric carcinoma is diagnosed on nuclear and structural criteria, even when invasion is absent. An appreciation of this difference is important for the interpretation of cancer statistics; thus, a united effort is required to reach consensus.

OESOPHAGEAL NEOPLASIA

Squamous cell carcinoma

It is important to identify a population at high risk, and the aetiological factors of squamous cell carcinoma are listed in Table 5.1. The geographical variation in the incidence of oesophageal cancer is remarkable for this tumour. Areas of high incidence (over 35 per 100 000) are found in Northern China, Northern Iran, Kazakhstan and in the

Table 5.1. Conditions in which to consider screening or surveillance to exclude squamous cell carcinoma of the oesophagus

- Tylosis
- Previous upper aero-digestive tract squamous cell cancer
- Previous caustic stricture
- Patterson–Kelly (Plummer–Vinson) syndrome
- Achalasia
- Coeliac disease

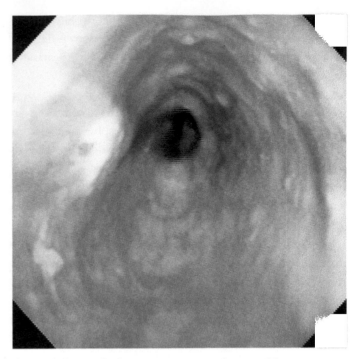

Figure 5.1. Dysplastic squamous oesophagus with hyperkeratotic areas of increased whiteness.

Transkei region of the Cape Province in South Africa. Patients with achalasia of the cardia of greater than 25 years' duration are at risk, with 7% of patients with this condition developing a squamous cell carcinoma in the upper oesophagus. Similarly, patients with a previous head neck squamous cell carcinoma are more prone to an oesophageal cancer, the cumulative risk being 25% at 5 years. This group of patients is receiving particular attention, and several centres in Europe are screening these patients with regular upper gastrointestinal endoscopy and also broncho-scopy. If a tumour is identified it is treated using endoscopic therapy [7]; this is important as part of the rationale of early detection is to allow early minimally invasive tissue-sparing endoscopic destruction.

The Patterson–Kelly (Plummer–Vinson) syndrome of iron-deficiency anaemia, glossitis and oesophagitis is associated with a 10% incidence of oesophageal or pharyngeal cancer and is more common in women. Following the identification in 1958 of two families from Liverpool in England with palmoplantar keratoderma at risk of oesophageal cancer, every high-risk group with the autosomal dominant disorder of tylosis oesophageal cancer (TOC) has been identified. Affected individuals have a 95% chance of developing oesophageal cancer by the age of 65. Recently, genetic studies have shown that the oesophageal cancer locus on 17q25.1 associated with TOC is commonly deleted in sporadic cancer. These patients may be identified early, and screening of their oesophagus becomes important [8].

The major group of patients that require screening endoscopy and endoscopic therapy are those identified as having oesophageal dysplasia (Fig. 5.1). It is clear that dysplasia is the earlier malignant lesion of the oesophagus and is associated with overexpression of the p53 protein [9]. The endoscopic detection of small and dysplastic lesions can be improved by spraying 2% Lugol's iodine. If detected early, cancers and regions of dysplasia can be treated endoscopically using the techniques of thermal laser ablation, photodynamic therapy and endoscopic mucosectomy. Following this it is essential to continue surveillance, as the rest of the oesophagus is at risk of transformation.

Barrett's oesophagus and adenocarcinoma

At present it is unlikely that there will be general population screening for patients at risk of developing adenocarcinoma of the oesophagus. However increasing numbers of patients are being identified at endoscopy with Barrett's oesophagus. This is defined as a condition in which the distal oesophagus becomes lined by metaplastic columnar epithelium and predisposes to the development of adenocarcinoma. Endoscopists have little problem detecting the characteristic red velvet-like epithelium (Fig. 5.2). Spechler *et al.* [10] have emphasized the importance of identifying specialized intestinal metaplasia as the hallmark of columnar lined oesophagus with the greatest malignant potential. They have also identified that it may be invisible and only present on biopsy of the gastro-oesophageal junction as ultra-short segment Barrett's oesophagus. This latter change is highly prevalent in

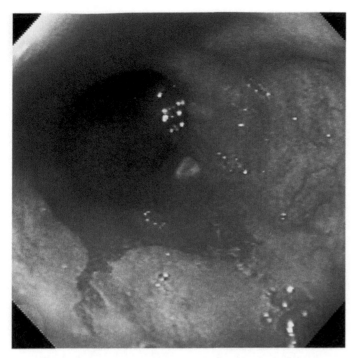

Figure 5.2. Velvet red appearance in the distal oesophagus with a linear streak typical of Barrett's oesophagus.

patients presenting for diagnostic endoscopy (9–36%), but if only investigated pathologically with haematoxylin and eosin stained tissue sections, it may be missed [11]. The endoscopic appearance of specialized intestinal metaplasia is identical to gastric-type columnar epithelium. However, certain endoscopic features increase the chance of finding intestinal metaplasia on biopsy. They are long segments of columnar lining, a jagged irregular squamocolumnar junction, a prominent squamocolumnar junction, discrete patches of columnar epithelium in the distal oesophagus, and vital staining with methylene blue [12].

Surveillance of Barrett's oesophagus

Most patients with Barrett's oesophagus will require minimal or no intervention for control of associated symptoms. The prevalence is variable but is being increasingly reported. Long-segment Barrett's oesophagus is found in 10–15% of patients who have endoscopy for gastro-oesophageal reflux symptoms. Provenzale *et al.* [13] estimated that 700 000 Americans had Barrett's oesophagus, and that annual endoscopic surveillance would cost $350 million. The increased risk of cancer is estimated to be of the overall frequency range (1 in 40 to 1 in 150 patient-years) and some are concerned by the poor yield from screening programmes [14]. There is a well-established progression from

Table 5.2. Risk factors for development of adenocarcinoma in patterns with Barrett's oesophagus

- Increased length of the Barrett's segment
- Smoking
- Males

metaplasia through to dysplasia and on to invasive carcinoma over a 4- to 5-year period. Thus, many advocate wide-scale endoscopic surveillance of all patients to detect dysplasia and early carcinoma, but these programmes are costly and only detect cancer once it is established. Certain high-risk groups have been identified (Table 5.2), and the search is on for biological or molecular markers to identify imminent malignant transformation [15]. In order to establish less costly surveillance methods, non-endoscopic balloon cytology is being explored and has been compared with biopsy and brush cytology. Essentially, balloon cytology detects 80% of patients with high-grade dysplasia and cancer, the cost being six times less than that of endoscopy and biopsy [16].

At present, surveillance should be performed on all patients with Barrett's oesophagus – as recommended by the 1990 Barrett's Esophagus Working Party [17]. A strategy for the management of patients with metaplastic Barrett's, and more importantly for those who develop worrying histological changes and cancer, is shown in Table 5.3. It is crucial that biopsy is performed according to a strict protocol, as dysplasia is heterogeneous and can be easily missed. The biopsy protocol involves four-quadrant biopsy specimens at 2-cm intervals (Fig. 5.3) throughout the columnar lined segment using 'jumbo' biopsy forceps with the 'suck and twist' approach (Fig. 5.4). In addition, specimens are obtained from any apparent lesions (Fig. 5.5) and additional specimens from known areas of dysplasia [18]. If we accept that the cancer risk is 1.3%, then a

Table 5.3. Recommendations for Barrett's surveillance endoscopy and therapy

Group	Frequency
All patients without significant co-morbidity	2 years
Confirmed dysplasia (start intensive antireflux therapy)	6-monthly
High-grade dysplasia	Surgery/endoscopic therapy
Carcinoma	Surgery

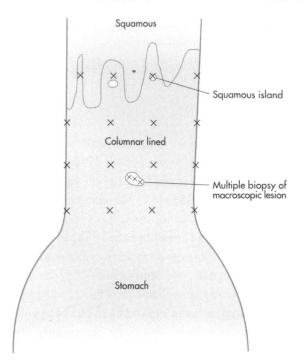

Figure 5.3. Four-quadrant biopsy technique aims to 'map out' the high-risk area.

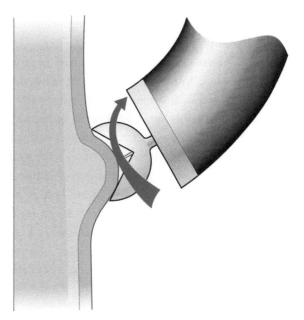

Figure 5.4. The 'suck and twist' technique of oesophageal biopsy.

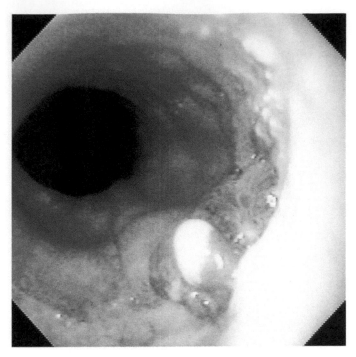

Figure 5.5. Area of macroscopic abnormality at the squamocolumnar junction, found to be dysplastic Barrett's oesophagus with no invasive cancer. This was treated using submucosal resection.

randomized trial designed to show the efficacy of endo-scopic surveillance would require 5000 patients to be followed for 10 years [13]. The logistics of such a trial are daunting and the ethics questionable [19], as there would be difficulty in entering patients in the no-surveillance arm.

Despite there being no absolute proof of efficacy of endoscopic surveillance, some studies support the practice. Streitz *et al.* [20] demonstrated that tumours found at surveillance were at an earlier stage and the 5-year survival rate (62%) was significantly better than for those who presented with cancer symptoms (20%; *P* = 0.007).

Strategies to prevent development of invasive carcinoma
Clearly, now that we have identified that Barrett's oesophagus is a pre-malignant condition, some thought must be given to cancer prevention. In particular, patients with high-grade dysplasia in Barrett's oesophagus present a very difficult clinical problem. Some advocate a policy of radical oesophageal resection as soon as high-grade dysplasia is confirmed. This approach is justified since a small previously undetected carcinoma may be found in the resected specimen in up to 45% of patients [21]. Others, concerned that half the patients are receiving a prophylactic operation with substantial morbidity and mortality, advocate intense endoscopic surveillance of dysplasia. Recently, with precise biopsy protocols, dysplasia can be distinguished from early cancer, and the risk of missing a small cancer can be reduced, but not eliminated. In a pathological study following

resection, the total area of Barrett's oesophagus was found to be 32 cm² with areas of high-grade dysplasia of 1.3 cm² and carcinoma 1.1 cm². In this series patients are more likely to be overstaged and diagnosed as having adenocarcinoma than a cancer being missed prior to surgery [22]. The problem of detection and surveillance may in part be resolved by endoscopic mucosal ablation [23]. If the mucosa can be destroyed and neo-squamous epithelium regenerated, the cancer risk may be reduced and small cancers destroyed endoscopically. At present it is clear that, following ablation, surveillance should continue as the pathological appearance suggests that there remain areas of Barrett's mucosa, and glands may be buried under the neo-squamous mucosa [24]. It is also unclear whether the neo-squamous epithelium is genetically stable and will not progress to cancer.

GASTRIC NEOPLASIA

Cancer of the cardia

Although much is known about gastric carcinogenesis, it is difficult to be clear as to which patients at risk of gastric cancer will eventually develop the condition. It is now apparent that different parts of the stomach are affected by different predisposing conditions. In particular, intestinal metaplasia and dysplasia at the Z line (Fig. 5.6) and short and ultra-short segments [11] of Barrett's oesophagus may be related to carcinoma of the cardia. However, many middle-aged people develop intestinal metaplasia and carditis at or just below the squamocolumnar junction. This is related to the same aetiological factors as Barrett's oesophagus, namely gastro-oesophageal reflux disease. The numbers appear of such a magnitude that screening or surveillance is not a realistic option [25].

Pre-malignant conditions
In this group are included conditions that if untreated become malignant, as well as disorders of the stomach that may predispose to gastric cancer. In particular patients with hypogammaglobulinaemia (50-fold excess) and pernicious anaemia (3- to 5-fold excess) are at high risk. Surveying patients is appropriate with hypogammaglobulinaemia, but at present is controversial for patients with pernicious anaemia and is not recommended.

Patients with hypogammaglobulinaemia and pernicious anaemia have chronic atrophic gastritis. Certainly,

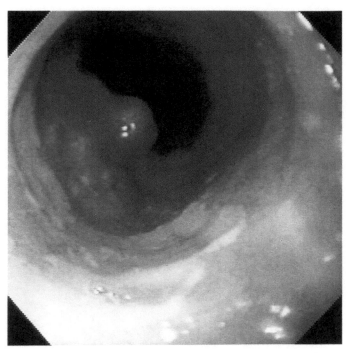

Figure 5.6. Early oesophageal cancer in segment of Barrett's oesophagus.

achlorhydria results from the chronic atrophic gastritis and 75% of patients with gastric carcinoma are achlorhydric. Strickland has divided chronic atrophic gastritis into two subgroups:

1. Type A, which is associated with pernicious anaemia, predominantly affects the fundus and body and is autoimmune in origin.
2. Type B gastritis affects the antrum and is related to environmental factors. It is also found in the stomach some years after gastrectomy for benign peptic ulcer disease. It may be regarded as a failure of the gastric mucosa to respond to repeated injury.

Both types predispose to cancer formation.

Helicobacter pylori, chronic atrophic gastritis and intestinal metaplasia
Intestinal metaplasia of the gastric mucosa is a common finding in association with gastric cancers, and epidemiological studies have confirmed that populations with a high incidence of carcinoma of the stomach also have a high incidence of intestinal metaplasia. Mucosal atrophy and intestinal metaplasia are common phenomena, their incidence increasing with increasing age, and they are particularly

common in elderly populations. It is becoming clear that the intestinal type of gastric cancer results in gastric mucosa that has undergone a sequence of mutations and defined histopathological changes that may start in the first decade of life. The first lesion is atrophic gastritis followed by progressive intestinalization of the mucosa to intestinal metaplasia, then dysplasia and finally carcinoma. *Helicobacter pylori* is the predominant cause of chronic gastritis and atrophic gastritis. This latter condition is a major risk factor for gastric cancer.

The epidemiological link between *H. pylori* infection and gastric cancer is now convincing. The World Health Organization consensus committee have concluded that there is sufficient evidence of the aetiological role. Virtually all infected patients will develop gastritis, leading to destruction and atrophy of gastric glands and other specialized cells. They are replaced by atrophic mucosa with intestinal metaplasia. The prevalence of atrophic gastritis increases by 2% annually in patients with *Helicobacter* infection, compared with 0.3% in the uninfected. There are many confounding factors, as treatment of patients who are infected with long-term acid suppression causes an increase in gastritis and intestinal metaplasia (Fig. 5.7). The hypothesis is that acid suppression changes the pattern of infection, with an antral gastritis being transformed to a gastric body gastritis, and this further suppresses acid secretion, increases inflammation and leads to atrophic gastritis. A large case control study in rural Japan showed by unconditional logistic regression analysis that *H. pylori* infection was associated with an increased odds ratio of 11 for men and 7 for women for the development of atrophic gastritis. In this study, diet, smoking and lifestyle were not related to atrophic gastritis. *H. pylori* infection also causes increased gastric cell proliferation and impaired secretion of vitamin C – factors that are improved after eradication of infection.

The particular subtype of *H. pylori* infection is becoming important. Subjects infected who have CagA antibodies were 5.8-fold more likely to develop gastric cancer, whereas those without CagA antibodies had an odds ratio of 2.2. The function of this immunodominant CagA protein is unknown. The CagA gene is the marker for a 40-kb pathogenicity island of *H. pylori*. The most important strain has been characterized further as being CagAvacAS1a positive. These bacteria increase proliferation and also

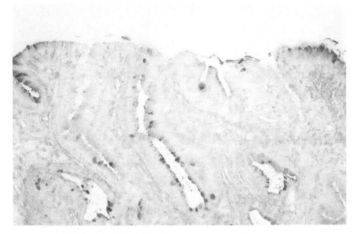

Figure 5.7. Mucin histochemistry of gastric intestinal metaplasia. Incomplete type IIb/III, stained with HIDAB (×100) to show sulphomucin expression.

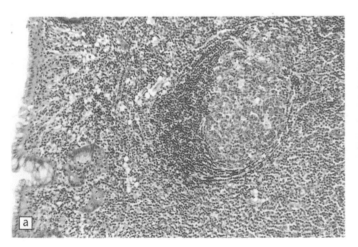

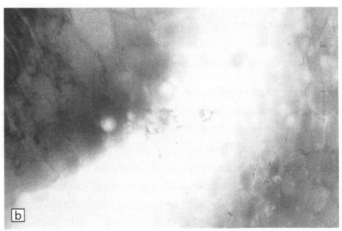

Figure 5.8. (a) A low-grade gastric MALT lymphoma which is centrocyte-like around a residual reactive lymphoid follicle and extending into the overlying epithelium to form a lymphoepithelial lesion. (b) *Helicobacter pylori* organisms on the surface of epithelial cells and the section has been stained by a modified Giemsa stain.

decrease apoptosis. However, those patients infected with CagA strains may be protected against the complications of gastro-oesophageal reflux disease, Barrett's oesophagus, dysplasia and carcinoma.

In the context of *H. pylori* and gastric malignancy, it is appropriate to discuss primary low-grade lymphoma of the mucosal-associated lymphoid tissue (MALT) of the stomach. MALT lymphoma is rare, accounting for between 1% and 5% of stomach malignancy. This tumour is strongly associated with *H. pylori* infection and may regress completely or be cured by *H. pylori* eradication (Fig. 5.8).

Screening and surveillance for H. pylori and intestinal metaplasia

Population screening for *H. pylori* remains controversial. It is clear that treatment may reduce the incidence of gastric cancer, and currently it is appropriate to test patients below the age of 45 with uncomplicated non-reflux dyspepsia for *H. pylori*, and to eradicate the organism if present. Older patients presenting with dyspepsia will need endoscopy to exclude neoplasia, though whether to test and treat these patients if no lesion is found is difficult to decide. Eradication of *H. pylori* in patients with non-ulcer dyspepsia does not improve symptoms, but may reduce subsequent gastric cancer risk. Since *H. pylori* infection is a cause of premature mortality, it would seem that testing and eradication of the bacterium in dyspeptic patients will be necessary. Screening the general population will have to wait for assessments of cost–benefit.

Surveillance of patients found to have *H. pylori* infection and intestinal metaplasia may be considered to detect early gastric cancer. Eradication of *H. pylori* at this stage may be too late to reverse progression to neoplasia, but nonetheless should be performed. General surveillance of patients with metaplasia cannot be recommended at present. Patients with certain histological changes such as dysplasia, or metaplasia characterized by tortuous crypts and abundant sulphomucins, are at greater risk, and should have endoscopic surveillance with widespread sampling as there is an increased detection of early gastric cancer.

Benign gastric and peptic ulcers

The relationship between benign gastric ulcer and gastric cancer is a controversial area, the debate being whether benign chronic gastric ulcers have malignant potential or not. The suggestion is that the regenerating mucosa around an ulcer is prone to become malignant. The issue is further clouded since some ulcerating gastric cancers can mimic benign gastric ulcers closely, sometimes healing in response to medical treatment. Approximately 4–10% of all gastric cancers behave in this way. In particular, 70% of early gastric cancers may heal as part of the 'life cycle of the malignant ulcer'. The great improvements in endoscopy with biopsy have improved detection of both benign and malignant disease, and it appears that the ulcer cancer (carcinoma developing in the edge of a benign gastric ulcer) is rare. The stable incidence of gastric ulcer with a decline in the incidence of gastric carcinoma supports the view that gastric ulcer is not a premalignant condition. Similarly, the location of benign and malignant disease is different, with most benign gastric ulcers (50–70%) occurring on the lesser curve. It is now accepted that the most important question on finding a gastric ulcer is to decide from the outset whether it is benign or malignant. A history of duodenal ulcer has emerged as having a significantly protective effect for gastric cancer. All patients with gastric ulcer should receive brushing and biopsy of the ulcer (10 biopsies) and endoscopic surveillance until the ulcer is healed. Failure to heal and dysplasia indicate the need for closer scrutiny.

Gastric polyps

Gastric polyps are found in 0.5% of postmortem examinations. Most (65–90%) are hyperplastic polyps that are regenerative, non-neoplastic lesions and usually smaller than 2 cm in size. Only two patients have been reported in whom a carcinoma was found in association with a hyperplastic polyp. There is no strong relationship with gastric carcinoma. An exception should be considered in patients with multiple hyperplastic polyps, as this may indicate a gastritis that suggests that the rest of the stomach needs to be inspected and biopsied for carcinoma.

In contrast, adenomatous polyps are truly premalignant (Fig. 5.9), often larger (80% are >2 cm in size), and are tubulovillous or villous on microscopic examination. The frequency of malignant change increases with increasing size. In a large series, 38% of patients with gastric adenomatous polyps had gastric carcinoma. Similarly, 34% of post-gastrectomy specimens for gastric cancer contained adenomatous polyps, and severe dysplasia with carcinoma *in situ* has been found in over 20% of removed polyps. It is important to survey these patients and to remove all polyps

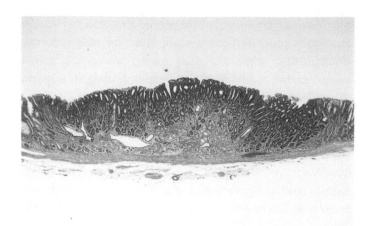

Figure 5.9. Histological section of a gastric adenoma. (Haematoxylin and eosin staining; original magnification, ×50).

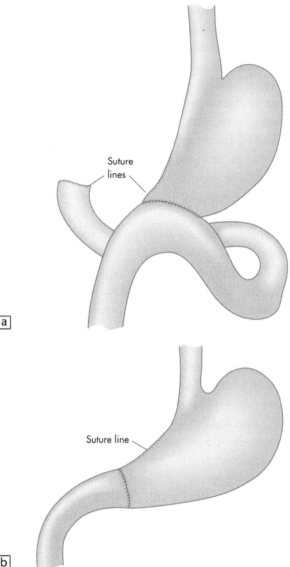

using laser therapy, endoscopic submucosal resection or surgery.

Previous gastric surgery

As early as 1922, Balfour reported a gastric cancer occurring in the residual stomach after surgery for benign peptic ulcer disease. The term 'stump cancer' was soon used, as carcinoma seemed to occur more frequently after Billroth I and II gastrectomy than after vagotomy with pyloroplasty or gastroenterostomy. A large postmortem study demonstrated that gastric cancer was less frequent in patients who had undergone gastric surgery 15 years before death, but six times greater in those who had surgery

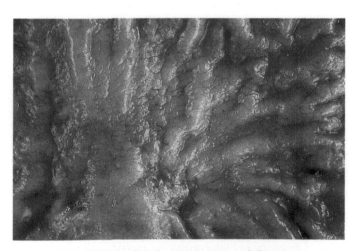

Figure 5.10. Depressed early gastric cancer following gastrectomy for benign ulcer disease 15 years previously. The patient had been undergoing surveillance as biopsy had shown dysplastic changes.

Figure 5.11. Common types of gastrectomy. (a) Polyagastrectomy. (b) Billroth gastrectomy.

25 years earlier. In a historical prospective cohort study in Denmark from 1955 to 1982, it was confirmed that the risk of gastric cancer immediately, and for 15 years after, peptic ulcer surgery, was less than expected (Fig. 5.10). This was explained because patients following gastrectomy have less gastric mucosa exposed to carcinogen. However, the risk of cancer was 2.1 times greater than the general population 25 years after surgery. The greatest risk (3.2 times) was in male patients who had had a Billroth II gastrectomy. The patients who had simple suture of a perforated ulcer had no increased risk, indicating that peptic ulcer disease was not a risk factor. The pathogenesis

of gastric 'stump cancer' has been shown experimentally to be related to operations that promote duodenogastric bile reflux, achlorhydria and atrophic gastritis. Overall, the risk of developing gastric cancer following gastrectomy has been reported as between 3% and 10%. The decline in surgery for peptic ulcer disease means that there is every prospect that in 20–30 years 'stump cancer' may become a rare phenomenon. Surveillance should be instituted for patients with worrying histological features to detect early gastric cancer (Fig. 5.11).

Menetrier's disease and hyperplastic gastropathy

Gastric carcinoma has been described as a complication of Menetrier's disease (Fig. 5.12), but the magnitude of risk is unknown. In Menetrier's disease there is giant hyperplasia of the gastric mucosal folds, and the condition can be difficult to distinguish from gastric polyposis or lymphoma. The mucosal abnormality associated with Menetrier's disease results in hyperplasia of mucous glands, whereas the parietal cell mass falls. Thus, the secretion is rich in protein and mucus, but often hypochlorhydric. Hypersecretory conditions including Zollinger–Ellison syndrome may be associated with hyperplastic rugal folds and excessive acid secretion without increased risk of gastric cancer.

Upper gastrointestinal cancer and familial adenomatous polyposis

The inherited autosomal dominant disease of familial adenomatous polyposis (FAP) induces hundreds of polyps, particularly of the colon and rectum, and has a gene locus on chromosome 5q21. Upper gastrointestinal and in particular periampullary carcinoma is a risk in these patients. Most duodenal and gastric adenomas progress, and particular attention must be paid to the ampulla of Vater. Endoscopic surveillance is recommended every 3–5 years. If polyps are found they should be treated with polypectomy, submucosal resection, laser or photodynamic ablation. Radical resection is required for progression to cancer. The use of vitamin C and/or non-steroidal anti-inflammatory drugs (Sulindac) should be used as chemo-prophylaxis [26]. Biopsy of the ampulla will often show microadenomas to be present (Fig. 5.13).

ENDOSCOPIC OPTICAL BIOPSY AND SPECTROSCOPIC DIAGNOSIS

Spectroscopic analysis of tissue depends on identifying a characteristic spectral emission from mucosa that can be used to differentiate between normal and abnormal areas. The main endoscopic goal is to identify early cancer or dysplasia, but it can be used to investigate physiological parameters. Systems are already available to the endoscopist

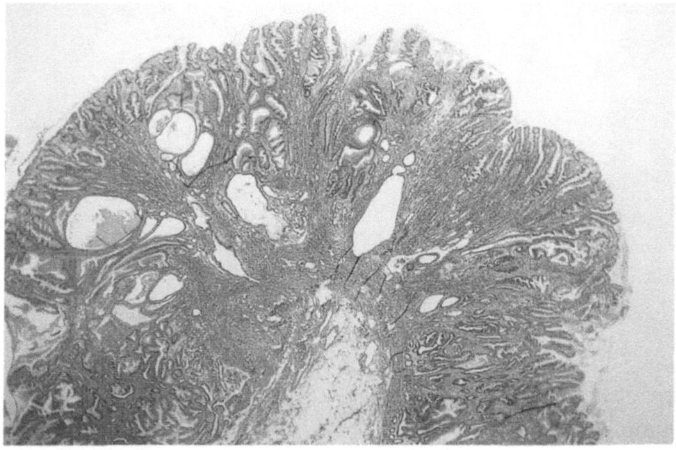

Figure 5.12. Menetrier's disease. The gastric mucosa is markedly increased in thickness. The gastric pits are elongated and some have a corkscrew appearance. The gastric glands are also elongated and several scattered cysts are present.

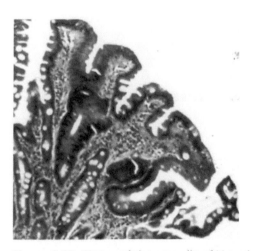

Figure 5.13. Biopsy of the ampulla of Vater in a patient with familial adenomatous polyposis, revealing a microadenoma. (Haematoxylin and eosin staining; original magnification, ×100.)

Table 5.4. Methods of endoscopic optical biopsy using tissue spectroscopy

Fluorescence spectroscopy
    Laser-induced tissue autofluorescence
    Laser-induced photosensitizer fluorescence
    Fluorescence polarization spectroscopy
    Time-resolved fluorescence spectroscopy
Elastic scattering spectroscopy
Optical coherence tomography
Raman spectroscopy

to improve and facilitate the early recognition of dysplasia [27,28]. Some of the methods under investigation are listed in Table 5.4.

Most techniques are at present concentrating on laser-induced fluorescence. Panjepour *et al.* [27] have successfully identified high-grade dysplasia in Barrett's oesophagus using this technique. Thirty-six patients were studied and the area of Barrett's oesophagus interrogated using a nitrogen-pumped dye laser emitting 410-nm light in 5-ns pulses. This was used to excite tissue autofluorescence which was collected by a fibre bundle and analysed by a spectrograph (Fig. 5.14). Both emitting and collecting fibres were included in a flexible fibreoptic probe (1.7 mm). The endoscopist passed this through the biopsy channel of the endoscope and placed the end just touching the tissue.

It must be noted that the fluorescence intensity is strongly affected by the probe placement against the tissue. Multiple measurements were taken and a histological biopsy was taken from the sites of spectral measurement. A mathematical model on differential normalized fluorescence was developed. Using this method, seven patients were detected to have high-grade dysplasia, and all correlated completely with the biopsy samples. All six patients with low-grade dysplasia were also correctly identified. Non-dysplastic Barrett's mucosa was identified in 16 of 23 patients (70%). An accompanying editorial [28] puts this paper in context, and suggests that a more user friendly system is required. It would be preferable if it was incorporated directly into the endoscope and real-time imaging and analysis required.

Another study of laser-induced fluorescence for the detection of adenocarcinoma in Barrett's oesophagus adopted a different approach [29]. Patients with adenocarcinoma were pre-treated with an intravenous photosensitizer and measurements performed immediately after resection of the oesophagus. Measurements were also taken during endoscopy in five patients to assess how applicable the technique was for clinical use. Fluorescence was excited using the nitrogen pumped dye laser connected to a 600-μm optical fibre. This fibre was used to collect light emitted from the tissue and connected to a charged coupled device camera; the fluorescence spectrum from 450 nm to 750 nm was analysed. A tumour demarcation function was

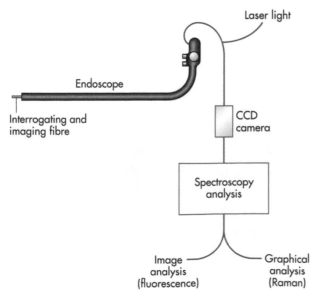

Figure 5.14. Optical biopsy technique.

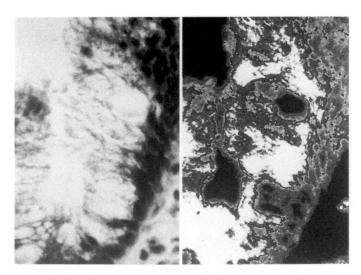

Figure 5.15. Mucosal fluorescence in dysplastic Barrett's oesophagus in a patient given 5-aminolaevulinic acid to generate protoporphyrin IX. The distribution is non-homogeneous.

established in the form of a fluorescence ratio: the quotient of porphyrins fluorescence at 630 nm divided by auto-fluorescence at 500 nm. Normal oesophageal mucosa had a fluorescence ratio of 0.1 ± 0.058, gastric mucosa 0.16 ± 0.073, Barrett's oesophagus 0.205 ± 0.17, severe dysplasia 0.79 ± 0.54 and adenocarcinoma 0.78 ± 0.56. Thus, this technique can characterize different histological changes in the oesophagus, which were not macroscopically evident. The problem which might occur in very early lesions was that uptake of a photosensitizer may not be homogeneous (Fig. 5.15). Our experience with 5-aminolaevulinic acid indicates that the uptake is high in preneoplastic lesions, but that there is such variability that more specific discriminators are necessary [30].

CONCLUSION

Virtually all gastrointestinal cancers present with surface abnormalities before becoming invasive tumours. These changes, which are invisible to white light illumination, must be detected before the development of invasive cancer if eradication and prevention are to be possible. There may be a prolonged period of some years between the detection of early precancer of the gastrointestinal tract and the development of invasive cancer. In addition, there is a dramatic rise occurring in the incidence of adenocarcinoma at the gastro-oesophageal junction. Although the precancerous changes are currently detected using rigorous biopsy protocols, which are both time-consuming and cumbersome, newly developed optical biopsy techniques may in future allow early diagnosis and permit screening protocols at endoscopy. Once such precancerous changes are detected, non-invasive endoscopic methods are now available for their eradication. Thus, over the next few years we are likely to see a revolution in endoscopic detection.

REFERENCES

1. Barr H, Greenall MJ. Carcinoma of the stomach. In: Morris PJ, Malt RA (eds) *Oxford Textbook of Surgery*. Oxford University Press, Oxford, 1994, pp. 931–943.

2. Spechler SJ. Barrett's esophagus. *Semin Oncol* 1994; 21: 431–437.

3. Blot WJ, Devesa SS, Fraumeni JF Jr. Continuing climb in rates of esophageal adenocarcinoma: an update. *JAMA* 1993; 270: 1320.

4. Barr H, Shepherd NA, Dix A *et al.* Eradication of high-grade dysplasia in columnar-lined (Barrett's) oesophagus by photodynamic therapy with endogenously generated protoporphyrin IX. *Lancet* 1996; 348: 584–585.

5. Suvakovic Z, Bramble MG, Jones R *et al.* Improving the detection rate of early gastric cancer requires more than open access gastroscopy: a five year study. *Gut* 1997; 41: 308–313.

6. Schlemper RJ, Itabashi M, Kato Y *et al.* Differences in diagnostic criteria for gastric carcinoma between Japanese and Western pathologists. *Lancet* 1997; 349: 1725–1729.

7. Grosjean P, Savary J-F, Wagnieres G *et al.* Tetra(m-hydroxyphenyl)chlorin clinical photodynamic therapy of early bronchial and oesophageal cancers. *Lasers Med Sci* 1996; 11: 227–235.

8. Iwaya T, Maesawa C, Ogasawara S, Tamura G. Tylosis esophageal cancer locus on chromosome 17q25.1 is commonly deleted in sporadic human esophageal cancer. *Gastroenterology* 1998; 114: 1206–1210.

9. Kitamura K, Kuwano H, Yasuda M *et al.* What is the earliest malignant lesion in the oesophagus? *Cancer* 1996; 77: 1614–1619.

10. Spechler SJ, Zeroogian JM, Antonioli DA *et al.* Prevalence of metaplasia at the gastroesophageal junction. *Lancet* 1994; 344: 1533–1536.

11. Nandurkar S, Talley NJ, Martin CJ *et al.* Short segment Barrett's oesophagus: prevalence, diagnosis and associations. *Gut* 1997; 40: 710–715.

12. Spechler SJ. Esophageal columnar metaplasia (Barrett's esophagus). In: Tytgat GNJ (ed.) *Gastrointestinal Endoscopy*. Vol. 7. Clinics of North America, 1997, pp. 1–18.

13. Provenzale D, Kemp JA, Arora S, Wong JB. A guide for surveillance of patients with Barrett's oesophagus. *Am J Gastroenterol* 1994; 89: 670–680.

14. MacDonald CE, Wicks AC, Playford RJ. Ten years experience of screening patients with Barrett's oesophagus in a university teaching hospital. *Gut* 1997; 41: 303–307.

15. Bailey T, Biddlestone L, Shepherd N *et al.* Altered cadherin and catenin complexes in the Barrett's esophagus-dysplasia-adenocarcinoma sequence. *Am J Pathol* 1998; 152: 1–10.

16. Falk GW, Chittajallu R, Goldblum JR *et al.* Surveillance of patients with Barrett's esophagus for dysplasia and cancer with balloon cytology. *Gastroenterology* 1997; 112: 1787–1797.

17. Dent J, Bremner CG, Collen MJ *et al.* Working party report to the World Congresses of gastroenterology, Sydney 1990: Barrett's oesophagus. *J Gastroenterol Hepatol* 1991; 6: 1–22.

18. Levine DS, Haggitt RC, Blount PL *et al.* An endoscopic biopsy protocol can differentiate high-grade dysplasia from early adenocarcinoma in Barrett's esophagus. *Gastroenterology* 1993; 105: 40–50.

19. Spechler SJ. Barrett's esophagus: should we brush off this ballooning problem. *Gastroenterology* 1997; 112: 2138–2152.

20. Streitz JM, Andrews CW, Ellis FH. Endoscopic surveillance of Barrett's esophagus: does it help? *J Thorac Cardiovasc Surg* 1993; 105: 383–388.

21. Altorki NK, Sunagawa M, Little AG, Skinner DB. High-grade dysplasia in columnar-lined esophagus. *Am J Surg* 1991; 161: 97–100.

22. Cameron AJ, Carpenter HA. Barrett's esophagus, high grade dysplasia and early carcinoma: a pathological study. *Am J Gastroenterol* 1997; 92: 586–591.

23. Barham CP, Jones RL, Biddlestone LR *et al.* Photothermal laser ablation of Barrett's oesophagus: endoscopic and histological evidence of squamous re-epithelialisation. *Gut* 1997; 41: 281–284.

24. Biddlestone LR, Barham CP, Wilkinson SP *et al.* The histopathology of treated Barrett's oesophagus: squamous re-epithelialisation following acid suppression, laser and photodynamic therapy. *Am J Surg Pathol* 1998; 22: 239–245.

25. Weinstein WM. Precursor lesions for cancer of the cardia. In: Tytgat GNJ (ed.) *Gastrointestinal Endoscopy.* Vol. 7. Clinics of North America, 1997, pp. 19–28.

26. Sawada T, Muto T. Role of upper gastrointestinal surveillance in patients with familial adenomatous polyposis. In: Tytgat GNJ (ed.) *Gastrointestinal Endoscopy.* Vol. 7. Clinics of North America, 1997, pp. 99–110.

27. Panjepour M, Overholt BF, Vo-Dinh T *et al.* Endoscopic fluorescence detection of high-grade dysplasia in Barrett's esophagus. *Gastroenterology* 1996; 111: 93–101.

28. Van Dam J, Bjorkman DJ. Shedding some light on high-grade dysplasia. *Gastroenterology* 1996; 111: 227–249.

29. Stael von Holstein C, Nilsson AMK, Andersson-Engels S *et al.* Detection of adenocarcinoma in Barrett's oesophagus by means of laser induced fluorescence. *Gut* 1996; 39: 711–716.

30. Barr H. Laser and photodynamic and therapy: endoscopic optical biopsy techniques. In: Cotton PB, Tytgat GNJ, Williams CB, Bowling TE (eds) *Annual of Gastrointestinal Endoscopy.* Rapid Science Publishers, Philadelphia 1997, pp. 171–176.

6 Acute non-variceal gastrointestinal bleeding

K.R. Palmer

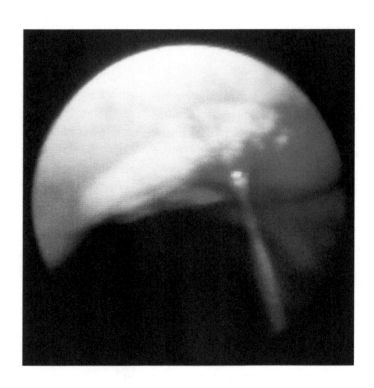

INTRODUCTION

Acute upper gastrointestinal haemorrhage accounts for approximately 25 000 hospital admissions each year in the United Kingdom. The annual incidence varies from 47 to 179 per 100 000 of the population and is higher in socioeconomically deprived areas. Although the hospital mortality rate has not improved over 50 years and remains at approximately 10%, older patients who have advanced cardiovascular, respiratory and cerebrovascular disease which puts them at increased risk of death, now comprise a much higher proportion of cases [1].

PRESENTATION

Haematemesis is the vomiting of blood from the gastrointestinal tract, as distinct from the expulsion of swallowed blood following epistaxis or haemoptysis. Melaena, the passage of black tarry stool, occurs when at least 200 ml of blood enters the upper gastrointestinal tract and is altered by the digestive process. The stool becomes purple or red when 1000 ml of blood abruptly enters the stomach or duodenum. Bleeding tends to be more severe in patients who have haematemesis and melaena than in those who have melaena only. There is little correlation between the cause of haemorrhage and whether haematemesis or melaena occurs, or whether vomitus is bright red or 'coffee grounds'.

Assessment

At the time of initial assessment it is important to define factors which have prognostic importance. A scoring system was derived from an assessment of 4701 cases of acute gastrointestinal bleeding admitted to 74 hospitals in England [2] (Table 1). Only a small minority had sustained variceal haemorrhage, and it is unlikely that the scoring system can be applied to that group of patients (see Chapter 7).

This (Rockall) scoring system involves five independent risk factors which are added to derive an overall score. In a British population the risk score, rebleeding and observed mortality were closely related although a score less than or equal to 2 was associated with 0.1% mortality.

An increasing score correlated with observed mortality. The system has also been tested in a Dutch population [3],

where it adequately predicted observed mortality but correlated poorly with risk of rebleeding. Further validation would be useful.

Patients at highest risk of death require intensive support and may be best managed in dedicated, high-dependency bleeding units. The most important factors predicting poor outcome include increasing age and co-morbidity, particularly renal insufficiency, hepatic failure or disseminated malignancy, and patients with these have a very poor prognosis. Hospital admission may be precipitated by gastrointestinal bleeding in many of these patients while death is often due to progression of the underlying condition rather than to bleeding. Patients who develop acute gastrointestinal bleeding after hospitalization for other serious illness have a much worse prognosis than those who are admitted because of bleeding, with a mortality rate of about 30%. Endoscopic stigmata of active, spurting haemorrhage, or a non-bleeding visible vessel within an ulcer are associated with significant risk of further bleeding (Figs 6.1, 6.2). The absence of these endoscopic findings implies little chance of rebleeding, and early discharge from hospital is planned.

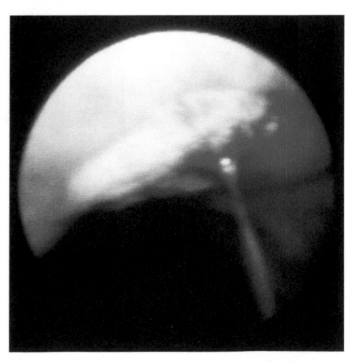

Figure 6.1. Spurting haemorrhage from a post-duodenal ulcer. This is associated with an 80% risk of continuing bleeding or rebleeding in shocked patients.

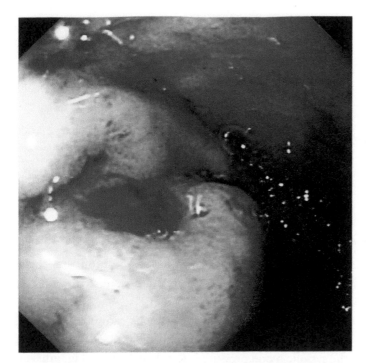

Table 6.2. Causes of acute upper gastrointestinal bleeding

Cause	%
Duodenal ulcer	24
Gastric/stomal ulcer	22
Gastric/duodenal erosions	18
Varices	10
Mallory–Weiss tear	7
Oesophagitis/oesophageal tear	8
Neoplasm	3
Vascular malformation	2
Others	6

Figure 6.2. A non-bleeding visible vessel. The appearances are due to a pseudoaneurysm of the damaged artery or to adherent blood clot. This endoscopic finding is associated with a 50% chance of rebleeding, usually within the first 24 hours of presentation.

CAUSES OF ACUTE GASTROINTESTINAL BLEEDING

Peptic ulcer disease

The most common cause of significant upper gastro-intestinal haemorrhage remains peptic ulcer (Table 6.2). A history of previous proven peptic ulcer or ulcer-like dyspepsia is absent in approximately 20% of cases. In these patients, consumption of aspirin or non-steroidal anti-inflammatory drugs is frequent. *Helicobacter pylori* infection is less prevalent in bleeding ulcers than in uncomplicated ulcer disease. Severe ulcer bleeding is due to arterial erosion by the ulcer, and the severity of bleeding is dependent upon the diameter of the artery and the size of the defect. Bleeding from an arterial defect >1 mm in size is unlikely to stop spontaneously, and does not respond to endoscopic therapy [4]. Large ulcers arising from the posterior part of the duodenal cap can erode the gastroduodenal artery and provoke brisk bleeding.

Table 6.1. Numerical scoring system for acute gastrointestinal bleeding. (From [2])

Variable	Score 0	Score 1	Score 2	Score 3
Age (years)	< 60	60–70	> 70	
Shock	None	Pulse > 100 b.p.m.	Systolic BP < 100.0 mmHg	
Co-morbidity	None	–	Cardiac disease	Renal or liver failure, advanced malignancy
Diagnosis	Mallory–Weiss tear: no SRH	–	Upper GI malignancy	–
Signs of recent bleeding	None, or black spots	–	Blood in lumen, active bleeding, visible vessel	–

BP = blood pressure; GI = gastrointestinal; SRH = stigmata of recent haemorrhage.

Oesophageal varices

Oesophageal varices account for a small proportion of cases, but have a disproportionate impact upon medical resources. Bleeding is often severe and other features of liver disease including fluid retention, hepatic encephalopathy, renal failure and sepsis often develop. Approximately one-third of patients will die, and prognosis is related to the severity of the underlying liver disease rather than to the magnitude of variceal bleeding (see Chapter 7).

Non-variceal oesophageal causes

Oesophagitis rarely causes significant acute haemorrhage. It more commonly presents with iron-deficiency anaemia. Mallory–Weiss tears are a consequence of retching, and most patients give a history of alcohol abuse, have features of other gastrointestinal disease such as peptic ulcer or gastroenteritis, or have non-gastrointestinal causes of vomiting. Bleeding usually stops spontaneously although endoscopic therapy is sometimes required.

Erosions and vascular anomalies

Bleeding from gastric erosions and vascular malformations usually stops spontaneously and is rarely life-threatening. However, anomalies such as the Dieulafoy malformation which may result in recurrent significant haemorrhage can be difficult to diagnose and therefore also to treat. Aortoduodenal fistula should be strongly considered in patients who develop severe bleeding after aortic graft insertion.

Upper gastrointestinal malignancy

Bleeding from upper gastrointestinal malignancy is not usually severe and the prognosis is dictated by the stage of the disease. Patients with extensive upper gastrointestinal cancer have a dismal prognosis, but death is not usually a consequence of gastrointestinal haemorrhage.

RESUSCITATION

The first priority is to support the circulation rather than to define the bleeding source. Endoscopy should not be

Table 6.3. Blood tests on admission

Test	Comments
Haemoglobin	May be normal until haemodilution
Urea and electrolytes	Elevated blood urea suggests severe bleeding
Cross match	Two units unless bleeding is severe
Liver function tests	
Prothrombin time	

undertaken until appropriate resuscitation has been undertaken. Standard blood tests are done at the time of initial assessment (Table 6.3).

At least one large-bore intravenous cannula is inserted. When the pulse rate is greater than 100 beats per min, or the systolic blood pressure is less than 100 mmHg, infusion with a plasma substitute is started. The rate of infusion is dependent upon the severity of shock. Blood is tranfused if the systolic blood pressure does not increase after administration of two units of plasma expander, or if the haemoglobin concentration is less than 10 g/dl. Rapid infusion of O-negative blood is occasionally necessary in extreme cases.

In shocked patients, and in those with a history of significant cardiac disease, insertion of a central venous catheter helps to define infusion requirements; a central venous pressure of 5–10 cm saline is ideal. A urinary catheter is also inserted. Many patients have other significant diseases affecting the heart, lungs, kidneys or central nervous system. This co-morbidity must be recognized and supported; for example, oxygen is required in most patients, and therapy for angina may be required in those with coronary artery disease. In anticoagulated patients, the International Normalized Ratio (INR) should be adjusted to 1.5 using fresh-frozen plasma [5].

It is most important when assessing any patient who presents with acute gastrointestinal bleeding to consider liver disease, because specific management is required (see Chapter 7). Circulatory support is crucial, but saline infusion is avoided since this exacerbates fluid retention. Specific therapies for hepatic encephalopathy, coagulopathy, renal failure and sepsis are frequently required.

DIAGNOSIS

Preparation and timing of endoscopy

When the patient has been resuscitated, endoscopy is undertaken. For the majority of patients, this is done electively on the next available routine list, but within 24 hours of admission. Only a minority of profusely bleeding patients need out-of-hours, emergency endoscopy, but there are no data to indicate that the timing of endoscopy is important. In severely bleeding patients endotracheal intubation is necessary to prevent aspiration into the bronchial tree.

Endoscopy should be done with the help of at least two trained assistants. Supplementary oxygen and pulse oximetry should always be used. The endoscopists must be experienced and have the ability to apply a range of therapeutic endoscopic modalities. Accessories including catheters to wash bleeding points and disposable injection needles are necessary. Intravenous sedation (midazolam or diazemuls) is often employed, but the combination of sedation plus anaesthetic throat spray is avoided because this predisposes to aspiration [6]. The minimal possible dose of sedation is chosen, particularly in patients who are hypotensive or have a history of cardiorespiratory or liver disease.

Endoscopy

Endoscopy is necessary to define the cause of bleeding, to provide prognostic information, and to apply haemostatic therapy.

Diagnosis

It is difficult to prove that diagnostic endoscopy improves outcome, but it is clearly important to define a precise diagnosis in order to plan therapy.

Prognosis

The endoscopic stigmata illustrated in Figures 6.1 and 6.2 are extremely useful in defining risk of further bleeding. The endoscopist should endeavour to see clearly the bleeding point, and this may involve washing away blood clots using endoscopically positioned catheters. Washing risks further bleeding, but this danger is outweighed by the importance of accurately defining the bleeding source, particularly since endoscopic therapy is then applied to appropriate cases.

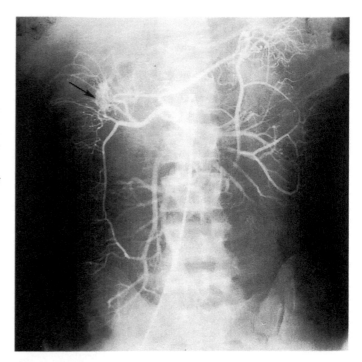

Figure 6.3. Selective angiography showing active bleeding (arrow) from a second part duodenal ulcer, not seen on endoscopy.

Therapy

A range of endoscopic therapies can be administered when endoscopic stigmata are identified (see below). When endoscopy does not yield a diagnosis and the patient is actively bleeding, urgent mesenteric angiography may show the site of bleeding (Fig. 6.3). In other patients, colonoscopy or a ^{99m}Tc-labelled red cell scan may be positive.

An algorithm for diagnosis and management is shown in Figure 6.4.

PRACTICALITIES

Choice of treatment

Approximately 80% of patients admitted to hospital because of acute gastrointestinal haemorrhage stop bleeding spontaneously [7,8], and endoscopic or surgical therapy is clearly unnecessary and meddlesome in this group. Patients at risk of uncontrolled bleeding tend to be elderly, present with hypotension, tachycardia and anaemia. Those who at endoscopy are found to be actively bleeding and who are shocked have an 80% risk of continuing to bleed or of rebleeding unless treatment is undertaken. The

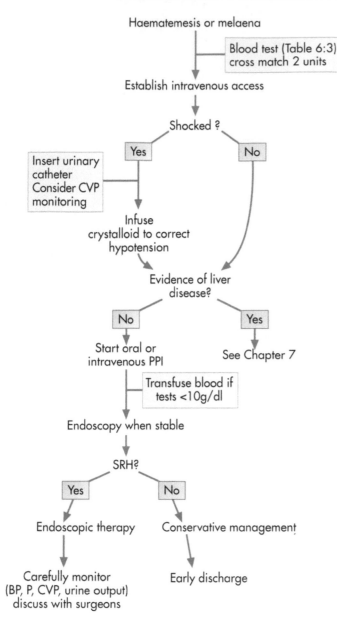

Figure 6.4. Algorithm for the management of upper gastrointestinal bleeding. CVP = central venous pressure; SRH = stigmata of recent haemorrhage; BP = blood pressure; P = pulse; PPI = proton pump inhibitor.

presence of a non-bleeding visible vessel is associated with a 50% chance of rebleeding. The visible vessel represents either a pseudoaneurysm of the damaged artery, or a sentinel blood clot. Adherent blood clot and oozing have been associated with a significant risk of rebleeding by some authors [9]; others suggest that rebleeding is uncommon and it is our practice not to treat endoscopically those patients who present with oozing or adherent blood clot from ulcers. A clean ulcer base is not associated with further bleeding.

Some enthusiasts have advocated the use of endoscopic Doppler probes to identify patent arteries within and around the ulcer, and suggest that only ulcers with a positive Doppler signal should be treated [10].

Drug therapy

There is conflicting evidence to support pharmacological therapy, and in general most experts have little enthusiasm for the view that oral or intravenous therapies are crucial in the treatment of major non-variceal haemorrhage.

Acid suppression therapy

Blood clot stability is improved when acid secretion is suppressed, and several studies have attempted to define the role of acid-lowering drugs. The largest of these showed no value for routine use of omeprazole as therapy in patients admitted to hospital because of acute bleeding; indeed, mortality tended to be higher in ulcer patients treated with omeprazole rather than placebo [11]. In contrast, a trial of 220 bleeding-ulcer patients reported from India concluded that high-dose oral omeprazole was associated with reduced rebleeding rates and need for urgent surgery [12]. It is our practice on the basis of this study to use omeprazole. There are no comparative studies of intravenous versus oral acid-suppressing therapy.

Somatostatin

Intravenous somatostatin and its synthetic analogue, octreotide, reduce splanchnic blood flow and suppress acid secretion. Anecdotal reports that these agents can stop active haemorrhage and meta-analyses have demonstrated overall benefit in terms of rebleeding and need for surgical intervention [13]. Most experts remain unconvinced and further studies are necessary.

Tranexamic acid

Although this antifibrinolytic drug enhances blood clot stability, and one trial suggests marginal benefit for ulcer bleeding [14], tranexamic acid is not widely used – possibly because of a fear of causing thrombosis at other sites.

Endoscopic therapy

It is now accepted that patients who are found to have major endoscopic stigmata should receive endoscopic therapy. Surgery is now reserved for the failures of endoscopic therapy, when access is impossible because of profuse, active haemorrhage, or when the patient continues to bleed despite apparently technically successful endoscopic therapy. The evidence that endoscopic treatment improves outcome in other causes of non-variceal acute bleeding is largely anecdotal. A range of approaches [15] have been used for vascular malformations and Mallory–Weiss tears, but none has been subjected to randomized clinical trials.

It is important that the endoscopist knows his or her limitations. Massive bleeding from a major artery does not respond to any form of endoscopic haemostatic treatment, and patients presenting in this way require emergency surgery. An operation should not be delayed by endoscopic therapy which has little chance of success. It follows that endoscopic treatments are only valuable in managing moderately severe cases. Minor bleeding will settle with conservative support, major haemorrhage requires an emergency surgical operation, while the intermediate group of patients benefit from endoscopic therapy. Endoscopic therapy may avoid the need for a surgical operation and reduce transfusion requirements, but because it has limited value in the most severely bleeding patients, its impact upon hospital mortality is only modest.

Table 6.4. Endoscopic therapy for bleeding ulcer

Principle	Treatment
Thermal modalities	Argon laser
	Neodymium YAG laser
	Heater probe
Electrocoagulation	BICAP
Injection	Adrenaline (1 : 10 000–1 : 100 000)
	Sclerosants (polidocanol, ethanolamine, sodium tetradecylsulphate)
	Alcohol
	Clotting factors (thrombin, fibrin glue)
Experimental	Mechanical devices (clips, rubber bands, sewing)
	Microwave coagulation

Principles of endoscopic treatment and evidence

The aim of haemostatic endoscopic therapy is to thrombose the bleeding artery. This may be achieved by thermal modalities, diathermy, injection or mechanical devices (Table 6.4).

Injection

Injection therapy for peptic ulcer bleeding is now widely used as first-line treatment. Clinical trials have shown that this approach is as effective as other options, and that it is safe and cheap (Fig. 6.5).

It is not entirely clear how injection therapy stops bleeding and prevents rebleeding. This is because operative specimens are rarely available and it is difficult to differentiate the effects of treatment from the histological characteristics of a chronic ulcer. Inflammation, vasculitis and thrombosis of vessels are an inherent feature of peptic ulcer. Furthermore, an appropriate reproducible animal model of bleeding peptic ulcer is unavailable. The efficacy of injection therapy is probably due to a combination of factors. These include a tamponade effect due to injection under high pressure into a fibrotic, rigid ulcer leading to compression of the bleeding artery, vasoconstriction (when dilute adrenaline is used), endarteritis (following injection with sclerosants), tissue dehydration (by alcohol injection), and stimulation of clotting factors (by thrombin or fibrin glue injection).

Controlled clinical trials

Relatively few studies have compared injection with conservative management, but these controlled trials have shown clear benefit for injected patients, and it can be argued that trials which include a no treatment arm have become unethical.

Dilute adrenaline

Most endoscopists inject appropriate ulcers with dilute adrenaline. Chung *et al.* showed that injection with 1 :10 000 adrenaline stopped active bleeding and reduced the need for urgent surgery [16]. Several groups subsequently performed trials in which adrenaline was combined with injection of sclerosants [17–20] (Table 6.5).

This was done because of the preconception – supported by experiments in animal models – that adrenaline would not cause thrombosis of the bleeding artery. While adrenaline might stop active haemorrhage by vasoconstriction,

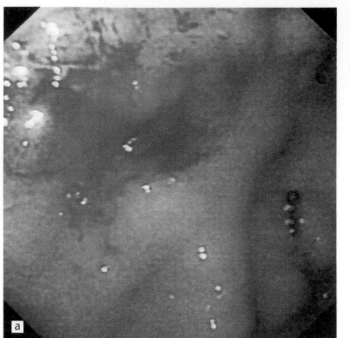 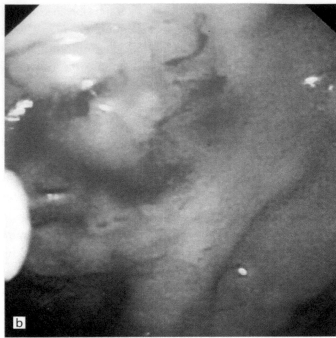

Figure 6.5. Endoscopic view of bleeding gastric erosion (a) before and (b) after injection with 1:10,000 adrenaline. Note blanching due to combination of tamponade and vasoconstriction.

a sclerosant was thought necessary to induce endarteritis leading to arterial thrombosis. To test this assertion, two clinical trials compared outcome in patients treated with dilute adrenaline or a combination of adrenaline plus a sclerosant. Chung *et al.* [21] randomized 200 actively bleeding ulcer patients to injection with 1 : 10 000 adrenaline or to adrenaline followed by 3% sodium tetradecylsulphate (STD). Initial haemostasis was achieved in almost all patients, and only two from each group rebled. Similar conclusions were reached by Choudari and Palmer [22], who randomized 107 patients with a range of endoscopic stigmata to injection with 1 : 100 000 adrenaline or to adrenaline plus 5% ethanolamine. Permanent haemostasis was achieved in 85% of patients in

both cases. These two trials thus showed that the addition of a sclerosant to an injection of adrenaline is unnecessary.

Adrenaline injection is remarkably safe with no reported serious complications.

Sclerosants

A range of sclerosing agents have been injected into and around bleeding ulcers to try and stop active haemorrhage and prevent rebleeding. These include 1% polidocanol, 5% ethanolamine and 3% STD. There are no controlled trials involving patients randomized to sclerosants or to conservative (no injection) treatment. Trials have shown that a combination of dilute adrenaline plus a sclerosant is superior to no endoscopic therapy in terms of reduction of the rate of rebleeding and need for surgery (Table 6.5).

Table 6.5. Controlled trials comparing endoscopic injection of adrenaline plus sclerosant versus conservative (no endoscopic) therapy

Reference	No. of patients	Uncontrolled bleeding: injected patients (%)	Uncontrolled bleeding: controls (%)	P-value
Chung *et al.* 1988 [16]	109	13	47	< 0.001
Panes *et al.* 1987 [18]	113	8	65	< 0.001
Balanzo *et al.* 1988 [19]	72	19	42	< 0.05
Oxner *et al.* 1992 [20]	93	17	47	< 0.05

However, the role of the sclerosant is difficult to interpret for two major reasons. First, because the trials suffer from the common problem of small sample size. Second, because the sclerosant has been injected with an agent which has proven therapeutic value. As already discussed, Chung *et al.* [21] and Choudari and Palmer [22] showed no advantage for combination therapy over injection with adrenaline alone. A third trial reported by Villanueva *et al.* [23] showed similar outcome following injection with adrenaline plus polidocanol or treatment with adrenaline alone (Table 6.6).

No study has compared haemostasis in patients treated by adrenaline with that achieved by injection of a sclerosant alone. Sclerosant injections have been associated with necrosis of the upper gastrointestinal tract, presumably due to extensive arterial thrombosis [24,25].

Alcohol

The efficacy of injection with 98% ethanol has been demonstrated in several clinical trials [26–28] (Table 6.7). The evidence that alcohol stops active bleeding and prevents rebleeding is more convincing than that for sclerosants. The potential for side effects following alcohol injection is similar to that for sclerosants, and many endoscopists are wary of its use.

Clotting factors

Two relatively large controlled trials have examined the efficacy of injection with agents which directly cause formation of a blood clot (Table 6.8).

Kubba *et al.* [29] randomized matched groups of bleeding ulcer patients to urgent endoscopic injection with a combination of 1 : 100 000 adrenaline plus 200 units of human thrombin, or to adrenaline alone. Rebleeding and hospital mortality were significantly lower in patients treated with the combination, although the need for emergency surgery was similar in the two groups. A large European multicentre trial [30] randomized patients to injection with 1% polidocanol, a single injection of fibrin glue, or to repeated glue injection. Fibrin glue comprises both thrombin and fibrinogen, injected into the bleeding point through a specially designed double-lumen needle. All patients underwent serial endoscopy at daily intervals, but only patients randomized to repeat injection were retreated with glue if the endoscopic stigmata persisted. Significant rebleeding was least in the group randomized to repeated glue injection, while outcome in those treated by a single glue injection was between that of the other two groups.

Although injection of clotting factors (thrombin or a combination of thrombin and fibrinogen) theoretically

Table 6.6. Controlled trials of endoscopic injection with adrenaline plus sclerosant versus adrenaline alone

Reference	No. of patients randomized	Uncontrolled bleeding: combination (%)	Uncontrolled bleeding: adrenaline controls (%)	P-value
Chung *et al.* 1993[21]	200	14	16	NS
Choudari *et al.* 1994 [22]	107	13	15	NS
Villaneuva *et al.* 1993 [23]	63	24	13	NS

NS = Not significant.

Table 6.7. Controlled trials comparing alcohol injection versus conservative treatment

Reference	No. of patients randomized	Uncontrolled bleeding: alcohol (%)	Uncontrolled bleeding: conservative (%)	P-value
Pasco *et al.* 1989 [26]	143	3	13	< 0.05
Lazo *et al.* 1992 [27]	39	4	57	< 0.05
Chiozzini *et al.* 1989 [28]	53	13	26	NS

NS = Not significant.

Table 6.8. Trials of clotting factors

Design (Reference)	No. of patients randomized	% Rebleeding: clotting factor once	% Rebleeding: clotting factor twice	% Rebleeding: control injection
Thrombin plus adrenaline versus adrenaline alone [29]	140	4	–	20 ($P < 0.05$)
Fibrin glue versus 1% polidocanol [30]	826	16	10 ($P < 0.05$)	18

risks causing thrombosis of mesenteric arteries, the safety of this approach appears excellent, and perforation or necrosis of the upper gastrointestinal tract is very rare even in patients receiving multiple glue injections.

Thermal modalities

Thermal methods comprise laser and the heater probe.

Laser

Photocoagulation for ulcer haemorrhage was first reported using the argon laser. Results were generally disappointing, possibly because of study design (small trials including low-risk patients) and probably because the depth and penetration of tissue damage was insufficient to cause arterial thrombosis. Subsequent trials used Nd-YAG lasers, and most studies (though not all) showed benefit in treated patients. A meta-analysis of controlled trials [31] showed a reduction in the need for urgent surgery, and reduced mortality. Laser therapy is expensive and the no-touch technique makes it more difficult than other endoscopic haemostatic methods. Even in expert hands, up to 19% of ulcers cannot be treated optimally because of technical difficulties [32].

For these reasons, laser therapy is no longer used routinely in the treatment of ulcer haemorrhage, though it does provide effective therapy for vascular malformations including gastric antral vascular ectasia [33], the Dieulafoy malformation [34] and other vascular lesions [35]. Argon plasma coagulation may prove to be superior to the laser as it causes comparable tissue damage, but is much easier to use.

Heater probe

The heater probe transmits predetermined amounts of energy to the mucosa through a Teflon-coated tip. Optimum therapy is best administered by the 3.2-mm probe, using firm tamponade, a power setting of 25–30 J, and repeated applications until the treated area blackens. The heater probe is relatively cheap and portable. The facility to apply forcible tamponade, a capacity to apply energy tangentially, and a powerful water jet which cleans and irrigates, are particular advantages.

Controlled trials [36] have shown that the heater probe reduces rebleeding and need for emergency surgery in bleeding ulcer patients. Further trials showed comparable efficacy for the heater probe and injection with adrenaline [37,38] and with alcohol [39] (Table 6.9).

Electrocoagulation

Electrocoagulation devices cause arterial thrombosis by passing an electric current through the mucosa. Monopolar units involve the application of ball-tipped probes, and the electrical circuit is completed through a plate attached to the patient. Tissue adherence and unpredictable mucosal

Table 6.9. Comparisons of heater probe and injection

Reference	No. of patients	Permanent haemostasis: heater probe (%)	Permanent haemostasis: injection (%)
Lin *et al.* 1990 [39]	78	95	71 ($P < 0.05$)
Chung *et al.* 1991 [37]	122	85	95 ($P < 0.05$)
Choudari *et al.* 1992 [38]	140	85	85

damage are particular problems, and the device has been superseded by other contact methods.

Multipolar coagulation works by passing an electrical current between probes applied to the mucosa. The multipolar elecrocoagulation pulse, known as BICAP, has three pairs of electrodes on its side and tip; electrocoagulation occurs if any pair of electrodes are in tissue contact, and this facilitates tangential treatment. The amount of energy applied to the area and the degree of tissue damage is therefore more predictable than with monopolar probes. Two prospective randomized trials [40,41] have shown that the BICAP is effective, both in achieving initial haemostasis and in preventing rebleeding from visible vessels. Best results are achieved using forceful application of the larger (3.2 mm) probe, a low wattage setting, and prolonged periods of coagulation.

Mechanical devices

Endoscopic haemostasis can be achieved using metal clips, clamps, rubber band ligation and sewing. The application of these approaches is technically demanding and none is established in clinical practice.

Combination endoscopic therapy

Combination of thermal and injection therapy for bleeding ulcer has been examined in several clinical trials, and a single device which combines bipolar coagulation and injection is commercially available.

Clinical trials do not generally show that the combination of heat and injection is superior to injection alone, though this may be due to relatively small sample sizes. One study has suggested that the combination of the heater probe plus dilute adrenaline injection is more effective therapy for actively bleeding ulcers than injection alone [42], but this needs to be confirmed by further studies. Although the combination of thermal treatment and injection (possibly with clotting factors) is theoretically attractive, the potential for complications (particularly perforation and mucosal necrosis) is probably increased by more aggressive approaches.

Failures of endoscopic therapy: when to operate

The endoscopist can adversely affect outcome in patients who fail to respond to endoscopic therapy. Repeated therapeutic endoscopy, excessive blood transfusion and delayed surgical operation in patients who ultimately fail endoscopic haemostasis all increase the risk of death. Unfortunately, it is not possible to predict the failures of endoscopic treatment. Clearly patients with the most active haemorrhage are the least likely to respond to non-operative approaches, both because massive bleeding can make administration of endoscopic therapy impossible and because large arterial defects cannot be sealed by these approaches. Studies have shown that patients who present with spurting haemorrhage from large posterior duodenal ulcers are the most resistant to any form of endoscopic haemostasis [43,44]. Even in these patients it is nevertheless possible to achieve endoscopic control in at least 50% of cases [44]. Repeat endoscopic treatment at 12- to 24-hours intervals improves the success rate in those patients who have persisting major stigmata [30].

The best policy in patients who rebleed after endoscopic treatment remains unclear. Many endoscopists attempt further endoscopic therapy in such cases, while others consider rebleeding to be an indication for urgent surgery. Clinical trials do not tell us when to operate, and indications for the timing of surgical intervention are not evidence-based; rather an operation is done on the basis of clinical judgement. A unit policy should be developed and adhered to; our own includes the option to re-treat endoscopically after a single rebleeding episode in a fit patient, while more frail patients undergo surgery after their first rebleed. Definitions of fitness and of rebleeding are difficult; the former are based upon anaesthetic criteria, the latter upon the development of fresh haematemesis or melaena with clinical shock or a fall in haemoglobin concentration of at least 2 g/dl over a 24-hours period.

No study has compared surgical with endoscopic treatment as first-line management. Most trials of endoscopic therapy define a need for surgical operation as treatment failure. On the other hand, endoscopic control of active haemorrhage may sometimes be used to facilitate semi-elective definitive surgery. A successful outcome depends upon a combination of endoscopic and surgical expertise and a team approach is essential.

REFERENCES

1. Laine L, Peterson WL. Bleeding peptic ulcer. *N Engl J Med* 1994; 33: 717–718.

2. Rockall TA, Logan RFA, Devlin HB, Northfield TC. Variation in outcome after acute gastrointestinal haemorrhage. *Lancet* 1995; 346: 346–350.

3. Vreeburg EM, Terwee CB, Snel P *et al.* Validation of the Rockall scoring system in upper gastrointestinal bleeding. *Gut* 1999; 44: 331–335.

4. Swain CP, Storey DW, Bown SG *et al.* Nature of the bleeding vessel in recurrently bleeding gastric ulcers. *Gastroenterology* 1986; 90; 595–608.

5. Choudari CP, Rajgopal C, Palmer KR. Acute gastrointestinal haemorrhage in anticoagulated patients: diagnosis and response to endoscopic therapy. *Gut* 1994; 35: 464–466.

6. Quine MA, Bell GD, McLoy RF *et al.* Prospective audit of upper gastrointestinal endoscopy in two regions of England: safety, staffing and sedation methods. *Gut* 1995; 36: 462–467.

7. Silverstein FE, Gilbert DA, Tedesco FJ. The National ASGE survey of upper gastrointestinal bleeding II. Clinical prognostic factors. *Gastrointest Endosc* 1981; 27: 80–93.

8. Branicki FJ, Coleman SY, Fok PF. Bleeding ulcer: a prospective evaluation of risk factors for rebleeding and mortality. *World J Surg* 1990; 14: 262–270.

9. Wara P. Endoscopic prediction of major rebleeding – a prospective study of stigmata of haemorrhage in bleeding ulcer. *Gastroenterology* 1985; 88: 1209–1214.

10. Kohler B, Reimann JC. The endoscopic Doppler. Its value in evaluating gastroduodenal ulcers after haemorrhage and as an instrument of control of endoscopic injection therapy. *Scand J Gastroenterol* 1991; 26: 471–476.

11. Daneshmend TK, Hawkey CJ, Langmann MJS *et al.* Omeprazole versus placebo for upper gastrointestinal bleeding: randomised double blind controlled trial. *Br Med J* 1992; 304: 143–147.

12. Khuroo MS, Yattoo GN, Javid G *et al.* A comparison of omeprazole and placebo for bleeding peptic ulcer. *N Engl J Med* 1997; 336: 1054–1058.

13. Imperiale TF, Birgissan S. Somatostatin or Octreotide compared with H$_2$ receptor antagonists and placebo in the management of acute non-variceal upper gastrointestinal haemorrhage: a meta-analysis. *Ann Intern Med* 1997; 127: 1062–1071.

14. Henry DA, O'Connell DL. Effects of fibrinolytic inhibitors on mortality from upper gastrointestinal haemorrhage. *Br Med J* 989; 298: 1142–1146.

15. Katz PO, Salas L. Less frequent causes of upper gastrointestinal bleeding. *Gastrointest Clin North Am* 1993; 22: 875–878.

16. Chung SCS, Leung JWC, Steele RJ *et al.* Endoscopic injection of adrenaline for actively bleeding ulcers: a randomised trial. *Br Med J* 1988; 269: 1631–1633.

17. Rajgopal C, Palmer KR. Endoscopic injection sclerosis: effective therapy for bleeding peptic ulcer. *Gut* 1991; 32: 727–729.

18. Panes J, Vivier J, Forne M *et al.* Controlled trial of endoscopic sclerosis in bleeding peptic ulcer. *Lancet* 1987; ii: 1292–1294.

19. Balanzo J, Sainz S, Such J. Endoscopic haemostasis by local injection of epinephrine and polidocanol in bleeding ulcer: a prospective randomised trial. *Endoscopy* 1988; 20: 289–291.

20. Oxner RBG, Simmonds NJ, Gertner DJ *et al.* Controlled trial of endoscopic injection for bleeding from peptic ulcers with visible vessels. *Lancet* 1992; 339: 966–968.

21. Chung SCS, Leung JWC, Leong HT *et al.* Adding a sclerosant to endoscopic epinephrine injection in actively bleeding ulcers: randomised trial. *Gastrointest Endosc* 1993; 39: 611–615.

22. Choudari CP, Palmer KR. Endoscopic injection therapy for bleeding peptic ulcer: a comparison of adrenaline alone with adrenaline plus ethanolamine oleate. *Gut* 1994; 35: 608–610.

23. Villaneuva C, Balanzo J, Espinos JC *et al.* Endoscopic injection therapy of bleeding ulcer: a prospective and randomised comparison of adrenaline with or without polidocanol. *J Clin Gastroenterol* 1993; 17: 195–200.

24. Levy J, Khakoo S, Barton R, Vicary R. Fatal injection sclerotherapy of a bleeding peptic ulcer. *Lancet* 1991; 337: 504.

25. Loperfids S, Patelli G, La Torre L. Extensive necrosis of gastric mucosa following injection therapy of bleeding peptic ulcer. *Endoscopy* 1990; 22: 285–286.

26. Pasco O, Draghici A, Acolvichi I. The effect of endoscopic haemostasis with alcohol on the mortality of non-variceal upper gastrointestinal haemorrhage: a randomised prospective study. *Endoscopy* 1989; 21: 53–55.

27. Lazo MD, Andrade R, Medina MC *et al.* Effect of injection sclerosis with alcohol on the rebleeding rate of gastroduodenal peptic ulcers with non bleeding visible vessels: a prospective controlled trial. *Am J Gastroenterol* 1992; 87: 843–846.

28. Chiozzini G, Bortoluzzi F, Pallini P *et al.* Controlled trial of absolute alcohol vs epinephrine as injection agent in gastroduodenal bleeding. *Gastroenterol* 1989; 96: A86.

29. Kubba AK, Murphy W, Palmer KR. Endoscopic injection for bleeding peptic ulcer: a comparison of adrenaline alone with adrenaline plus human thrombin. *Gastroenterol* 1996; 111: 623–628.

30. Rutgeerts P, Rawes E, Wara P, Swain P *et al*. Randomised trial of single and repeated fibrin glue compared with injection of polidocanol in treatment of bleeding ulcer. *Lancet* 1997; 350: 692–696.

31. Cook DJ, Gruyatt GH, Salendra BJ, Laine L. Endoscopic therapy for acute non-variceal gastrointestinal haemorrhage: a meta-analysis. *Gastroenterol* 1992; 102: 139–148.

32. Swain CP, Kirkham JS, Salmon PR *et al*. Controlled trial of Nd-Yag laser photocoagulation in bleeding peptic ulcers. *Lancet* 1986; 1; 1113–1117.

33. Gostout CL, Ahlquist DA, Radford CM *et al*. Endoscopic laser therapy for watermelon stomach. *Gastroenterol* 1989; 96:1462–1465.

34. Reilly HF, Al-Kawas FH. Dieulafoyls lesion: diagnosis and management. *Dig Dis Sci* 1991; 37: 1702–1707.

35. Cello JP, Grendell JH. Endoscopic laser treatment for gastrointestinal vascular ectasias. *Ann Intern Med* 1986; 104: 352–354.

36. Fullarton GM, Birnie GG, MacDonald A, Murray WR. Controlled trial of heater probe treatment in bleeding peptic ulcers. *Brit J Surg* 1989; 76: 541–544.

37. Chung SCS, Leung JWC, Sung JC. Injection or heat probe for bleeding ulcer. *Gastroenterol* 1991; 100: 33–37.

38. Choudari CP, Rajgopal C, Palmer KR. A comparison of endoscopic injection therapy versus the heater probe in major peptic ulcer haemorrhage. *Gut* 1992; 33: 1159–1161.

39. Lin HJ, Lee FY, Kang KW. Heat probe thermocoagulation and pure alcohol injection in massive peptic ulcer haemorrhage: a prospective, randomised controlled trial. *Gut* 1990; 31: 753–757.

40. Laine L. Multipolar electrocoagulation in the treatment of active upper gastrointestinal tract haemorrhage. *New Eng J Med* 1989; 99: 1303–1306.

41. Laine L. Multipolar electrocoagulation in the treatment of ulcers with non bleeding visible vessels. *Ann Intern Med* 1989; 110: 510–514.

42. Chung SCS, Lau YW, Sung JJY *et al*. Randomised comparison between adrenaline injection alone and adrenaline injection plus heater probe treatment for actively bleeding ulcers. *Brit Med J* 1997; 314: 1307–1314.

43. Villaneuva C, Balanzo J,Espinoz JC. Prediction of therapeutic failure in patients with bleeding peptic ulcer treated with endoscopic injection. *Dig Dis Sci* 1993; 38: 2062–2070.

44. Choudari GP, Rajgopal C, Elton RA, Palmer KR. Failures of endoscopic therapy for bleeding peptic ulcers: an analysis of risk factors. *Am J Gastroenterol* 1994; 89: 1968–1972.

Endoscopic therapy of oesophageal and gastric varices

A. Gimson

With acknowledgement to J. Collier

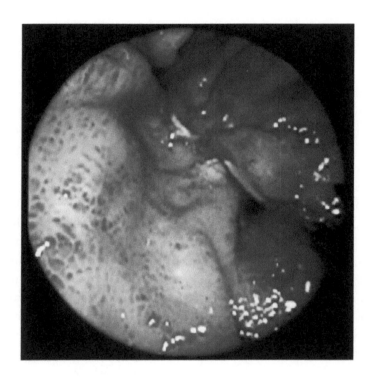

INTRODUCTION

In the natural history of chronic liver disease, approximately 30% of patients will sustain a variceal haemorrhage with a mortality rate of up to 50% for the index bleed [1,2]. Subsequently up to 70% will rebleed if no definitive treatment is undertaken with an in-hospital mortality rate of between 15% and 30% [3]. The management of variceal bleeding continues to be an area of controversy and, despite numerous randomized clinical trials, some aspects of therapy await clarification.

PRESENTATION

Haemorrhage from oesophageal varices usually presents as haematemesis or melaena, when bleeding is substantial and dramatic. Presentation as iron-deficiency anaemia is very rare, and other gastrointestinal sources of blood should be excluded. The majority of cases with variceal haemorrhage have a clear history of excess alcohol consumption or chronic liver disease with coexistent stigmata of chronic liver disease, jaundice, ascites and encephalopathy. Occasionally, patients with well-compensated cirrhosis may have no such features, similar to those with a portal vein thrombosis where the only clue to the presence of portal hypertension may be splenomegaly. Nevertheless, the risk of variceal haemorrhage is related to the severity of liver disease (Childs–Pugh grade C), and the presence of these features should strongly suggest the possibility of variceal haemorrhage.

Clinical assessment

The initial examination must seek evidence for chronic liver disease (splenomegaly, cutaneous stigmata) as well as complications of portal hypertension including ascites and encephalopathy. Components of the Childs–Pugh score (ascites, encephalopathy, albumen, prothrombin time and bilirubin) are important as it closely relates to prognosis after variceal haemorrhage. Possible precipitating factors for the haemorrhage include alcohol consumption, non-steroidal anti-inflammatory drug use, development of portal vein thrombosis or hepatocellular carcinoma and acute alcoholic hepatitis. Sepsis as either bacteraemia or spontaneous bacterial peritonitis may also precipitate

Table 7.1. Clinical assessment of patients presenting with variceal haemorrhage

Initial resuscitative measures after acute variceal haemorrhage

Intravenous access: CVP monitoring

Initial colloid then transfuse with packed RBC to CVP 6–12 cm H_2O and Hb >10 g/dl

Platelet infusion if <50 × 10^9/dl

FFP if prothrombin time >20 s

Cryoprecipitate if fibrinogen <0.25 g/l

10 ml 10% calcium gluconate after 4 units RBC

Prophylactic antibiotics

CVP = central venous pressure; FFP = fresh-frozen plasma; RBC = red blood cells.

haemorrhage, and appropriate cultures must be taken. All such factors may be important in assessing prognosis and aiding therapeutic decisions in individual cases.

Haemodynamic monitoring and resuscitation

Clinical assessment of volume status during variceal haemorrhage is difficult as patients may have an associated cardiomyopathy, autonomic neuropathy or already be on β-blockers. Central venous pressure (CVP) monitoring is mandatory for significant variceal bleeding along with pulse, arterial pressure and urine output. Conscious level needs monitoring in those with encephalopathy (Table 7.1).

Adequate venous access with large-bore cannulae allows rapid transfusion, as aggressive resuscitation is necessary before endoscopic therapy can be undertaken [4].

Central volume replacement, to avoid tissue hypoxia and maintain organ perfusion, is required with colloid and blood when available, aiming to keep the haemoglobin concentration above 10 g/dl. Patients with a coagulopathy (prothrombin time > 20 seconds) and thrombocytopenia (platelets < 50 × 10^9/l) secondary to chronic liver disease and/or splenomegaly should receive fresh-frozen plasma (FFP) and platelets. In cases of massive blood transfusion (> 2.5 litres), platelets and FFP should be given, as well as cryoprecipitate if multiple blood transfusions are required. In massive transfusion, hypothermia should be avoided by warming blood, hypocalcaemia due to citrate toxicity managed with 10 ml of 10% calcium gluconate given after every 3 units of blood, and hyperkalaemia treated with insulin and dextrose. The aim is to maintain CVP at 6–12 cmH$_2$O, as higher values may disproportionately elevate right-sided vascular pressures and be transmitted to portal and varix pressure.

At presentation with a variceal bleed, some patients already have a bacteraemia and/or spontaneous bacterial peritonitis [5], and are at risk of aspiration pneumonia or other septic events in subsequent days [6]. Prophylactic antibiotics, which cover Gram-negative organisms, have been shown in randomized trials to reduce this risk of infection following a variceal bleed [7].

Endoscopic diagnosis

Early upper gastrointestinal endoscopy is crucial to make the diagnosis of variceal haemorrhage. Up to 25% of patients with portal hypertension may be bleeding from non-variceal lesions [8], including peptic ulceration, Mallory–Weiss tears, gastritis, portal hypertensive gastropathy (Fig. 7.1) or gastric antral vascular ectasia (Fig. 7.2), although the bleeding is usually less severe than from varices. The site of gastric variceal (greater curve versus lesser curve) haemorrhage must be recorded [9]. Endoscopy in these circumstances can be difficult if the patient is confused or encephalopathic.

Protection of the airway and scrupulous avoidance of tracheal aspiration must be ensured. Occasionally, tracheal intubation and positive-pressure ventilation is necessary, but may have beneficial effects on lowering portal pressure. As vision may be severely limited during acute variceal

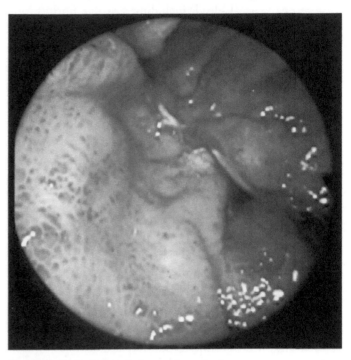

Figure 7.2. Gastric antral vascular ectasia.

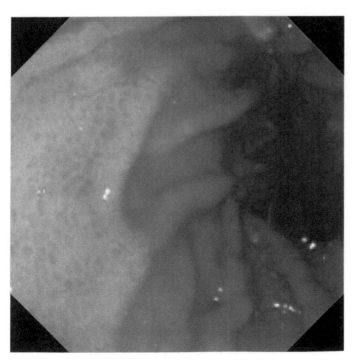

Figure 7.1. Retroflexed view into fundus showing moderate portal hypertensive gastropathy.

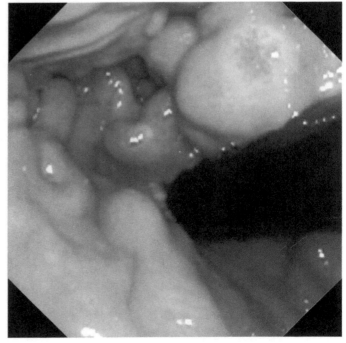

Figure 7.3. Large greater curve and anterior wall gastric varices.

haemorrhage a dual-channel endoscope has advantages in allowing suction and washing at the same time as endoscopic therapy.

Up to 60% of patients will have stopped bleeding by the time of endoscopy [8], so it is important to identify stigmata of a recent variceal bleed, including a visible fibrin/nipple sign on a varix. In those without evidence of fresh or altered blood in the upper gastrointestinal tract the absence of any other mucosal abnormality usually points to varices as the cause. In these circumstances distinguishing between a prior gastric or oesophageal source can be difficult. Gastric varices usually only bleed when they are large, on the greater curve and with high-risk stigmata on them (Fig. 7.3). In the presence of active bleeding a spurting varix may be seen, but fundal varices can bleed and be hidden beneath a fundal pool of blood in the stomach.

Prognostic factors

Various trials have demonstrated important prognostic factors in these patients, including the presence of an active spurting vessel at index endoscopy, Childs–Pugh score and portal pressure. The first two are most easily monitored and have a clear relationship to survival and risk of variceal rebleeding.

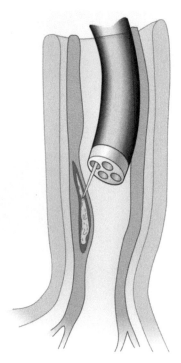

Figure 7.4. Injection sclerotherapy, intravariceal technique.

THERAPEUTIC TECHNIQUES

Endoscopic methods

Injection sclerotherapy

The technique of injection sclerotherapy has been developed over many years from using rigid oesophagoscopes to the present flexible endoscopes (Fig. 7.4). A wide range of sclerosants has been used including ethanolamine, sodium morrhuate, polidocanol and alcohol. There is no good evidence of a significant advantage with any one agent. Similarly, differences in injection technique, paravariceal or intravariceal, while requiring different volumes of sclerosant (small volumes with paravariceal injection) do not demonstrate significant differences in efficacy or complication rates. In Europe, intravariceal ethanolamine is the most commonly used technique.

After the endoscope (end or oblique viewing) is placed at the gastro-oesophageal junction, an injection needle is inserted down the instrument channel. The needle is protruded from the cannula, inserted into the varix column, and the sclerosant injected. It is rare to need more than 2 ml per injection – which is stopped immediately the varix blanches. All variceal columns are injected starting at the gastro-oesophageal junction and moving up for 2–4 cm.

In some cases, during massive variceal haemorrhage, vision is obscured by blood, and use of an overtube has been recommended with a side-port through which the varix can appear, to isolate it from others (Fig. 7.5). This technique is not used routinely.

Sclerotherapy arrests active variceal haemorrhage in 85–95% of cases, and if used as secondary prevention of recurrent variceal bleeding must be undertaken at weekly intervals until varices are obliterated. This usually takes five to six sessions, and oral sucralfate (1 g q.d.s.) given until that time has been shown to be of benefit in preventing recurrent bleeding from sclerotherapy-induced mucosal damage [10].

Variceal band ligation

Band ligation of oesophageal varices was first described by van Steigmann *et al.* [11] (Fig. 7.6). The banding device consists of a short plastic sleeve on the tip of a forward-viewing endoscope, preloaded with stretched elastic bands each attached to a trip wire passing up the instrument channel to a winch apparatus (Fig. 7.7). The device allows water to be injected down the endoscope to improve vision.

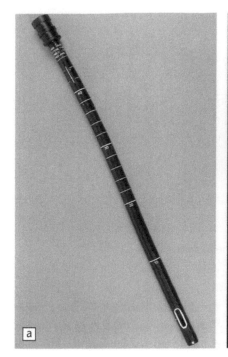

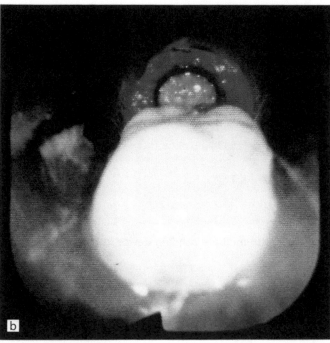

Figure 7.5.
(a) Overtube for variceal injection. Note the slot in the distal end of the tube through which the varices prolapse, facilitating injection. (b) Varix prolapsing through the slot.

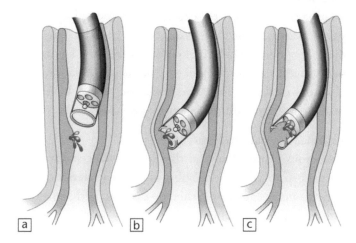

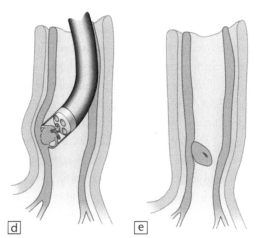

Figure 7.6. Variceal band ligation; aspiration of varix into hood, firing of band, ligation of varix.

Recently developed banding devices hold five or more bands, obviating the use of an overtube and withdrawal of the endoscope after each band is applied.

Bands should be applied to each varix, starting at the oesophageal/gastric junction. They should not be applied to varices within the stomach other than just below the gastrooesophageal junction. When a varix to be banded has been identified (Fig. 7.8a), the endoscope and banding device is angled onto the varix, which is then sucked into the outer hood until a 'red-out' occurs (Fig. 7.8b) when the band is fired using the trip wire. Suction is only released after a few seconds to allow the band to constrict the varix (Fig. 7.8c,d). Further bands can then be applied to the varices proximally for up to 2–4 cm. The bands fall off over the next 3–5 days, leaving superficial ulceration that rarely bleeds (Fig. 7.8e).

Banding ligation arrests active variceal haemorrhage with similar rates as sclerotherapy (85–95%) and can be repeated weekly until varices are eradicated. Five to six bands are usually applied at the first session, which is repeated weekly until varices are obliterated after a mean of three sessions.

Difficulty may be encountered in using banding ligation when the varices are small, or when they have been partially thrombosed by prior sclerotherapy. There is no evidence of benefit in combining sclerotherapy and band ligation.

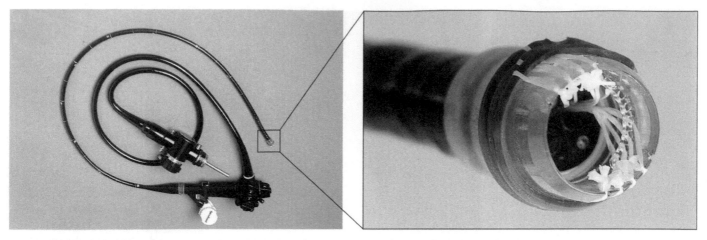

Figure 7.7. End-viewing endoscope with multiple banding device attached and winch mechanism.

Injection sclerotherapy variants

Two other sclerotherapy variations, using tissue adhesive [12,13] or thrombin [14], deserve special mention. The former has been reported to be highly effective in arresting variceal haemorrhage from both large oesophageal and gastric varices. The material, 2-cyanoacrylate, solidifies immediately on contact with blood or other tissue fluids. A standard varix injection needle is primed by flushing with radio-opaque contrast medium and the adhesive is diluted 1 : 1 with contrast. Care must be taken to avoid any adhesive being applied to the endoscope tip. The technique is similar to that for standard sclerotherapy, although aliquots of 1 ml are usually injected.

While impressive results have been reported in high-risk cases, the technique requires some expertise and may be best reserved for rescue therapy and large greater curve gastric varices. Embolization of the solidified material into both pulmonary and cerebral circulations has been recorded.

Balloon tamponade (Table 7.2)

Balloon tamponade correctly placed is highly effective in stemming bleeding, but should be reserved for those cases with massive uncontrollable and life-threatening haemorrhage in order to stabilize the situation [15]. Expertise is required to insert the balloon safely, and even in experienced hands the method carries a high complication rate in Childs–Pugh grade C liver disease. Balloon tamponade should be used for the minimum time possible before instituting some other more definitive therapy as it causes significant mucosal damage.

Three types of tube are available. The Sengstaken–Blakemore and Minnesota tubes both have gastric and oesophageal balloons, whereas the Linton tube has a single large gastric balloon. With all types, inflation of the gastric balloon alone, anchored to the side of the mouth with tape so as to compress varices against the crus of the diaphragm, is usually sufficient to control both oesophageal and gastric varices. The Minnesota tube has the advantage over the Sengstaken–Blakemore tube of having an oesophageal aspirate channel that allows continual clearance of oesophageal secretions whereas gastric variceal bleeding is better controlled with the larger Linton gastric balloon.

Pharmacological intervention

Numerous pharmacological therapies have been advocated for the control of acute bleeding as primary haemostasis, in order to make endoscopic therapy easier to perform and to prevent early rebleeding.

The principal pharmacological therapies are the vasoconstrictor vasopressin, and glypressin (a synthetic analogue of vasopressin), vasopressin combined with nitroglycerine (to prevent the systemic side effects of vasopressin) and octreotide (a synthetic analogue of somatostatin). Dosages and administration are described in Table 7.3. Most evidence suggests that pharmacological therapy is better than no therapy in terminating haemorrhage [3], but initial trials with vasopressin had significant side effects. These can be partially abolished by adding a nitroglycerine infusion or using glypressin [16]. Octreotide, with few side effects, is also effective when administered over 5 days to try to avoid early rebleeding [17]. Trials comparing pharmacological with endoscopic therapy will be described below.

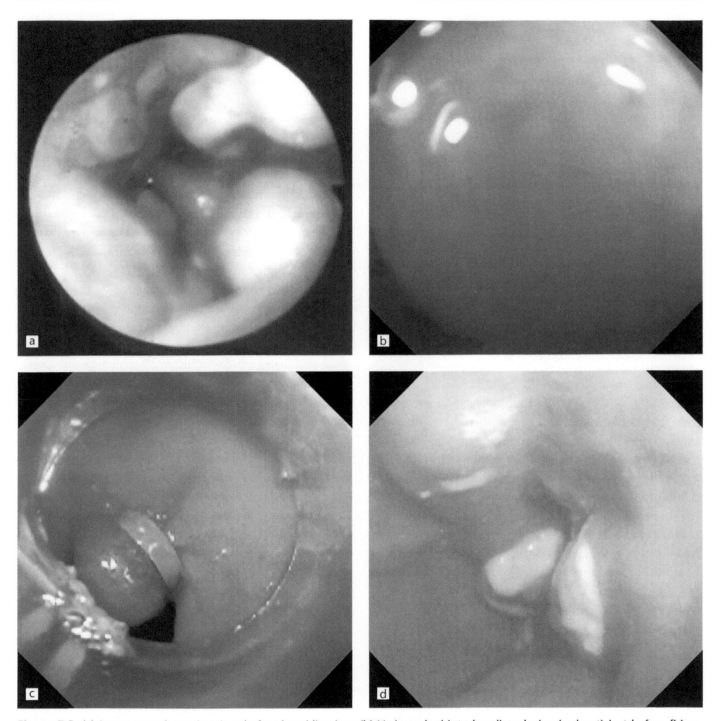

Figure 7.8. (a) Large oesophageal varices before band ligation; (b) Varix sucked into banding device (red out) just before firing band; (c) band constricting varix; (d) ligation-induced ulcers 7 days after banding session.

MANAGEMENT OF ACUTE VARICEAL HAEMORRHAGE

Once the initial assessment, haemodynamic monitoring and diagnosis have been made, optimal management depends on the site of the haemorrhage (oesophageal or gastric), and the cause of the portal hypertension. Initial management to control bleeding is then followed by secondary prevention of further bleeds. Bleeding from gastric varices or in the presence of extrahepatic portal vein obstruction will be dealt with separately.

Table 7.2. Balloon tamponade

Use of balloon tamponade during acute variceal haemorrhage
Keep tamponade balloons in refrigerator to maintain stiffness
Prepare clamps and water/contrast solution for gastric balloon
Explain procedure to patient if conscious
Insert balloon and check tip in stomach by auscultation while injecting 20 ml air down gastric aspirate
Inflate gastric balloon with 200 ml (Minnesota) or 400 ml (Linton/Nachlas), and clamp
Pull back firmly to mark on balloon shaft approximately 2–5 cm shorter than distance from teeth to gastro-oesophageal junction assessed at endoscopy
Tape to side of mouth
Aspirate stomach, oesophageal ports regularly
Keep in place for minimum time before undertaking definitive therapy

A management algorithm for acute variceal haemorrhage (Fig. 7.9) would start with appropriate resuscitation and only use balloon tamponade to arrest massive life-threatening bleeding. The importance of very early pharmacological therapy has been highlighted by Levacher et al. who demonstrated that terlipressin and glyceryl trinitrate significantly improved haemostasis and reduced transfusion requirements and mortality [18]. Studies comparing pharmacological therapy with endoscopic variceal injection have demonstrated that both therapies are highly effective in achieving haemostasis [19–22]. Although Westaby et al. [19] achieved initial haemostasis in 88% using endoscopic injection sclerotherapy and only 65% (P <0.05) with vasopressin and nitroglycerine, two more recent studies have demonstrated that both modalities are equally effective, with sclerotherapy achieving haemostasis in 90% and 83%, compared with 84% and 80% after pharmacological therapy [20,21]. No one form of therapy is conclusively superior, each having disadvantages. While sclerotherapy requires endoscopic expertise, it carries a higher complication rate than somatostatin, whereas pharmacological therapy has the disadvantage that, if it fails, control of variceal haemorrhage with endoscopic injection sclerotherapy becomes less effective. Shemesh et al. demonstrated that early emergency sclerotherapy was associated with a lower in-hospital rebleeding rate (5%) compared with those treated with pharmacological therapy [23].

More recently, studies have compared the combination of long-acting somatostatin analogue plus endoscopic therapy with endoscopic therapy alone. Early rebleeding, transfusion requirements and mortality have been improved in some of these trials using a 5-day infusion of octreotide with urgent endoscopic therapy [16,21].

In all the randomized trials of sclerotherapy and band ligation similar haemostasis rates have been observed in the range 85–95% when used for active variceal bleeding, with the exception of the trial by Lo et al. which found better haemostasis for ligation, particularly for actively spurting varices [24]. Band ligation has the advantage that varices are subsequently obliterated sooner than with sclerotherapy, and complications of therapy including oesophageal ulceration, stricture and perforation are lower in some, but not all, studies.

An important aspect of this algorithm is the early recognition of failure of therapy. If haemorrhage continues

Table 7.3. Pharmacological intervention

Drug	Dose	Route	Comments
Vasopressin	20 units in 100 ml 5% dextrose bolus 20 units/h	Central	Severe side effects in 25%
Terlipressin	2–4 mg bolus, then 2 mg every 4–6h	i.v.	Side effects less common
Nitroglycerine	100–400 mg/min titrated to systolic BP >100 mmHg; then 5–10 mg every 4 h	i.v. sublingual/transdermal patch	Reduces side effects of vasopressin
Octreotide	50 mg bolus and 50 mg/h for 5 days	i.v.	Few side effects

BP = Blood pressure.

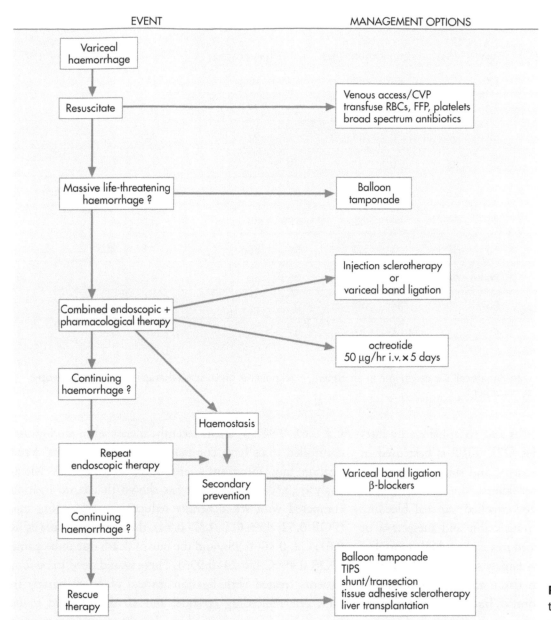

Figure 7.9. Algorithm for the management of variceal haemorrhage.

over the first 24 hours, further endoscopic therapy can be repeated once only. Attempting endoscopy for a third session is not beneficial and only serves to delay moving on to rescue therapy.

Rescue therapy

Once it is clear that continuing haemorrhage persists despite combined octreotide and two sessions of endoscopic therapy (approximately 5–10% of cases), a range of options is available and their use will depend on local expertise. It is important not to delay such therapy until the patient is moribund, and to intervene early. In these circumstances coagulation deficits must be corrected once the source of the bleeding is accurately identified. Abdominal paracentesis may help to reduce portal pressure. In most centres a transjugular intrahepatic portal-systemic stent shunt (TIPS) is the preferred rescue therapy (Fig. 7.10). This radiological procedure creates a channel with an expandable metal stent between the portal and hepatic vein and is able to reduce portal pressure by approximately 50%. It has been shown to be highly effective as rescue therapy in arresting haemorrhage [25,26]. Nevertheless, its disadvantage is a high stenosis rate requiring regular shunt cannulation and

Table 7.4. Randomized trials comparing injection sclerotherapy (EIS) with variceal band ligation (EVL)

Study	n	Rebleeding (%)		Survival (%)		Complications (%)		Acute haemostasis (%)		Session to obliteration (%)	
		EVL	EIS	EVL	EIS	EVL	EIS	EVL	EIS	EVL	EIS
[11]	129	36	48	72	55	2	22	86	77	4	5
[28]	103	30	53	52	37	0	11	91	92	3.4	4.9
[30]	77	26	44	89	85	0	33	89	89	4.1	6.2
[29]*	57	42	73	17	26	3	22	87	41	–	–
[30]	134	19	42	81	91	4	22	100	88	3.5	4.6
[33]	120	33	51	16	32	3	19	94	80	3.8	6.5
[35]	95	9.4	21	94	94	0	11	86	80	4.2	5.2
[36]**	77	17	27	80	79	35	60	–	–	3.7	5.8
[24]+	71	17	33	81	65	5	29	97	76	–	–

*All patients actively bleeding with hepatocellular carcinoma at enrolment; **All patients given sclerotherapy at index endoscopy; +All patients actively bleeding at enrolment.

dilatation in subsequent months and encephalopathy rates of up to 30% in some series [27]. TIPS is best used in Childs–Pugh grade A and B cases, and should be avoided in those with more severe liver failure.

Surgical approaches to uncontrolled variceal bleeding have included oesophageal transection and mesocaval or portocaval shunts. Such procedures carry a high mortality in this context and have been largely superseded by TIPS.

Use of sclerotherapy with tissue adhesive or thrombin may also have a role in this context, but there are impressive technical difficulties in performing them accurately in the face of uncontrolled bleeding. Balloon tamponade may also buy time in such cases before more definitive therapy is undertaken.

Secondary prevention of variceal haemorrhage

Once haemorrhage has stopped, secondary prevention measures can be instituted. Meta-analyses have clearly demonstrated that long-term endoscopic injection sclerotherapy is of proven benefit compared with no therapy, with a reduction in both variceal rebleeding rates (pooled odds ratio (POR) 0.63; 95% C.I. 0.49–0.79) and mortality, irrespective of Childs grade (POR 0.78; 95% C.I. 0.61–0.94) [3]. More recently, at least seven randomized controlled trials have compared endoscopic variceal band ligation and injection sclerotherapy [11,28–36]. Meta-analysis [37] of these trials has shown that band ligation compared with sclerotherapy reduces the rebleeding rate (POR 0.52; 95% C.I. 0.37–0.74), the mortality rate (POR 0.67; C.I. 0.46–0.98), and the rate of death due to bleeding (POR 0.49; C.I. 0.24–0.996). There would need to be four patients treated with ligation instead of sclerotherapy to avert one rebleeding episode, and 10 would need to be treated with ligation instead of sclerotherapy to prevent one death. Oesophageal strictures occurred less frequently with ligation (POR 0.10; 95% C.I. 0.03–0.29). Furthermore, ligation requires approximately two fewer sessions to achieve obliteration compared with sclerotherapy. One study has also suggested that, although the rate of variceal recurrence is higher after banding ligation than after sclerotherapy, the development of portal hypertensive gastropathy is less frequent [35], but this awaits confirmation.

Meta-analyses of the numerous trials of β-blockade have demonstrated that, compared with no therapy, they are highly effective in preventing recurrent variceal bleeding (POR 0.40; 95% C.I. 0.30–0.53), but their effect on survival is equivocal (POR 0.70; 95% C.I. 0.48–1.02) [3].

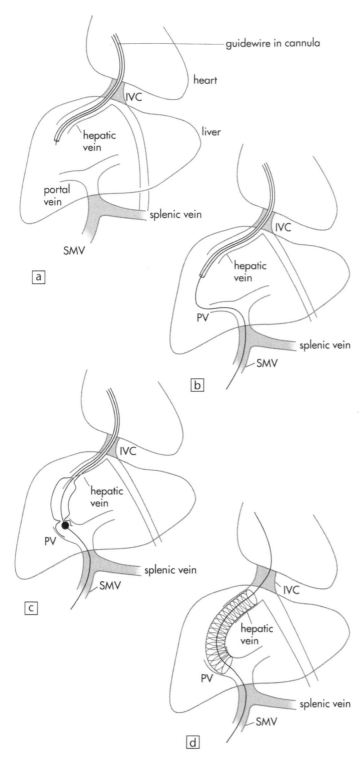

This may be due to the relatively small proportion of cases that have a significant fall in portal pressure with β-blockade. In the series by Feu *et al.*, 41% of cases had a reduction in portal pressure of less than 10% and had a 53% rebleed rate in the follow-up period. In contrast, of the 25% who had a reduction in portal pressure of >20% only 12% rebled [38]. Other pharmacological approaches including long-term octreotide and combination therapy with nitrates require further study.

Comparison of sclerotherapy with β-blockers in nine trials involving over 700 patients has shown no clear benefit for either modality in rebleeding rate or mortality [3]. Similarly, the combination of both compared to one modality alone is not clearly beneficial.

Four randomized trials have compared TIPS with endoscopic sclerotherapy for the prevention of rebleeding from oesophageal varices [25,26,39,40]. In two studies, patients were randomized after the initial haemorrhage had been controlled endoscopically. Cello *et al.* reported that although varices were more likely to be obliterated by TIPS, and less likely to rebleed, there was no beneficial effect on survival [25]. In contrast, Sanyal *et al.* showed a higher mortality in the TIPS groups and no difference in rebleeding rates when patients were followed for 1000 days [26]. Hepatic encephalopathy is also more common following TIPS (33%) than following endoscopic therapy (9%) [40].

The evidence therefore seems to suggest that variceal banding ligation is the preferred endoscopic technique for secondary prevention of variceal rebleeding, and that TIPS should be reserved for patients with uncontrolled acute variceal haemorrhage, bleeding gastric varices and failure of endoscopic therapy when liver transplantation is not appropriate.

CONTROVERSIAL ISSUES

Gastric variceal haemorrhage

Haemorrhage from gastric varices occurs in approximately 10% of all cases, but carries a higher mortality than bleeding from oesophageal varices. Large fundal varices and those with red spots are at greatest risk of bleeding. Although gastric varices may disappear in up to 60% of cases after sclerotherapy of oesophageal varices, they should always be considered – particularly with haemorrhage in

Figure 7.10. Principle of TIPS procedure. (a) The guidewire and cannula is introduced via the jugular vein and inferior vena cava (IVC) into the hepatic vein, (b) a passage is created through the liver parenchyma to the portal vein (PV). (c) The passage is dilated with a balloon and (d) the self-expanding endoprosthesis is deployed to achieve a shunt.

any patient following eradication of oesophageal varices. Accurate assessment of the site of gastric variceal bleeding is important. Lesser curve varices or those within a hiatus hernia can be injected with a similar efficacy to oesophageal varices (as described above) using similar sclerosants [41]. In contrast, sclerotherapy of isolated fundal varices is less effective and has been associated with gastric perforation [42]. Initial haemostasis here is probably best achieved with balloon tamponade (Linton tube).

Other treatments that have been proposed for achieving primary haemostasis in fundal varices include cyanoacrylate polymer injection [12,13] thrombin [14], endoscopic snares [43], intravascular balloon occlusion [44] and TIPS [45]. All the endoscopic techniques for fundal varices are difficult if haemorrhage is continuing, and may require endoscopy in the right lateral position to remove the pool of blood accumulating in the fundus. Surgery with a gastric devascularization, high gastric transection or shunt may be considered, but only in those with well-maintained liver function (Childs–Pugh grade A or B liver disease). TIPS has been used successfully to arrest bleeding from gastric varices [45] with a reported rebleeding rate of only 15% and is probably the treatment of choice, although others have reported disappointing results in isolated fundal varices [27].

Extrahepatic portal vein obstruction

These cases require special consideration because of their near-normal liver function and otherwise excellent long-term prognosis. Patients are often younger and tolerate bleeding better than in the presence of cirrhosis, although gastric variceal and in particular fundal variceal haemorrhage may be more prevalent. Endoscopic techniques and pharmacological therapy are still effective and remain the first line. Although TIPS has been used in these cases it is usually considered a relative contraindication. Surgery is better tolerated in these cases, and in those with isolated splenic vein thrombosis is curative and the treatment of choice. Accurate anatomical assessment of the portomesenteric and splenic venous drainage by angiography is essential.

Orthotopic liver transplantation

Despite improvements in the management of variceal bleeding through better endoscopic therapy and TIPS, the overall mortality following variceal bleeding has not improved. Predictors of increased early mortality in patients with chronic liver disease following variceal bleed include active variceal bleeding at the time of the index endoscopy and poor liver function as indicated by a Childs–Pugh grade C score. All cases with these adverse prognostic features should be considered for liver transplantation in the absence of contraindications. TIPS may be useful in certain cases to prevent early rebleeding as a bridge to liver transplantation.

Duration of endoscopic therapy

The aim of all endoscopic trials has been to achieve variceal obliteration with regular review for varix recurrence, thereby reducing rebleeding rates and mortality. Such an intensive regime of endoscopic surveillance may not be necessary, as recent trials have suggested that similar rebleeding and mortality rates may be achieved with less intensive regimes of endoscopic therapy at the time of haemorrhage only [46,47].

Prophylactic endoscopic therapy

Many trials have been performed assessing the value of endoscopic therapy in the primary prevention of variceal haemorrhage. Unfortunately meta-analyses have demonstrated significant heterogeneity both with respect to the magnitude of the effect as well as the direction [3]. Most trials have examined the use of injection sclerotherapy, and some have demonstrated worse survival with this therapy. Three trials have recently compared the use of prophylactic band ligation against sclerotherapy in one [48], and against no therapy in the others [49,50] in cases with varices at high risk of bleeding. The lower rebleeding rate and improved survival seen in the ligation group is provocative, but will need to be confirmed in larger series.

REFERENCES

1. Baker L, Smith C, Liebram G. The natural history of oesophageal varices. *Am J Med* 1956; 26: 228–231.

2. North Italian Endoscopy Club for the Study and Treatment of Oesophageal Varices. Prediction of the first Variceal Haemorrhage in patients with cirrhosis of the liver and oesophageal varices. *N Engl J Med* 1988; 319: 983–987.

3. Pagliaro L, Bosch J, Politi F *et al*. Prevention and treatment of variceal bleeding: overview. In: Holstege A, Scholmeric J, Hahn A (eds), *Portal Hypertension*. Kluwer Academic, Dordrecht 1985, pp. 235–266.

4. Gimson AES, Vlavianos T. Resuscitative measures in acute variceal haemorrhage. *Gastrointest Endosc Clin North Am* 1992; 38: 31–41.

5. Bleicher G, Boulanger R, Squara P *et al*. Frequency of infections in cirrhotic patients presenting with acute gastrointestinal haemorrhage. *Br J Surg* 1986; 73: 724–726.

6. Rolando N, Gimson A, Philpott-Howard J *et al*. Infectious sequelae after endoscopic sclerotherapy of oesophageal varices: role of antibiotic prophylaxis. *J Hepatol* 1993; 18: 290–294.

7. Rimola A, Bory F, Teres J *et al*. Oral non-absorbable antibiotics prevent infection in cirrhotics with gastrointestinal haemorrhage. *Hepatology* 1985; 5: 463–467.

8. Mitchell K, Theodossi A, Williams R. Endoscopy in patients with portal hypertension and upper gastrointestinal bleeding. In: Westaby D, MacDougall B, Williams R (eds), *Variceal Bleeding*. Pitman, London, 1982, pp. 62–67.

9. Sarin SK, Lahoti D, Saxena SP *et al*. Prevalence, classification and natural history of gastric varices: a long-term follow-up study in 568 portal hypertensive patients. *Hepatology* 1992; 16: 1343–1349.

10. Polson R, Westaby D, Gimson A *et al*. Sucralfate for the prevention of early rebleeding following injection sclerotherapy for oesophageal varices. *Hepatology* 1989; 10: 279–282.

11. Stiegmann GV, Goff JS, Michaletz-Onody PA *et al*. Endoscopic sclerotherapy as compared with endoscopic ligation for bleeding esophageal varices. *N Engl J Med* 1992; 326: 1527–1532.

12. Soehendra N, Grimm H, Nam VC *et al*. N-butyl-2-cyano-acrylate: a supplement to endoscopic sclerotherapy. *Endoscopy* 1986; 18: 25–26.

13. Oho K, Iwao T, Sumino M *et al*. Ethanolamine oleate versus butyl cyanoacrylate for bleeding gastric varices: a nonrandomised study. *Endoscopy* 1995; 25: 349–354.

14. Williams SG, Peters RA, Westaby D. Thrombin – an effective treatment for fundal gastric varices. *Gut* 1993; 34: S48.

15. Panes J, Teres J, Bosch J. Efficacy of balloon tamponade in treatment of bleeding gastric and oesophageal varices. *Dig Dis Sci* 1988; 33: 454–459.

16. Gimson AES, Westaby D, Hegarty J *et al*. A randomized trial of vasopressin and vasopressin plus nitroglycerin in the control of acute variceal haemorrhage. *Hepatology* 1986; 6: 410–413.

17. Besson I, Ingrand P, Person B *et al*. Sclerotherapy with and without octreotide for acute variceal bleeding. *N Engl J Med* 1995; 333: 555–560.

18. Levacher S, Letoumelin P, Pateron D *et al*. Early administration of terlipressin plus glyceryl trinitrate to control active upper gastrointestinal bleeding in cirrhotic patients. *Lancet* 1995; 346: 865–868.

19. Westaby D, Hayes P, Gimson A *et al*. A controlled trial of injection sclerotherapy for active variceal haemorrhage. *Hepatology* 1989; 9: 274–277.

20. Planas R, Quer JC, Boix J *et al*. A prospective randomized trial comparing somatostatin and sclerotherapy in the treatment of acute variceal bleeding. *Hepatology* 1994; 20: 370–375.

21. Sung J, Chung S, Lai C-W *et al*. Octreotide infusion or emergency sclerotherapy for variceal haemorrhage. *Lancet* 1993; 342: 637–641.

22. Shields R, Jenkins SA, Baxter JN *et al*. A prospective randomized controlled trial comparing the efficacy of somatostatin with injection sclerotherapy in the control of bleeding oesophageal varices. *J Hepatol* 1992; 16: 128–137.

23. Shemesh E, Czerniak A, Klein E *et al*. A comparison between early and delayed endoscopic sclerotherapy of bleeding oesophageal varices in non-alcoholic portal hypertension. *J Clin Gastroenterol* 1990; 12: 5–9.

24. Lo GH, Lai KH, Cheng JS *et al*. Emergency banding ligation versus sclerotherapy for the control of active bleeding from esophageal varices. *Hepatology* 1997; 25: 1101–1104.

25. Cello JP, Ring EJ, Olcott EW *et al*. Endoscopic sclerotherapy compared with percutaneous transjugular intrahepatic portosystemic shunt after initial sclerotherapy in patients with acute variceal haemorrhage. A randomized controlled trial. *Ann Intern Med* 1997; 126: 858–865.

26. Sanyal AJ, Freedman AM, Luketic VA *et al*. Transjugular intrahepatic portosystemic shunts compared with sclerotherapy for the prevention of recurrent variceal haemorrhage. A randomized controlled trial. *Ann Intern Med* 1997; 126: 849–857.

27. Sanyal AJ, Freedman AM, Luketic VA *et al.* The natural history of portal hypertension after transjugular portosystemic shunts. *Gastroenterology* 1997; 112: 889–898.

28. Gimson AE, Ramage JK, Panos MZ *et al.* Randomised trial of variceal banding ligation versus injection sclerotherapy for bleeding oesophageal varices. *Lancet* 1993; 342: 391–394.

29. Lo GH, Lai KH, Cheng JS *et al.* Emergency banding ligation versus sclerotherapy for the control of active bleeding from esophageal varices. *Hepatology* 1997; 25: 1101–1104.

30. Laine L, el-Newihi HM, Migikovsky B, Sloane R, Garcia F. Endoscopic ligation compared with sclerotherapy for the treatment of bleeding esophageal varices. *Ann Intern Med* 1993; 119: 1–7.

31. Hashizume M, Ohta M, Ueno K *et al.* Endoscopic ligation of esophageal varices compared with injection sclerotherapy: a prospective randomized trial. *Gastrointest Endosc* 1993; 39: 123–126.

32. Hou MC, Lin HC, Kuo BI *et al.* Comparison of endoscopic variceal injection sclerotherapy and ligation for the treatment of esophageal variceal hemorrhage: a prospective randomized trial. *Hepatology* 1995; 21: 1517–1522.

33. Lo GH, Lai KH, Cheng JS *et al.* A prospective, randomized trial of sclerotherapy versus ligation in the management of bleeding esophageal varices. *Hepatology* 1995; 22: 466–471.

34. Bhargava DK, Pokharna R. Endoscopic variceal ligation versus endoscopic variceal ligation and endoscopic sclerotherapy: a prospective randomized study. *Am J Gastroenterol* 1997; 92: 950–953.

35. Sarin SK, Govil A, Jain AK *et al.* Prospective randomized trial of endoscopic sclerotherapy versus variceal band ligation for esophageal varices: influence on gastropathy, gastric varices and variceal recurrence. *J Hepatol* 1997; 26: 826–832.

36. Avgerinos A, Armonis A, Manokopoulos S *et al.* Endoscopic sclerotherapy versus variceal ligation in the long-term management of patients with cirrhosis after variceal bleeding. A prospective randomized study. *J Hepatol* 1997; 26: 1034–1041.

37. Laine L, Cook D. Endoscopic ligation compared to sclerotherapy for treatment of oesophageal variceal bleeding. A meta-analysis. *Ann Intern Med* 1995; 123: 280–287.

38. Feu F, Garcia-Pagan JC, Bosch J *et al.* Relation between portal pressure response to pharmacotherapy and risk of recurrent variceal haemorrhage in patients with cirrhosis. *Lancet* 1995; 346: 1056–1059.

39. Cabrera J, Maynar M, Granados R *et al.* Transjugular intrahepatic portosystemic shunt versus sclerotherapy in the elective treatment of variceal haemorrhage. *Gastroenterology* 1996; 110: 832–839.

40. Merli M, Salerno F, Riggio O *et al.* Transjugular intrahepatic portosystemic shunt versus endoscopic sclerotherapy for the prevention of variceal bleeding in cirrhosis: a randomized multicenter trial. Gruppo Italiano Studio TIPS (G.I.S.T.). *Hepatology* 1998; 27: 48–53.

41. Gimson AE, Westaby D, Williams R. Endoscopic sclerotherapy in the management of gastric variceal haemorrhage. *J Hepatol* 1991; 13: 274–278.

42. Ng EK, Chung SC, Leong HT, Li AK. Perforation after endoscopic injection sclerotherapy for bleeding gastric varices. *Surg Endosc* 1994; 8: 1221–1222.

43. Yoshida T, Hayashi N, Suzumi N *et al.* Endoscopic ligation of gastric varices using a detachable snare. *Endoscopy* 1994; 26: 502–505.

44. Koito K, Namieno T, Nagakawa T, Morita K. Balloon-occluded retrograde transvenous obliteration for gastric varices with gastrorenal or gastrocaval collaterals. *Am J Roentgenol* 1996; 167: 1317–1320.

45. Stanley AJ, Jalan R, Ireland HM *et al.* A comparison between gastric and oesophageal variceal haemorrhage treated with transjugular intrahepatic portosystemic stent shunt (TIPSS). *Aliment Pharmacol Ther* 1997; 11: 171–176.

46. Moreto M, Zaballa M, Ojembarrena E *et al.* Combined (short-term plus long-term) sclerotherapy v. short-term only sclerotherapy: a randomized prospective trial. *Gut* 1994; 35: 687–691.

47. Parikh SS, Desai HG. What is the aim of esophageal variceal sclerotherapy – prevention of rebleeding or complete obliteration of veins? *J Clin Gastroenterol* 1992; 15: 186–188.

48. Baroncini D, Milandri GL, Borioni D *et al.* A prospective randomized trial of sclerotherapy versus ligation in the elective treatment of bleeding oesophageal varices. *Endoscopy* 1997; 29: 235–240.

49. Sarin SK, Guptan RK, Jain AK, Sundaram K. A randomized controlled trial of endoscopic variceal band ligation for primary prophylaxis of variceal bleeding. *Eur J Gastroenterol Hepatol* 1996; 8: 337–342.

50. Lay CS, Tsai YT, Teg CY *et al.* Endoscopic variceal ligation in prophylaxis of first variceal bleeding in cirrhotic patients with high-risk esophageal varices. *Hepatology* 1997; 25: 1346–1350.

Enteral nutrition

8

P. A. O'Toole

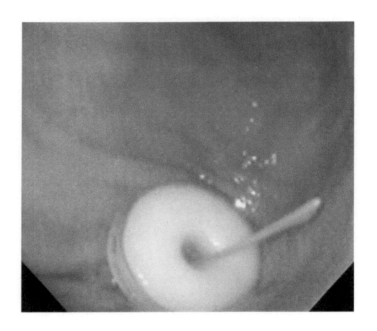

INTRODUCTION

In recent years, endoscopists have found themselves playing an increasingly prominent role in nutritional support. There have been many technical advances allowing endoscopic placement of feeding tubes in a variety of different circumstances. At the same time, the importance of nutrition in assisting recovery from disease has become more widely recognized and there has been a move away from parenteral nutrition to enteral feeding whenever possible. Consequently, the list of patient groups being referred for feeding tubes has grown considerably.

INDICATIONS

In general terms, enteral tube feeding is indicated whenever there is a functioning gastrointestinal tract but adequate nutrition cannot be maintained through oral feeding alone [1]. This may be due to decreased consciousness, difficulty with swallowing (mechanical or neurological), impaired gastric function, loss of appetite or an excessive nutritional demand (Table 8.1).

Neuropathic

Neurological dysphagia is the most common indication at most centres, chiefly as a result of cerebrovascular accidents. Following acute stroke, the incidence of dysphagia is 30–40%. Many patients recover their ability to swallow, but after 4 weeks persistent dysphagia is found in about 6% of survivors. The duration of artificial feeding required following brain damage from head injury is more variable

Table 8.1. Indications for enteral nutritional support

	Common	Uncommon	Rare
Neuropathic	Cerebrovascular disease Head injury Prolonged coma (any cause) Postoperative gastroparesis Post-traumatic gastroparesis Motor neurone disease Multiple sclerosis Cerebral palsy	Parkinson's disease Alzheimer's disease Intracerebral malignancy Chronic idiopathic gastroparesis Polyneuropathies Huntington's chorea Persistent vegetative state Hyperemesis gravidarum	Multiple system atrophy Other dementias Encephalitis/TB/meningitis Diabetic gastroparesis Myotonic dystrophy Inflammatory myopathies Steele-Richardson syndrome Hereditary childhood neurological diseases
Oesophagopharyngeal pathology	Oropharyngeal cancer Oesophageal cancer Postoperative maxillo-facial/ENT surgery Postoperative oesophago-gastric surgery Oesophageal perforation	Oesophageal dysmotility Benign oesophageal stricture Facial injury During radiotherapy to oesophagus/head & neck Oesophagotracheal fistula	Cricopharyngeal dysmotility Caustic oesophageal injury Severe stomatitis
Gastrointestinal pathology	Cystic fibrosis Crohn's disease Acute pancreatitis	Short bowel syndrome Enteric fistulas Severe coeliac disease Scleroderma Low output enterocutaneous fistulas	Whipple's disease Radiation enteritis Tropical sprue Lymphangectasia Amyloidosis Chronic diarrhoea of childhood
Systemic pathology	Acute trauma, sepsis or critical illness Burns Acute/chronic liver failure Acute/chronic renal failure Chemotherapy/radiotherapy Preoperative malnutrition AIDS	Bone marrow transplantation Anorexia nervosa Severe depression Severe protein/energy malnutrition – any cause	

and unpredictable. In degenerative neurological disorders such as motor neurone disease, Huntington's chorea and Alzheimer's disease, where progressive deterioration and death are inevitable, the role of artificial nutritional support is much more controversial.

Gastric stasis, whether chronic (as in diabetes) or acute (following trauma or surgery), may be so severe as to prevent adequate nutrition through the oral route. In this situation, tube feeding distal to the pylorus is indicated, usually in conjunction with a gastric venting tube. In chronic gastroparesis, a surprisingly short period of such treatment may produce long-lasting symptomatic improvement [2].

Oesophagopharyngeal pathology

Intractable obstructive dysphagia is most often due to malignancy. Dysphagia from oesophageal cancer can usually be overcome to an extent (see Chapters 3 and 4), but tumours of the oropharynx are much less amenable to palliation. Moreover, attempts at curative surgery may disrupt swallowing mechanisms, sometimes permanently. This group of patients have a particular need for nutritional support as they have frequently lost a good deal of weight before presentation. Enteral feeding is the rule following surgery for oropharyngeal cancer, and in some centres it is routinely commenced preoperatively [3]. Likewise, where surgery or chemotherapy/radiotherapy are undertaken for oesophageal or gastric cancer, pretreatment nutritional support can improve outcome [4]. In the past, this often meant total parenteral nutrition (TPN), but nowadays there are few obstructions that the experienced endoscopist is unable to negotiate.

Gastrointestinal pathology

Although, by definition, enteral feeding requires a functioning gastrointestinal tract, there are situations where it can be used to compensate for relative inadequacy of digestion or absorption. Patients with short-gut syndrome, cystic fibrosis and extensive small bowel Crohn's (or other rare causes of malabsorption) may require a higher calorie intake than can be achieved by oral feeding alone. Overnight gastrostomy feeding allows such individuals to make up the additional nutritional requirements with minimum disruption to their lives [5].

Enteral nutrition is making in-roads into territory that was hitherto the preserve of TPN. Instrumental oesophageal perforations have been successfully managed by jejunal feeding, sometimes coupled to sump-tube drainage at the site of perforation. Patients with acute pancreatitis can be fed enterally, provided that feed is delivered beyond the duodenum [6]. Early jejunal feeding is also possible after gastrointestinal surgery. The so-called postoperative 'ileus' is a phenomenon largely restricted to the stomach and colon; normal peristaltic function in the small intestine returns quickly. The same is often true of post-traumatic ileus in the intensive care unit (ICU), where nasojejunal feeding is increasingly used as an alternative to TPN.

Systemic pathology

Serious systemic illness results in an increased metabolic demand. At the same time, anorexia may prevent sufficient energy intake to meet the increased requirements [7]. This occurs not only in acute illnesses such as burns or major trauma but also in chronic diseases characterized by cachexia, such as malignancy and AIDS. Artificial feeding can limit deterioration in nutritional status in the acute situation and can improve well-being and prolong survival in chronic wasting diseases. In other situations, anorexia may have a psychological rather than physical cause. Here the decision to institute enteral feeding, often against the individual's wishes, is more difficult and requires close collaboration with colleagues in psychiatry.

DIAGNOSIS AND DECISION MAKING

Before undertaking endoscopic feeding tube placement, five questions should be considered:

1. What is the current or predicted nutritional status?
2. Is there a genuine need for artificial nutritional support?
3. Is enteral feeding the correct approach?
4. Which is the best route for tube feeding in this particular situation?
5. Is endoscopy the preferred approach for placement of the tube?

Table 8.2. Nutritional assessment

History	Examination	Anthropometric measurements	Biochemical measurements	Functional assessments
Recent weight loss	Weight loss > 10%	BMI < 20	Serum albumin	Hand grip strength
Loss of appetite	Loss of subcutaneous fat	Weight/age (children)	Serum prealbumin	Respiratory muscle strength
Difficulty swallowing	Muscle wasting	Triceps skinfold thickness	Serum transferrin	Adductor pollicis stimulation response
Other GI symptoms	Oedema	Mid arm circumference	Creatinine/height index	Delayed hypersensitivity reaction
Disease state (stress factor)	Signs of specific micronutrient deficiency	Body fat estimation (impedance analysis)	Micronutrient levels	In-vitro T-cell responses

BMI = Body mass index; GI = gastrointestinal

Choice of feed formula and feeding regimens are beyond the scope of this chapter.

What is the current or predicted nutritional status?

A variety of nutritional assessment tools have been developed. These range from questionnaires about recent weight loss and dietary intake, through scoring systems based on anthropometric measurements, to more complex tools incorporating biochemical and physiological markers of malnutrition (Table 8.2). Unfortunately, no system is ideal and there is no agreement as to which single tool performs best in clinical practice. Dietary history by recall is unreliable unless undertaken by a skilled interviewer. Changes in weight are difficult to quantify unless serial measurements are available and, even then, oedema or ascites may hinder interpretation. Simple biochemical markers such as serum albumin do not reliably reflect nutritional state in the presence of disease and can be remarkably normal when starvation occurs without other illness (such as in anorexia nervosa).

These difficulties should not discourage attempts to detect malnutrition in routine practice. Surveys have shown that up to one-third of hospital patients are malnourished, and that even the most elementary measurements such as height and weight are performed far too infrequently [8]. In practice, the most powerful diagnostic tools are a comprehensive history and physical examination undertaken with an awareness that poor nutritional status may be a problem. Despite the plethora of tests available, this subjective global assessment remains the most reliable method of detecting patients in need of artificial nutritional support.

Is there a genuine need for artificial nutritional support?

Not all patients needing nutritional support require tube feeding. This sounds obvious but, in practice, patients with oesophageal strictures are often referred for tube placement before any attempt has been made at liquid oral feeding. Likewise, patients with neurological dysphagia can often manage with thickened fluids. In such cases a supervised swallow, performed by a trained observer, is usually sufficient to confirm that oral feeding is safe, but a formal speech therapy assessment is helpful if there is uncertainty. A water-soluble contrast swallow using videofluoroscopy is useful for studying swallowing mechanisms in detail, but failure to demonstrate penetration of contrast into the trachea does not exclude the possibility of aspiration occurring at other times.

Verifying a genuine necessity for enteral feeding is particularly important where the indication is a chronic upper gastrointestinal motility disorder. These conditions can be mimicked by, or coexist with, significant psychopathology and tube feeding, rather than solving the problem, may become a new focus for neurosis. Objective evidence of oesophageal or gastric dysmotility should always be sought using physiological studies or scintigraphy.

Table 8.3. Contraindications to artificial enteral feeding

Absolute

Complete mechanical bowel obstruction

High-output enterocutaneous fistula

Severe, uncontrollable diarrhoea

Necrotizing enterocolitis in the neonate

When not desired by the patient

When not warranted by prognosis

When the patient will derive no benefit from feeding

When an enteral feeding route cannot be safely established

Relative

Acute ileus following trauma/surgery (see text)

Severe acute pancreatitis (see text)

When gut function is inadequate (intestinal failure)

(may be combined with parenteral nutrition)

Is enteral feeding the correct approach?

Having established the need for artificial feeding, the next step is to choose between the enteral and parenteral route. The golden rule of nutritional support is 'if the gut works, use it!' Enteral nutrition is cheaper, requires less intensive monitoring, and has a lower complication rate than parenteral feeding. Moreover, it does not carry the increased risk of sepsis at distant sites that is a feature of TPN [9]. This is probably because enteral nutrition maintains integrity of the gut mucosa which acts as a barrier against infection. Should enteral nutrition fail, it may be necessary to substitute TPN, but attempts at tube feeding should not be abandoned too readily. Contraindications to enteral nutrition are given in Table 8.3.

Which is the best route for tube feeding in this particular situation?

Tubes passing via the nose are difficult to tolerate for long periods. They irritate the nasopharynx, carry an increased risk of respiratory complications, and are frequently dislodged. These are also cosmetically unacceptable and may hamper psychological rehabilitation following illness. For all these reasons, gastrostomy feeding is clearly preferable when it is anticipated that nutritional support will be required for longer than 4 weeks [10]. Since its introduction in 1980, percutaneous endoscopic

gastrostomy (PEG) has become well established as the procedure of choice in virtually all patients requiring long-term enteral nutrition [11]. The superiority of PEG over nasogastric tube feeding in acute stroke [12] and persisting neurological dysphagia [13] has been clearly demonstrated, both in terms of the quality of nutritional support provided and overall survival.

For shorter periods, fine-bore nasogastric tubes are still preferred because of the ease with which they can be passed at the bedside, and their low complication rate. Nonetheless, it must be accepted that nasogastric feeding is frequently interrupted by tube displacement and, because of this, maintenance of adequate nutritional support can be difficult [10].

Indications for post-pyloric tube feeding are given in Table 8.4. As with intragastric feeding, tubes can be placed through the nose or percutaneously, the choice being determined by the likely duration of feeding. Nasojejunal feeding has proven advantages over intragastric feeding in patients on ICU, where it results in better delivery of nutrition and a lower rate of pneumonia. This probably reflects the high rates of gastroparesis in such patients. Double-lumen nasoenteral tubes, allowing gastric aspiration at the same time as post-pyloric feeding, are particularly useful in this situation.

Table 8.4. Indications and techniques for post-pyloric feeding

Indications

Gastric outflow obstruction

Gastroparesis – acute or chronic

Persistent gastro-oesophageal reflux of feed

Recurrent aspiration pneumonia

Acute pancreatitis

Following gastric surgery

Techniques

Nasojejunal tube (endoscopically or radiologically assisted)

PEG + Jejunal extension tube (JET-PEG or J-Tube)

Direct percutaneous endoscopic jejunostomy (D-PEJ)

Radiological percutaneous gastrojejunal tube

Radiological direct percutaneous jejunostomy

Surgical jejunostomy

Surgical needle-catheter jejunostomy

Laparoscopically inserted jejunostomy

Combined laparoscopic/endoscopic jejunostomy

Long-term post-pyloric feeding is most commonly achieved using a jejunal extension tube inserted via a gastrostomy (JET-PEG). These tubes were introduced in the hope of reducing pulmonary aspiration caused by gastro-oesophageal reflux [14]. Initial enthusiasm was dampened by studies suggesting that they do not eliminate aspiration and have a high rate of technical failure. This conclusion is based on small numbers, however, and needs to be re-evaluated in the light of recent improvements in tube design [15]. Direct percutaneous jejunostomy is now well described but generally reserved for patients in whom PEG is not an option [16].

Is endoscopy the preferred approach for placement of the tube?

When an enteral feeding tube is required, endoscopy is not always the most appropriate method for tube placement. Nasogastric tubes can usually be passed at the bedside. If bedside placement fails, direct visualization of the larynx using a laryngoscope or flexible nasopharyngoscope is often all that is required in patients with an impaired swallowing reflex. Where the passage of a nasogastric tube is impeded by oesophageal obstruction, the endoscopist has the advantage of being able to dilate the stricture to facilitate tube placement, but an experienced radiologist can achieve similar success rates, less invasively, using hydrophilic guidewires.

Gastrostomy tubes can also be placed radiologically. Percutaneous radiological gastrostomy (PRG), using fluoroscopy and/or ultrasound, has advantages over PEG in that it does not require sedation and the catheter is uncontaminated by passage through the mouth. Despite series suggesting equivalent complication rates for the two techniques, there is a higher rate of tube displacement following PRG, and it cannot be recommended as a first-line approach [17]. It is, nonetheless, useful in situations where sedation is contraindicated, where gastric access is not possible, or where a safe gastric puncture site cannot be identified at gastroscopy.

For nasoduodenal or nasojejunal feeding, the choice is between 'blind' intubation at the bedside or assisted placement using fluoroscopy or endoscopy. In expert hands, nasoenteral tubes can be manoeuvred blindly into the duodenum in up to 90% of cases. In routine practice, however, satisfactory placement cannot be guaranteed by this method and failed attempts produce delays in starting feeding. Fluoroscopic screening offers a better guarantee of duodenal intubation but still fails in 10–15% of cases. It also requires frequent patient repositioning, which can be difficult in the ICU setting. Endoscopic placement is probably the most reliable technique, but whether this or the radiological approach is chosen as first line will depend on local expertise and enthusiasm.

Some of the alternative methods for placing long-term jejunal feeding tubes are listed in Table 8.4. Non-surgical methods are preferred whenever possible but consideration should always be given to needle-catheter jejunostomy at the time of surgery if prolonged postoperative nutritional support is likely to be needed. Success rates and complications of JET-PEG and the corresponding radiological equivalent have not been compared in randomized trials, but manoeuvring a tube into the jejunum is probably easier using X-ray screening.

Where the stomach is not available for percutaneous gastrostomy, a direct jejunostomy may be possible under endoscopic or radiological control. If there is an oesophagojejunostomy or small gastric remnant, endoscopic access to the small bowel is often easier. This improves the success rate for direct percutaneous endoscopic jejunostomy (direct PEJ). If the stomach is intact, direct PEJ is more difficult and a radiological approach may be preferred. Again, the two techniques have not been compared directly in a randomized study.

PRACTICAL ASPECTS

Patient preparation

Informed consent

A high proportion of PEGs placed for neurological dysphagia are in patients unable to give informed consent. The implications of the procedure go far beyond its immediate risks and complications since artificial feeding in people with neurological damage raises important ethical and legal issues. Relatives, carers and medical staff may have different views about the appropriateness of PEG feeding for a particular individual. In all cases it is vital that consensus is achieved through multidisciplinary team discussion, with the views of relatives and carers given due consideration. Input from primary care physicians regarding the patient's pre-morbid quality of life is particularly helpful when a·PEG is being considered following acute stroke.

Sedation

The patient is prepared with pharyngeal anaesthesia, and intravenous benzodiazepine sedation is given as required. Additional opiate analgesia is rarely necessary even for PEG insertion, provided that local anaesthetic is used for the skin incision.

Position

For endoscopic placement of nasogastric or nasojejunal feeding tubes the patient is usually placed in the left lateral position. PEG insertion requires the patient to be supine. Some operators prefer to perform the preliminary endoscopy with the patient on their left side, although intubation and inspection are quite satisfactory in the supine position with the benefit that it avoids rolling the patient mid-procedure. One of the important consequences of the supine position is the greater risk of aspiration of gastric contents. Assiduous pharyngeal suction is required and gastric juice should be removed from the stomach at the first opportunity.

Antibiotics

Intravenous antibiotics given before PEG placement reduce the rate of wound infection by almost 25% [18]. A second dose given 6 hours later is common practice. There is no evidence that attempting to reduce the bacterial flora of the mouth with antiseptics has any effect on the infection rate.

Anticoagulants

Significant coagulopathy precludes PEG insertion, but can usually be corrected – PEG should be considered as a semi-elective procedure and can always be delayed for a day or two while coagulation status is improved. Patients on warfarin should omit the drug for 3–5 days until the INR falls below 1.3. If the indication for anticoagulation is strong (for example, a prosthetic heart valve), heparin can be substituted during this period and discontinued 5 hours before the procedure. Recommencing heparin 2 hours after the procedure does not seem to increase the risk of significant bleeding. Warfarin therapy can generally be resumed on the night of the procedure. Patients on drugs that inhibit platelet function should ideally have these stopped, but experience has shown that PEG can be performed safely in patients on low-dose aspirin.

Preliminary endoscopy

Whatever type of tube is being placed, a preliminary inspection of the oesophagus, stomach and duodenum is important. It is not uncommon to discover incidental pathology. Oral cancer has many risk factors in common with stomach cancer, and although an early gastric malignancy does not necessarily prevent PEG placement, it is better to delay the procedure while treatment options are considered. Stroke and ICU patients have a high incidence of peptic ulceration. Unless there is a large ulcer in the stomach situated over the only available puncture site, PEG or nasal tube placement can go ahead. Pyloric stenosis rules out any form of intragastric tube and may make tube passage into the jejunum impossible. Oesophageal varices produce anxiety when passing nasogastric tubes, but in practice there is rarely a problem. Of more concern is the possibility that variceal bleeding could be precipitated by a PEG retention disc as it is pulled through the oesophagus. In the presence of significant varices a 'push' method of PEG placement is preferred, but remains hazardous because of the increased risk of bleeding asssociated with portal hypertension. Occasionally, previously unsuspected gastric surgery is encountered, and this may make PEG placement difficult. A particular problem arises when attempting to place a nasojejunal tube in a patient who has had a gastroenterostomy or Polya gastrectomy: it is not always possible to tell from the endoscopic appearance which is the efferent and which the afferent limb. Tube placement in this situation is best left to the radiologist.

TECHNIQUES

Endoscopically assisted nasoenteric tube placement

Whether nasogastric or nasojejunal access is required there are three basic techniques: tubes may be passed beside the scope, through the scope, or over a guidewire. In the description below, the emphasis is on nasojejunal intubation as this is the most technically demanding.

'Beside-the-scope' technique

For this technique, a fine-bore feeding tube is first modified by creating a loop of thread (or suture) at its distal end so that it can be grasped by endoscopic forceps. The alternative is to use one of the commercially available tubes which have a small knob at the end designed for this purpose.

The feeding tube is passed gently through the nose and guided into the oesophagus under direct vision from an endoscope positioned in the hypopharynx (Fig. 8.1a). The tube is advanced until either resistance is met against an oesophageal obstruction or sufficient tube has been inserted to reach the stomach. The endoscope is then passed into the oesophagus and the tip of the feeding tube located. The thread (or knob) is grasped with endoscopy forceps (Fig. 8.1b) and the tube is carried down by carefully advancing the endoscope. If the tube has a stiffening wire stylet this is withdrawn before attempting to steer the tube around acute angles. When the tube has reached a satisfactory position, the endoscope is slowly withdrawn while at the same time advancing the forceps so that the tip of the tube, still held by the forceps, is maintained in position (Fig. 8.1c). This prevents the tube from sliding back with the scope. When the handle of the forceps reaches the biopsy channel and further insertion is impossible, the forceps are

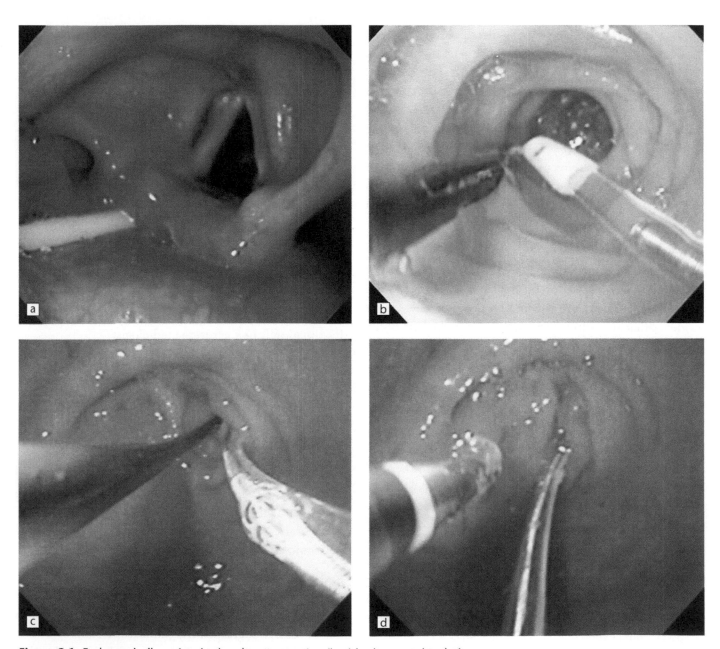

Figure 8.1. Endoscopically assisted tube placement using 'beside-the-scope' technique.

opened and gently agitated to release the thread (Fig. 8.1d). They are then withdrawn into the endoscope. Withdrawal of the endoscope continues with gentle rotational movements to prevent the tube from being dragged back by friction with the scope.

Tips and precautions

Advancement of the endoscope with the forceps protruding must be performed very carefully with the lumen clearly in view at all times. Blind negotiation of bends should *never* be attempted as there is a high risk of perforation. If the wire stylet is withdrawn it should not be reinserted as it may penetrate the fine-bore tube and result in perforation of the oesophagus or duodenum.

Careful coordination is required when withdrawing the scope over the forceps, particularly when the tip of the forceps is lost to sight around bends. Advancing the forceps too fast drives them distally and risks perforation.

'Through-the-scope' technique

This technique requires an endoscope with a 3.2-mm working channel and an 8 F feeding tube with a removable feeding attachment at its proximal end (Fig. 8.2). The tube must be long enough to allow the endoscope to be removed over it once it is in place. For nasojejunal placement, using a standard gastroscope, a tube of 250 cm works well.

The tube is prepared by passing a lubricated 2.6-m hydrophilic guidewire along its length to reinforce it. The wire should be marked with tape at 240 cm so that it stops short of the end of the tube. In this way, the last 10 cm of

the tube remains floppy and the risk of perforation is reduced. Endoscopy is performed in the usual way and the scope is advanced as far as possible into the small bowel. The well-lubricated feeding tube, with its stiffening guidewire *in situ*, is then passed down the endoscope channel until it appears at the distal end. It is then gently advanced into the intestine until resistance is met. The endoscope is then withdrawn while the tube is simultaneously advanced through the biopsy channel so that the distal end of the tube stays in the same position (Fig. 8.3). As soon as the endoscope reaches the mouth, the emerging tube is grasped by the nursing assistant and the scope is pulled off it. The mouth guard is then removed.

The feeding tube must now be re-routed from mouth to nose. This is achieved using an oronasal transfer technique: a short, soft, Ryles-type tube is passed through the nose to the back of the mouth (suitable tubes are provided in some commercial kits) (Fig. 8.4). Using a gloved finger, the tube is swept forward and delivered out of the mouth. Alternatively, dental forceps can be used to retrieve the Ryles tube from the nasopharynx. The feeding tube, still

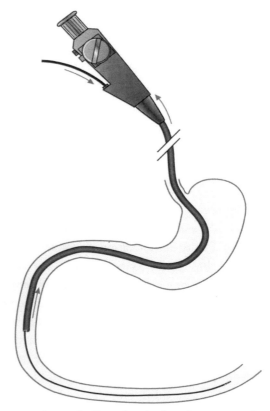

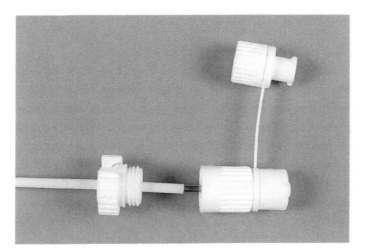

Figure 8.2. A naso-jejunal feeding tube suitable for 'through-the-scope' placement.

Figure 8.3. Endoscopically assisted tube placement using 'over-the-wire' technique.

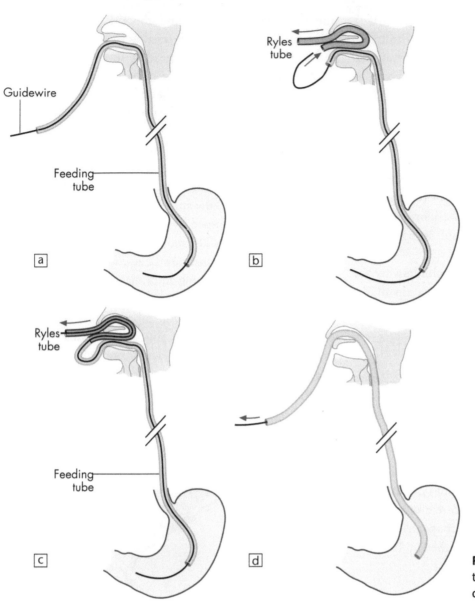

Figure 8.4. Conversion of oropharyngeal to naso-pharyngeal tube passage, as described in text.

with its reinforcing guidewire, is inserted into the oral end of the Ryles tube and pushed through until it emerges from the nose end. Plenty of lubrication is required. The feeding tube is pulled through the Ryles tube until the loop of tube coming out of the mouth is reduced to a few centimetres.

Then, with a finger in the patient's mouth to control the loop, both the Ryles tube and the fine-bore tube are pulled together through the nose so that the loop in the mouth disappears completely. The nasojejunal tube now passes directly from the nose into the oesophagus. The Ryles tube is pulled off and discarded, and the guidewire is removed and the feeding attachments connected to the end of the tube.

Tips and precautions

Plenty of lubrication is required to pass the tube through the instrument channel of the endscope. Silicon-based lubricant, in spray or liquid form, should be applied liberally. Oronasal transfer requires practice, but is a useful technique to master (it is also used for nasobiliary tubes; see Chapter 9). The most common beginners' mistake is failing to take the mouth-guard *completely off* the tube and guidewire before starting the transfer. This results in the mouth-guard becoming incorporated in the oronasal loop, and there is no alternative but to start again!

The Ryles tube should be left in position until the final stage of the transfer. It protects the soft palate from damage as the loop is pulled through. This is particularly important when this technique is being used to re-route a guidewire.

Occasionally, the guidewire cannot easily be removed from the feeding tube. Rather than pulling hard and risking damage to the tube, the feeding attachments can be fitted with the wire still *in situ* and water forced down the tube to lubricate it. The guidewire can then usually be removed.

'Over-the-wire' technique

This technique is best performed with X-ray screening facilities available. Endoscopy is performed on a screening trolley with the patient in the endoscopic retrograde cholangiopancreatography (ERCP) position to facilitate fluoroscopy. The scope is passed as far as possible into the small bowel.

A Teflon-coated, floppy-tipped ERCP guidewire is passed through the biopsy channel until it appears at the distal end. The wire is then carefully advanced into the intestine until resistance is encountered and its position is confirmed by fluoroscopy. In case of difficulty, an ERCP catheter can be passed over the wire and, with alternate advancement of wire and catheter, a position distal to the ligament of Treitz can nearly always be achieved. The catheter is then withdrawn, the endoscope is withdrawn over the wire and screening is used to confirm that the wire has not moved. The wire is then re-routed to the nose using the oronasal transfer technique described above. Care must be taken to ensure that the wire has not looped at the back of the mouth. The nasojejunal tube is lubricated and passed through the nose over the wire. Judicious tension applied to the wire by the nursing assistant will ensure that the tube passes smoothly to its desired position in the jejunum. Progress can be monitored by screening. Finally, water is injected down the tube and the guidewire is removed.

Tips and precautions

If the nasojejunal tube is impeded in its passage and the endoscopist continues to push, the tube will loop, usually in the mouth or stomach. This tends to drag the tip of the guidewire proximally. Once a loop has started to form, it is difficult to straighten it while maintaining a distal guidewire position. Loop formation can be avoided by keeping the correct degree of tension on the wire at all times and by screening frequently – particularly at the sites where the advancing tube is likely to be held up such as the oesophagogastric junction, the pylorus or at any obstructing lesion.

Although advisable, X-ray screening is not mandatory for this technique. With experience, a satisfactory position can be achieved by 'feel', especially in patients who have undergone gastrectomy where access to the jejunum is more direct.

Beside-the-scope technique (Fig. 8.5)

A modification of the over-the-wire technique is to start by passing the feeding tube through the nose into the stomach. The endoscope is then introduced into the stomach in the usual way. A guidewire is passed down the nasojejunal tube into the stomach, where it is picked up by forceps passed through the endoscope channel. The endoscope is then advanced into the jejunum, carrying the wire down with it. The endoscope is carefully withdrawn while advancing the

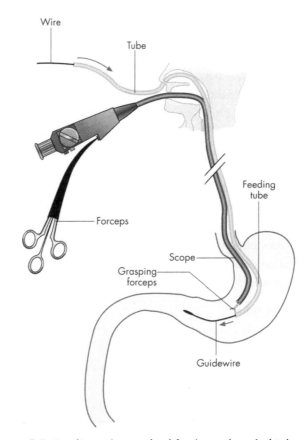

Figure 8.5. An alternative method for 'over-the-wire' tube replacement. The feeding tube is passed into the stomach through the nose with the endoscope alongside it. A guidewire is passed through the feeding tube and picked up by forceps passed through the endoscope channel. The wire is carried down into the small bowel and the endoscope withdrawn back to the stomach. The feeding tube is advanced over the wire.

forceps so that the tip of the guidewire remains in position. When the endoscope is back in the stomach the forceps are opened, gently agitated to release the guidewire, and withdrawn into the scope. The nasojejunal tube is then advanced over the wire with X-ray screening to monitor its progress and direct endoscopic vision within the stomach to control loop formation. When the tube is in a satisfactory position the endoscope is carefully withdrawn.

This modification has the advantage of not requiring an oronasal transfer, but its drawbacks are that very distal guidewire placement is more difficult and there is a risk that the tube will be pulled back as the endoscope is withdrawn.

Choice of technique

The 'beside-the-scope' method is simplest and quickest because it does not require oronasal transfer. Distal tube placement is often difficult, however, because the endoscope becomes less easy to manoeuvre with a tube held alongside it. Nonetheless, it is a useful method for placing nasogastric tubes beyond an oesophageal obstruction.

The 'through-the-scope' technique has the advantage of not requiring fluoroscopy. This is useful in the ICU where X-ray screening can be difficult. The biggest drawback is that the diameter of the feeding tube is limited by the size of the endoscope's working channel.

In expert hands, the 'over-the-wire' technique has the highest success rate for intubation beyond the ligament of Treitz. It is more difficult to master, however, and requires competent nursing assistance. It is the technique of choice for passing double-lumen tubes if sump drainage or gastric decompression is required at the same time as feeding.

Choice of tube

There is little to choose between the various nasogastric tubes available. They are generally made from soft polyurethane or silicone elastomer with a diameter of 3 mm or less.

Nasojejunal tubes are made from similar materials but are longer, usually 110–120 cm. A wide variety of tube designs are available, incorporating weighted tips and modified side holes intended to prevent blockage or retrograde migration into the stomach. None of these has been shown to offer a particular advantage in controlled trials. Many of the elaborate tip adaptations prohibit passage over a guidewire. The choice of tube for 'through-the-scope' placement is even more limited, as few are long

or thin enough or have feeding attachments that can be removed.

Complications

A number of potential procedural difficulties have already been discussed. Others include an inability to expel the feeding tube from a sharply angulated endoscope tip, and kinking of the guidewire. Serious complications relating to tube insertion are very rare with good technique, but perforation by the guidewire was reported in 0.8% in one series. Following successful placement the most frequent and disheartening complication is accidental removal of the tube by the patient or nursing staff. This occurs in more than half of all tubes inserted. Tube dysfunction due to blockage or kinking occurs in about 9% of cases. Double-lumen tubes may occasionally cause necrosis of the nasal septum if left in place for long periods.

Percutaneous endoscopic gastrostomy

As well as the general contraindications to enteral feeding (Table 8.3), there are specific circumstances in which PEG should not be attempted. The most commonly encountered is an inability to bring the anterior walls of the stomach and abdomen into close apposition. This may be due to interposed organs, partial gastrectomy, or an impacted hiatus hernia. Only rarely can failure be predicted without endoscopy; a safe puncture site can often be found in patients with only a small post-surgical gastric remnant. Other absolute contraindications include uncorrected coagulopathy, sepsis anywhere along the proposed path of the puncturing needle, and the presence of gastric ulceration in the field of puncture. Relative contraindications are given in Table 8.5, but there are isolated case reports describing successful PEG placement in all these situations. Despite concerns about abscess and fistula formation, PEG appears to be quite safe in Crohn's disease [19].

The 'pull-through' technique

The Ponsky–Gauderer 'pull-method' is described in detail as it is the most popular technique. With the patient supine and the abdomen exposed, the stomach is fully inflated with air to displace neighbouring organs and to bring the gastric and anterior abdominal walls into apposition. Digital pressure is applied to the left upper quadrant. This is seen as an indentation of the stomach wall in the

Table 8.5. Contraindications to PEG insertion

Absolute

Uncorrected coagulopathy

Inability to appose the stomach and anterior abdominal wall

Distal gastrointestinal tract obstruction

Gastric ulceration within the field of needle puncture

Complete pharyngeal or oesophageal obstruction

Severe respiratory disease or other contraindication to endoscopy

Relative

Ascites

Obesity

Pregnancy

Portal hypertension

Neoplastic and infiltrative disease of gastric wall

Previous subtotal gastrectomy

Marked hepatic or splenic enlargement

Sepsis anywhere along the path of needle puncture

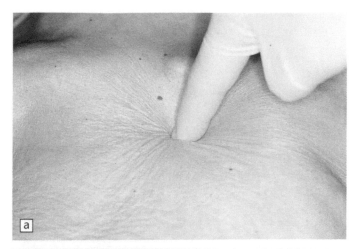

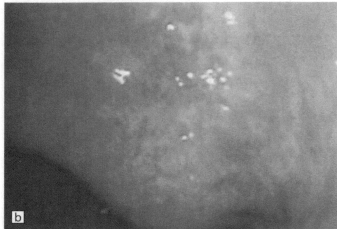

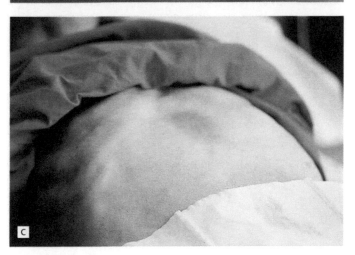

Figure 8.6. Finding an insertion site: (a) external indentation with finger (b) should be visible by the endoscopist and (c) transillumination from within can also be helpful.

endoscopic view. By pressing sharply over this region of the abdomen the site of optimal indentation can be established (Fig. 8.6a,b). When a suitable site is obtained, the endoscope is brought close to the point of indentation, the theatre lights are dimmed, and the abdomen is inspected for a bright red transillumination (Fig. 8.6c) (the transillumination facility on modern endoscopy light-sources is useful to boost the light, especially when the patient is more obese). The position at which finger indentation is best defined and transillumination is brightest is then marked on the skin. This typically lies about one-third of the way along a line drawn between the mid-point of the left inferior costal margin and the umbilicus, but sites more medially and higher than this are perfectly acceptable. If transillumination is not seen it is unsafe to proceed. Conversely, however, good transillumination does not completely exclude the possibility of a bowel loop interposed between the stomach and abdominal wall.

The chosen site is prepared with a suitable antibacterial, sterile drapes are applied, and the skin is anaesthetized with lignocaine 2%. A 21-G needle, with the lignocaine-containing syringe still attached, is then passed perpendicularly through the abdominal wall while pulling back on the syringe (Fig. 8.7a). Air should bubble into the syringe at the same moment the tip of the needle appears in

the stomach. If the needle cannot be seen in the stomach, another viscus may have been entered and a new insertion site must be found. (Inadvertent puncture of small bowel or

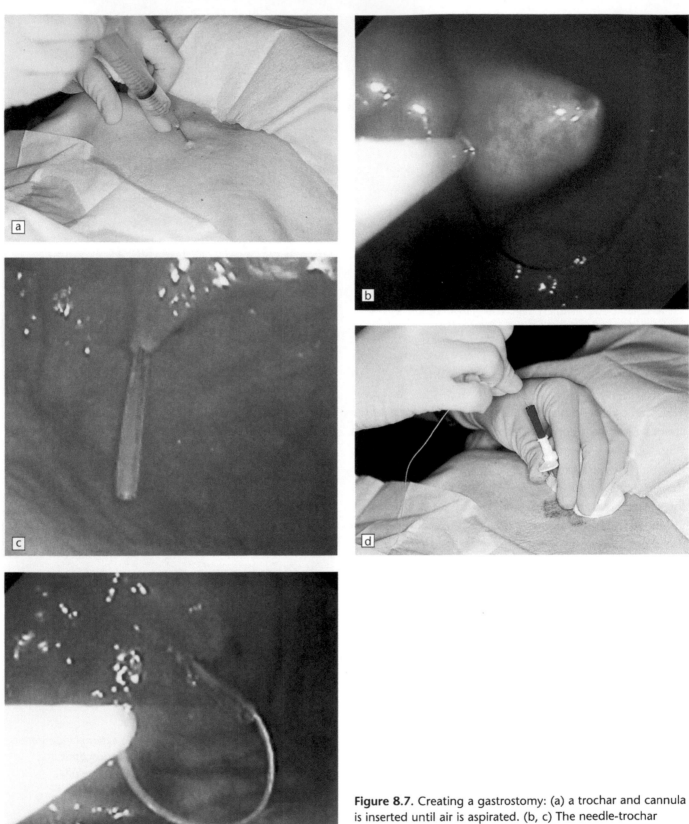

Figure 8.7. Creating a gastrostomy: (a) a trochar and cannula is inserted until air is aspirated. (b, c) The needle-trochar should be visualized by the endoscopist. (d) A guide string is inserted through the cannula and (e) grasped with a forceps by the endoscopist.

colon with a small-gauge needle is surprisingly well tolerated.) The needle is then withdrawn, while infiltrating the deeper tissues with lignocaine. Next, a stab incision is made in the skin with a number 11 blade. In very malnourished subjects it is important to ensure that the blade does not puncture the stomach. A trochar needle is then inserted through the abdominal wall into the stomach (Fig. 8.7b) and is lassoed by a snare passed down the endoscope channel. This will prevent the trochar becoming dislodged in the event of the patient coughing or moving. The needle is withdrawn, leaving the cannula in place (Fig. 8.7c), and a guidewire or string is passed through it into the stomach (Fig. 8.7d). Releasing the snare slightly allows it to slip off the cannula and over the string. It is then closed tightly (Fig. 8.7e) and withdrawn a short distance into the endoscope channel to maintain a firm hold. The scope is then slowly withdrawn and the string emerges from the patient's mouth. The tapered end of the PEG tube is secured to the end of the string/wire, and by carefully pulling the abdominal end of the string it is drawn through the mouth, oesophagus and stomach until resistance is felt as the tapered end of the PEG tube abuts against the trochar cannula in the stomach. At this point the cannula is pulled back with the string and the PEG tube emerges through the abdominal wall, dilating the track as it comes (Fig. 8.8a).

The PEG tube is pulled out until the internal retention device (or 'bumper') reaches the gastric wall and prevents further withdrawal of the tube. The distance between the inner gastric bumper and the surface of the skin can be judged by markings on the tube. It is often necessary to push the tube back in by a few millimetres, as excessive pressure from the retention device can lead to necrosis of the gastric wall. When the tension is correct, the tube should rotate freely and there should be a small degree of 'play' to allow for increases in abdominal wall thickness as nutrition is improved.

When learning the technique of PEG placement it is essential to repeat the endoscopy at this point to confirm that the position of the bumper is satisfactory and that the surrounding mucosa is not blanching because of excessive tension (Fig. 8.8b). The experienced operator soon develops a feel for the appropriate degree of tension and, provided that the tube rotates freely, the second-look endoscopy has been shown to add little to the success or safety of the procedure [20]. Despite this, check endoscopy

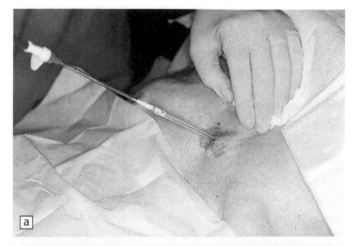

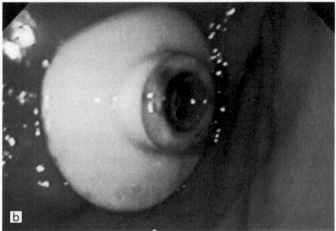

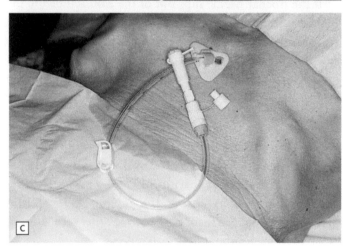

Figure 8.8. Inserting the PEG tube: the tube is attached to the string exiting from the stomach and (a) pulled through until (b) the internal button abuts the gastric wall. (c) The external fixing device is attached and secured.

is still recommended by many authorities as a useful precaution [21]. The external fixation device is then fitted, the tube is trimmed to the desired length, and the site covered with a dry dressing (Fig. 8.8c).

Tips and precautions

The key to success lies in selecting the best possible puncture site, and it is worth spending time over this part of the procedure.

Occasionally, there are problems entering the stomach with the trochar needle because of excessive 'tenting' of the gastric mucosa. An additional risk in this situation is that the needle may puncture the posterior wall of the stomach. This is most likely to happen if the insertion site is at the inscisura or high in the gastric body where rugal folds are prominent and more readily stretched. If possible, a different insertion site should be found. Alternatively, gentle pressure can be applied with an open snare to oppose elongation of the fold. Great care is needed to avoid damaging the mucosa.

If a good site for insertion was established initially but the needle does not appear in the stomach, this may mean that continued air insufflation has overinflated the stomach and displaced it from its usual position. Removing some air from the stomach may help.

If the trochar needle slips out of the stomach before the passage of the string, the puncture site is lost and there is a risk of gastric contents leaking into the peritoneum. In this situation the best approach is to complete PEG insertion as quickly as possible through an adjacent puncture site so that the stomach and abdominal walls are pulled together and the leak sealed.

Sachs–Vine push method

This is very similar to the Ponsky (pull) technique described above except that, in place of a string, a stiffer guidewire is brought out of the mouth. A long, firm gastrostomy tube is then pushed over the wire until it emerges from the abdominal wall.

Russell introducer method

In this approach a suitable puncture site is identified as above, but needle puncture is used to pass a flexible J-wire rather than a thread. Over this, one or more dilators are passed to enlarge the tract followed by an introducer in a peel-away sheath. The introducer is then removed and a Foley balloon or Malecot catheter is inserted into the stomach. The peel-away catheter is then split and peeled away.

The great difficulty with this technique is in maintaining apposition of the gastric and abdominal walls during passage of the dilator. This can be ensured by using nylon anchor sutures (also known as T-fasteners). Four of these are placed by needle puncture around the insertion site. They are expelled from their needles, unfold to take up the T-shape, and then remain in the stomach after the needles are withdrawn. By fixing them at skin level the stomach is held firmly against the abdominal wall. Once the PEG is established, the T-fasteners can be cut and the end pieces allowed to pass safely through the gastrointestinal tract (Fig. 8.9).

Choice of technique

The Ponsky-pull technique is almost universally adopted. There is little to commend the push technique as an alternative. However, the drawback of both these approaches is that the PEG tube has to pass through the mouth, where it may become contaminated. This is avoided with the introducer method. While bacterial contamination is rarely a problem when antibiotics are used routinely, there is an argument for avoiding tube contamination if the patient's mouth is infected with *Candida* or resistant organisms such as methicillin-resistant *Staphylococcus aureus* (MRSA). Unfortunately, the introducer method results in a larger abdominal wall defect so the tube fits less snugly and is more likely to leak.

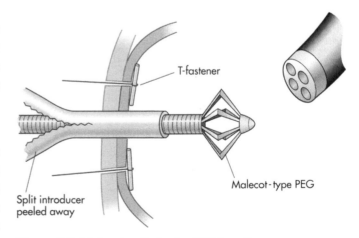

Figure 8.9. Malecot catheter for PEG insertion.

Post-procedure management

Research has shown that prolonged fasting after PEG insertion is not necessary. Feeding can begin after 4 hour if all appears well and bowel sounds are present. It is probably wise to confirm first that sterile water passed down the tube does not produce pain, as this might indicate primary tube displacement.

After 24 hours the dry dressing may be removed and the site is cleaned daily using mild soap and warm water.

A fistulous track into the stomach usually develops within 7–14 days. Before this there is the possibility that feed or gastric contents may leak into the peritoneal cavity, and disturbance of the tube should be minimal. It is also advisable to avoid bathing or immersing the site in water during this period, although showering is permitted. After 2 weeks the patient may bathe normally and should be encouraged to rotate the tube once a week as part of the cleaning process to promote development of a healthy fistula. The tube must be flushed with at least 50 ml of water after each feed to prevent blockage.

Choice of tube

A bewildering variety of tubes have arrived on the market in recent years, but they differ from one another in only a few important respects: tube diameter, the materials from which they are made, the external fixing device and, most important, the type of internal retention device used. In general, thinner diameter tubes (down to 9 F) have a similar blockage rate to larger ones and are preferred for their better tolerability. The choice of material is chiefly between silicone elastomers and polyurethane. The former is softer, but such a tube has a larger external diameter in relation to its lumen. Both materials are durable; polyurethane tends to split if left kinked for long periods, whereas silicon can become stretched and distorted with time. Experience with polyurethane tubes indicates that they can last up to 6 years. External fixation is achieved with either a simple disc or a more sophisticated device which positions the tube at a 90° angle, keeping it flat against the abdominal wall.

There are four basic types of internal retention device (Fig. 8.10). The simplest is a soft silicon-rubber disc. This is very reliable and longlasting, but requires endoscopy for removal. The others are all designed for 'traction removal'; that is, they can be pulled out through the anterior abdominal wall without endoscopy. The most common of these is a silicon-rubber dome which, when pulled

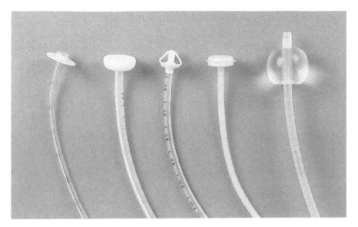

Figure 8.10. Examples of PEG tube internal retention devices. From left to right: simple silicone disc (not traction removable); silicone dome (traction removable); Malecot-type flange arrangement (removable with obturator); semi-deflatable disc (traction removable after tube is cut) and balloon retained PEG (easily removed when balloon is deflated).

hard, will collapse sufficiently to pass through the fistula. Others use a balloon or hollow bolster that can be partially deflated to aid removal. The final group employ a Malecot or 'mushroom' arrangement which can be stretched with an obturator to make them narrower before removal. With all traction-removable catheters there is a higher risk of inadvertent removal by the patient or staff. This is not common, but if it occurs before the fistula has matured, then peritonitis may result. All available designs reflect a compromise between ease of removal and safety: the less likely they are to be accidentally removed, the harder they are to remove intentionally when the time comes, and vice versa. It is important to suit the tube to the patient. Patients likely to pull at their tubes, or those in whom swallowing function is never likely to return, are probably better served by non-traction removal retention discs.

Complications and their management (Table 8.6)

PEG placement is successful in 95% of patients [22]. The reported 30-day mortality rate varies widely depending on the population studied, and tends to reflect the underlying disease process rather than complications of the procedure. Mortality rates around 10% are typical, and reports of much higher mortality (up to 35%) probably reflect inappropriate patient selection [23]. Procedure-related mortality is between 1 and 2% and major complications occur in 5% of cases. Minor complications are more frequent, the most common being minor infection or

Table 8.6. Complications of PEG (after [24])

Major complications	Considerations for prevention
Aspiration	Avoid feeding supine. Feed by continuous infusion.
	Prokinetic drugs. Jejunal extension tube.
Peritonitis (without displacement)	Use anchor sutures in high-risk patients, i.e. severe malnutrition, low albumin, on corticosteroids or impaired wound healing.
Early displacement (before tract mature)	Avoid traction removable tubes in confused/elderly.
	Cover tube with dressing. Avoid tube manipulation.
Tube migration through gastric wall	Avoid excessive tension on internal bumper.
	Reduce tension as patient puts on weight.
Perforated viscus	Use 'safe tract' technique (see below and text).
Gastrocolocutaneous fistula	Ensure transillumination and that air aspiration is simultaneous with needle's appearance in stomach during gastric puncture.
Haemorrhage	Correct coagulopathy. Careful preliminary inspection OGD.
Necrotizing fasciitis	Prophylactic antibiotics. Adequate scalpel skin incision.
	Avoid excessive tension on internal bumper.
Tumour implantation at PEG site	Avoid pull-through technique for preoperative PEG placement in oropharyngeal cancer

Minor complications

Peristomal wound infections	Prophylactic antibiotics. Careful wound hygiene.
	Avoid pull-through technique if MRSA in mouth.
Tube blockage	Flush tube well after all food and drugs. Use formula feeds only.
	Avoid very sticky liquid medications.
Tube fracture	Avoid kinking.
	Do not leave C-clamps or gate-clamps closed for long periods.
Leakage around tube	Limit tube manipulation.
	Avoid large diameter tubes.
Late tube displacement	Avoid traction removable tubes in confused/elderly.
	Limit tube manipulation.
Tube migration into small bowel	Keep external fixation device in appropriate position.

MRSA = methicillin-resistant *Staphylococcus aureus*; OGD = oesophago-gastro-duodenoscopy.

leakage at the stoma site. Of the early complications, generalized peritonitis is the most serious. This can occur during the first week before the fistula is mature and may result from displacement of the internal fixation bolster into the peritoneal cavity or leakage around the gastric puncture site. PEG displacement can be confirmed by injection of water-soluble contrast down the PEG (a 'PEGogram') (Fig. 8.11). Surgery is usually required and mortality rates are high. Leakage into the peritoneum around a non-displaced PEG usually results in only minor, localized peritonitis which settles quickly with antibiotics and suspension of feeding. More significant leakage is seen rarely, usually in extremely malnourished patients or those on corticosteroids in whom the gastric puncture site may fail to seal itself because of impaired wound healing. Anecdotal reports suggest that using anchor sutures (T-fasteners) for the first 2 weeks to maintain close apposition of gastric and abdominal walls may help prevent this [24].

Tube displacement after the first 7–10 days is usually uneventful. The priority in this eventuality is to prevent the fistula from closing over. This starts to happen within 24 h, so prompt action is necessary. A small Foley catheter passed through the stoma with the balloon inflated in the stomach will maintain intragastric access for a few days while arrangements are made for PEG replacement (Fig. 8.12).

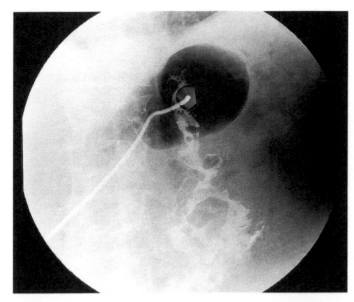

Figure 8.11. PEGogram demonstrating leakage into the peritoneal cavity.

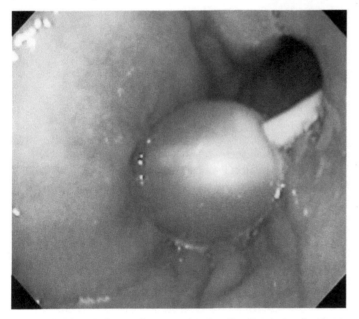

Figure 8.12. A Foley catheter maintains the fistula inadvertent PEG removal.

Foley catheter balloons perish very quickly in contact with gastric acid, so this is not a long-term solution.

There is considerable variation in the reported rates of aspiration pneumonia following PEG insertion in patients unable to protect their airway. Some series fail to distinguish between aspiration of gastric contents and penetration of the airway by oropharyngeal secretions. Clearly, a PEG tube cannot influence the latter. Nevertheless, gastro-oesophageal reflux with the attendant risk of aspiration is undoubtedly a major problem in patients with neurological dysphagia. Adding methylene blue to colour the feed is a useful way of confirming that there is regurgitation to the mouth. The initial approach to this problem is to use continuous infusion rather than bolus feeding, to avoid feeding in the supine position, and to use prokinetic drugs. If these measures fail, a jejunal extension (J-tube) can be added to the PEG to allow feeding beyond the ligament of Treitz (but see the discussion above).

Two other complications that merit special mention are necrotizing fasciitis and gastrocolonic (or colocutaneous) fistula formation. Necrotizing fasciitis appears to be very rare, but if not recognized and treated early, then mortality is high. It usually becomes apparent 3–14 days after the procedure and is characterized by high fever, oedema of the skin around the PEG, cellulitis and eventually crepitus. Treatment is by surgical debridement. By contrast, colonic fistula formation is often not recognized until many months after PEG placement. The first sign may be diarrhoea following PEG replacement as a result of feeding directly into the colon. The fistula will usually close spontaneously when the tube is removed.

PEG removal

PEG removal should never be attempted until the gastrocutaneous fistula is mature. The technique for traction removal will depend on the type of PEG used, and familiarity with the tube type is essential before attempting removal. Some, but not all, have an internal fixation device that can be deflated or collapsed, allowing the PEG to be removed by pulling firmly on the tube, close to its insertion, while the other hand is placed on the abdomen with fingers either side of the tube. Before attempting this, it is necessary to establish that the internal retention device is freely mobile in the stomach by pushing it in a short distance and rotating it. If this is not possible, or causes pain, the bolster may have migrated into the submucosal tissues and traction removal may be hazardous (see below). Despite manufacturers' claims to the contrary, traction removal can be painful and analgesia or sedation is required for some patients. If the PEG does not come out easily it is better to resort to endoscopic removal rather than pulling harder. This is particularly important for devices that rely on stretching with an obturator where difficulty may be due to technical failure.

PEG tubes with rigid internal fixation discs require endoscopic removal – a procedure which is quick and easy. A snare is placed over the retention disc and closed around the tube above it, though care must be taken to avoid including a fold of gastric mucosa within the snare. The external part of the tube is then cut close to skin level and allowed to slip into the stomach as the endoscope is withdrawn. Retrieval of the internal disc in this way is much better than simply cutting the tube and letting it fall into the stomach in the hope that it will pass uneventfully through the gastrointestinal tract. Although this is often successful, there are a growing number of reports of obstruction caused by retained bumpers.

Occasionally, a disc retention device will be found to have migrated into the submucosal tissues so that it cannot be seen at endoscopy (the 'buried bumper syndrome'). The site of the PEG is then marked by a heaped-up area of gastric mucosa with a central depression. This is more likely to occur if a PEG tube has been fixed too tightly or has not been slackened off to allow for increased adipose tissue in the abdominal wall with improved nutrition. Removal of the disc may require surgical exploration, but a recently described alternative is to use a small-calibre dilatation balloon to push the disc back into the stomach at the same time as dilating the track (Fig. 8.13).

PEG replacement

PEG tubes may need to be replaced because of accidental displacement or tube fracture. Replacement is possible without endoscopy using a balloon or Malecot-type PEG tube. These are passed through the existing fistula and inflated (or otherwise deployed) in the stomach. Inserting the obturator-dependent 'mushroom'-type retention device without endoscopic control can no longer be recommended. Some force is needed to push them through the stoma, and there are reports of this causing separation of the stomach and anterior abdominal wall leading to unrecognized intra-peritoneal PEG placement with disastrous consequences.

If endoscopy is required to remove an old PEG tube, a new one can be placed through the existing fistula using the 'pull'-technique described above. This can be achieved with a single pass of the endoscope if the thread is delivered from the mouth at the same time as the old PEG retention disc. Passing a thread through the old tube so that it will be held by the snare as it closes above the disc is sometimes successful, but more often the thread slips out of the snare

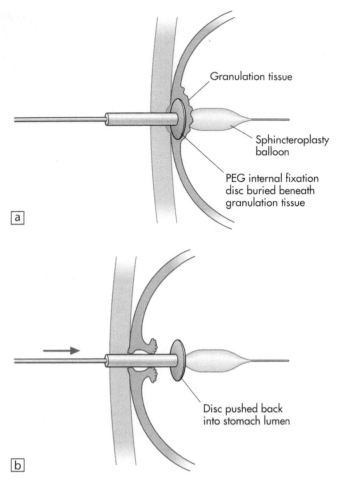

Figure 8.13. Push technique for removing impacted PEG discs. (a) The balloon is passed into the PEG tube and inflated. (b) Pushing the balloon delivers the PEG retention disc back into the stomach.

en route to the mouth. A method of avoiding this is shown in Figure 8.14. The alternative is to stitch the thread to the stump of the old tube after it is cut.

Buttons

When a PEG fistula has fully matured (which may take up to 8 weeks), there is the option of replacing the tube with a low-profile or skin-level device (more commonly referred to as a 'button'). These are preferred by younger, more active people because they are easily concealed and interfere less with lifestyle. Designs vary but, as with non-endoscopic PEG replacements, the choice is between balloon-retained buttons and those that use an obturator to stretch a mushroom-shaped retention device to allow its passage through the fistula (Fig. 8.15). Balloon-retained buttons are easier (and safer) to pass, but have a shorter life

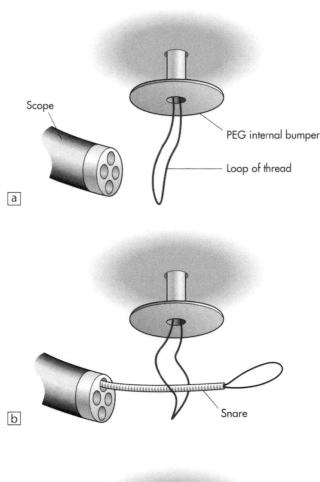

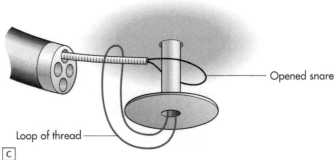

Figure 8.14. Securing a thread during PEG replacement. (a) The loop of thread is passed through the PEG. (b) The closed snare is passed through this loop. (c) The snare is opened and placed over the PEG bumper, securing it and the thread at the same time.

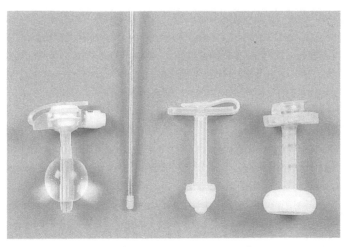

Figure 8.15. Types of button device. From left to right: balloon retained button; button using mushroom-shaped retention device which can be stretched and narrowed by the obturator (also shown) to facilitate insertion; button formed by conversion of an existing PEG using the Bard Genie ® system.

expectancy and require regular checks to ensure that the balloon is properly inflated. Those with 'mushroom'-shaped retaining devices tend to last longer and require less maintenance, but greater care is required to fit them.

The first step is to find the distance from skin to gastric mucosa using a measuring device. A button of the correct length can then be selected. Balloon buttons are simply passed through the fistula and the balloon inflated with water in the stomach. 'Mushroom' buttons are better inserted under endoscopic control in view of their potential for causing separation of the stomach and abdominal wall layers during passage (see above). The endoscope can verify that the retention device has reached the stomach before the obturator is removed to allow it to take up its preformed mushroom shape. A further safeguard against disruption of the tract is to pass a guidewire through the fistula into the stomach. The wire can be kept taught by grasping it within the stomach by endoscopic forceps. The button can then be passed over the wire so that, even if tract disruption occurs, safe access to the stomach is maintained.

A recent development is a PEG tube which can be converted into a button by cutting it flush with the skin and fitting an external feeding attachment containing a non-return valve. This has much to recommend it for those patients who express a clear preference for a button at the outset, though how durable they will be prove to be in clinical use remains to be determined.

Jejunal extensions (JET-PEG or PEG-J tubes)

A great variety of approaches are described for placing jejunal extension tubes through PEGs (JET-PEGs or J-tubes), implying that no one technique is perfect [15].

The two basic methods are parallels of the 'beside-the scope' and 'over-the-wire' techniques for nasojejunal tube placement. The first step with either approach is to replace the existing PEG with one of larger diameter so that a J-tube of 8–12 F can be accommodated.

In the 'beside-the-scope' method, the J-tube is passed through the PEG and picked up in the stomach using endoscopic forceps (most have a terminal knob or thread for this purpose). It is then carried down with the scope as far into the intestine as possible and the scope is withdrawn, taking precautions to prevent the tube being dragged back with the scope. The disadvantage of this technique, as for nasojejunal tube placement, is that positioning the tube beyond the duodenum is difficult.

For 'over-the-wire' methods, there are at least three approaches described for positioning the wire. The simplest is to pass a wire through the PEG, using a valve to prevent air escaping from the stomach. This is carried down into the small intestine with grasping forceps (Fig. 8.16). Dragging a wire down in this way affects the manoeuvrability of the endoscope much less than pulling a tube alongside it.

In the second method, the endoscope is inserted as far as possible into the intestine and a wire is passed through its working channel. The scope is then withdrawn back into the stomach over the wire. A small loop of wire is formed in the stomach by feeding more of it through the endoscope. Grasping forceps are passed through the PEG and used to grab the wire loop. The proximal end is then drawn through the PEG using the forceps while feeding more wire through the endoscopy channel. Great care is required to prevent displacement of the distal tip of the wire during this manoeuvre, as it is not always easy to tell which is the proximal and which the distal end of the loop (Fig. 8.17a). In the third method, a 'skinny' endoscope is passed directly through a 28 F PEG tube and manoeuvred

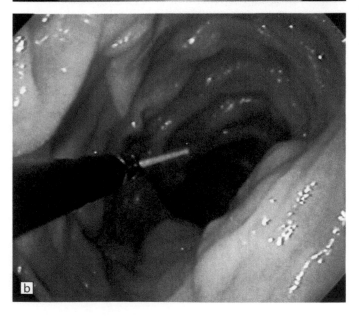

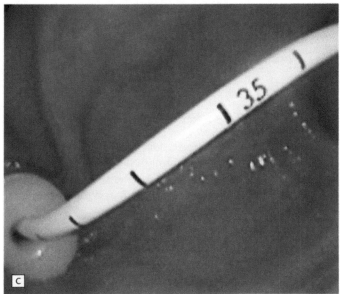

Figure 8.16. Jejunal extension to a previously placed PEG tube. (a) A fine-bore tube is inserted through the PEG, (b) grasped with an endoscope forceps and (c) pushed through the pylorus into place in the jejunum.

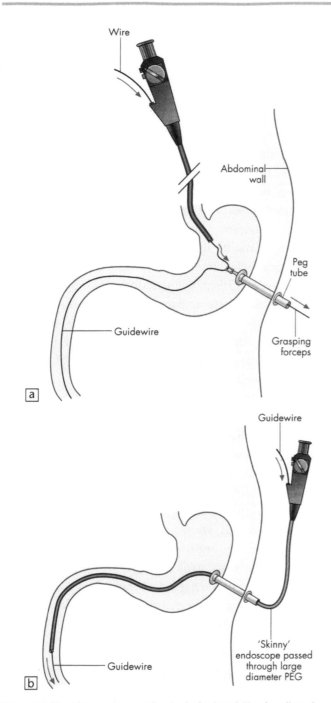

Figure 8.17. Alternative method of placing PEJ tube directly.

into the jejunum. The wire is then passed through the biopsy channel and the endoscope removed over the wire. This has the disadvantage of requiring a much larger PEG tube than the other techniques and uses a specialist endoscope which is unlikely to be available in most units (Fig. 8.17b).

Once wire placement has been achieved, by whichever method, a J-tube is fed over the wire, with X-ray screening

if preferred, until a satisfactory position is obtained. Progress of the tube is monitored endoscopically from the stomach to prevent gastric loop formation.

Direct percutaneous endoscopic jejunostomy (direct PEJ)

This technique employs the pull method for PEG placement, except that the tube is placed directly into the jejunum. It relies upon there being a superficial loop of jejunum, within reach of the endoscope or enteroscope, which can be identified by transillumination. A number of minor modifications to the PEG technique are required. First, peristalsis is inhibited with hyoscine or glucagon. Second, the initial pass with a 21-G needle needs a short, sharp stab to enter the small bowel – gradual pressure results in the bowel moving away from the needle. Third, it may be advisable to grasp the 21-G needle with an endoscopic snare as soon as it appears. The needle is then disconnected from the syringe and left in place while the trochar needle is passed parallel to it. This maintains apposition of bowel and abdominal wall during passage of the thicker trochar needle (although it can limit the endoscopic view). Finally, great care is needed to prevent the PEJ from being pulled too tight, as the jejunum is very susceptible to pressure necrosis. Endoscopic confirmation of the internal bumper position is recommended in every case. An 86% success rate has been reported using this technique in a large series of 150 patients, nearly half of whom had not had previous gastric surgery. Major complications requiring surgery occurred in only 0.6% [16].

CONTROVERSIAL ISSUES

Evidence-based practice?

The benefits of nutritional support are often regarded as self-evident. While this may be reasonable where long-term feeding is concerned, there are many situations where short-term enteral nutrition is used without good evidence of benefit. It may prevent weight loss, but does it influence clinical outcome in critical illness, or during cancer therapy? And if so, do all patients benefit or only those with pre-morbid nutritional impairment? In many conditions weight loss is a result of the disease process itself rather than nutritional deficiency. Does delivering extra calories by artificial nutrition make any sense in such circumstances [25]? There is a pressing need for good prospective randomized trials to answers these questions.

PEG placement by a nurse practitioner

A major constraint determining whether PEG insertions can be readily accommodated within routine endoscopy lists is not the procedural time but the limited availability of skilled assistance. Although the assistant requires no specific endoscopic skills and works under the direct guidance of the endoscopist, it has been generally regarded that he or she should be medically qualified. Frequently, the only medical personnel available are relatively junior, with limited experience of the technique and its potential complications. For this reason nursing staff have been trained to perform gastric puncture for PEG as an extension of their role as endoscopy nurse practitioners. They carry out gastric puncture under the supervision of a medical endoscopist who retains responsibility for selecting an appropriate site. A non-randomized study has demonstrated that a nurse–doctor team can perform the procedure just as well as two doctors without compromising safety and with less disruption to other endoscopy services [26]. Furthermore, by incorporating pre-procedure visits by the nurse, there may be advantages in terms of continuity and quality of care for the patient.

Paediatric practice

The emphasis of this chapter has been on enteral feeding in adults. Many of the indications for long-term nutritional support, such as intestinal failure and neurological impairment, are equally common in children. PEG insertion can be performed safely in children, but is more technically demanding as the 'target area' is smaller [27]. Furthermore, endoscopy in children generally requires general anaesthetic, so one of the potential advantages of the non-surgical approach is lost. Some paediatricians prefer to rely on surgical gastrostomies so that a fundoplication can be performed at the same time to prevent gastro-oesophageal reflux, which is a particular problem in neurologically impaired children. Others

choose to use PEG because of its lower procedural complication rate.

Timing of PEGs following cerebrovascular accident

The dilemma following dysphagic stroke is whether to insert a PEG tube within the first week to avoid nutritional deficiency in the early stages of recovery or to wait several weeks until it becomes clear which patients are likely to suffer long-term dysphagia. Early intervention undoubtedly results in 'unnecessary' PEG procedures in those patients who are destined to recover their swallowing before 4 weeks. Others will deteriorate and die within the first few weeks whatever happens, and they too will have been subjected to an unnecessary invasive procedure. Patients who survive but make little recovery from their stroke may face the prospect of continued PEG feeding, despite a very poor quality of life.

On the other hand, delaying PEG insertion compromises the nutrition of the much larger group of patients who have dysphagia in the first few weeks. The usual approach is to use nasogastric feeding for the first 3–4 weeks but, in practice, repeated tube displacement seriously reduces nutritional delivery by this route. To what extent this relative starvation impairs recovery from stroke is not known. PEG feeding from 14 days onwards certainly improves the 6-week mortality rate compared with nasogastric feeding [12], but earlier PEG placement may have even greater benefit. Large-scale clinical trials are currently ongoing in the hope of answering these questions.

Ethical issues in nutritional support

Over the last two decades, there has been great progress in overcoming the technical problems of PEG placement, but these have been replaced by ever more complex ethical dilemmas. Unlike most medical interventions, nutrition is regarded as a basic human right and its withdrawal from a patient, even in the terminal stages of their life, produces a strong emotional response. Without intervention, a terminally ill patient will reach a point where they become unable to eat or drink or are simply uninterested in food. If a PEG is *in situ*, the temptation is to continue administering food, water and medication right up until the end. The consequent postponement of the inevitable is rarely in the patient's interests. Likewise, it is possible to keep patients in persistent vegetative states or in the terminal stages of senile dementia alive for long periods with PEG feeding. Pressure to insert a PEG tube in such situations often comes from nursing staff or distressed family members who are concerned about aspiration pneumonia and progressive weight loss. In these circumstances, it is important to consider the ethical issues very carefully before proceeding since it is unlikely that a decision to discontinue feeding will ever be made once the PEG is in place (although in law there is no distinction between withholding tube feeding and withdrawing it once started) [28].

Quality of life should be the principal concern when deciding whether to prolong survival by gastrostomy feeding, but this is notoriously difficult to measure or define. If the patient is able to express their wishes, these should be given paramount importance, even if contrary to the 'medical' view. Where the patient is not competent to give consent, consensus should be obtained among all concerned parties before proceeding. During discussion with family and carers it is important to emphasise that a PEG does not abolish the risk of aspiration, nor does it always improve the patient's functional status. Expectations of survival benefit should also be realistic. An 18-month follow-up of PEG insertion in nursing home residents showed that 20% were dead within one month and 90% of those designated 'not for resuscitation' at the time of PEG placement died during the study period [29].

PEG insertion, like any other medical intervention, can be justified only if there is evidence of its clinical effectiveness [25]. In dementia and in terminal illness the true impact of PEG on survival and quality of life is not known. In the few areas where prospective studies have been attempted (in AIDS, for example, and to a limited extent in motor neurone disease [30]), there is at least some evidence on which recommendations can be based; in other situations health professionals must face decisions which have formidable ethical and legal implications, armed with nothing but speculation and individual prejudice. Many of the present ethical dilemmas might be resolved if we knew more about the true clinical effectiveness of PEG feeding in these difficult situations.

REFERENCES

1. Duncan HD, Silk DB. Diagnosis and treatment of malnutrition. *J R Coll Physicians* 1997; 31: 497–502.

2. Kim CH, Nelson DK. Venting percutaneous gastroscopy in the treatment of refractory idiopathic gastroparesis. *Gastrointest Endosc* 1998; 47: 67–70.

3. Gibson S, Wenig BL. Percutaneous endoscopic gastrostomy in the management of head and neck carcinoma. *Laryngoscope* 1992; 102: 977–980.

4. Daly J, Weintraub F, Shou J *et al.* Enteral nutrition during multimodality therapy in upper gastrointestinal cancer patients. *Ann Surg* 1995; 221: 327–338.

5. Klein S, Kinney J, Jeejeebhoy K *et al.* Nutrition support in clinical practice: review of published data and recommendations for future research directions. *J Parenteral Enteral Nutr* 1997; 21: 133–156.

6. McLave SA, Greene LM, Snider HL *et al.* Comparison of the safety of early enteral vs parenteral nutrition in mild acute pancreatitis. *J Parenteral Enteral Nutr* 1997; 21 :14–20.

7. Payne-James JJ. Enteral nutrition. *Eur J Gastroenterol Hepatol* 1995; 7: 501–506.

8. McWhirter J, Pennington C. Incidence and recognition of malnutrition in hospital. *Br Med J* 1994; 308: 945–948.

9. Moore F, Feliciano D, Andrassy R *et al.* Early enteral feeding, compared with parenteral, reduces postoperative septic complications. The result of a meta-analysis. *Ann Surg* 1992; 216: 172–183.

10. Wicks C, Gimson A, Vlavianos P *et al.* Assessment of the percutaneous endoscopic gastrostomy feeding tube as part of an integrated approach to enteral feeding. *Gut* 1992; 33: 613–616.

11. Gauderer M, Ponsky J, Izant R. Gastrostomy without laparotomy: a percutaneous endoscopic technique. *J Pediatr Surg* 1980; 15: 872–875.

12. Norton B, Homer-Ward M, Donnelly M *et al.* A randomised prospective comparison of percutaneous endoscopic gastrostomy and nasogastric tube feeding after acute dysphagic stroke. *Br Med J* 1996; 312: 13–16.

13. Park R, Allison M, Lang J *et al.* Randomised comparison of percutaneous endoscopic gastrostomy and nasogastric tube

feeding in patients with persisting neurological dysphagia. *Br Med J* 1992; 304: 1406–1409.

14. DeLegge MH, Duckworth F, McHenry L *et al.* Percutaneous endoscopic gastrojejunostomy: a dual center safety and efficacy trial. *J Parenteral Enteral Nutrition* 1995; 19: 239–243.

15. Kirby D, DeLegge M, Fleming CR. American Gastroenterological Association technical review on tube feeding for enteral nutrition. *Gastroenterology* 1995; 108: 1282–1301.

16. Shike M, Latkany L, Gerdes H, Bloch AS. Direct percutaneous endoscopic jejunostomies for enteral feeding. *Gastrointest Endosc* 1996; 44: 536–540.

17. Elliott L, Sheridan M, Denyer M, Chapman A. PEG – Is the E necessary? A comparison of percutaneous and endoscopic gastrostomy. *Clin Radiol* 1996; 51: 341–344.

18. Jain NK, Larson DE, Schroeder KW *et al.* Antibiotic prophylaxis for percutaneous endoscopic gastrostomy: a prospective, randomised, double-blind clinical trial. *Ann Intern Med* 1987; 107: 824–828.

19. Mahajan L, Oliva L, Wyllie R *et al.* The safety of gastrostomy in patients with Crohn's disease. *Am J Gastroenterol* 1997; 92: 985–988.

20. Sartori S, Trvisani L, Neilsen T *et al.* Percutaneous endoscopic gastrostomy placement using the pull-through techniques: is the second pass of the gastroscope necessary? *Endoscopy* 1996; 28: 686–688.

21. Mellinger J, Ponsky J. Percutaneous endoscopic gastrostomy: state of the art, 1998. *Endoscopy* 1998; 30: 126–132.

22. Larson DE, Burton DD, Schroeder KW, DiMagno EP. Percutaneous endoscopic gastrostomy: indications, success, complications and mortality in 314 consecutive patients. *Gastroenterology* 1987; 93: 48–52.

23. Tham T, Taitelbaum G, Carr-Locke D. Percutaneous endoscopic gastrostomies: are they being done for the right reasons? (Editorial) *Q J Med* 1997; 90: 495–496.

24. Schapiro GD, Edmundowicz SA. Complications of percutaneous endoscopic gastrostomy. *Gastrointest Endosc Clin North Am* 1996; 6: 409–422.

25. Rabeneck L, McCullough LB, Wray NP. Ethically justified, clinically comprehensive guidelines for percutaneous endoscopic gastrostomy tube placement. *Lancet* 1997; 349: 496–498.

26. Sturgess R, O'Toole P, McPhillips J *et al.* Percutaneous endoscopic gastrostomy: Evaluation of insertion by an endoscopy nurse practitioner. *Eur J Gastroenterol Hepatol* 1996; 8: 631–634.

27. Berrens R, Lang T, Muschweck H. Percutaneous endoscopic gastrostomy in children and adolescents. *J Pediatr Gastroenterol Nutr* 1997; 25: 487–491.

28. Goodhall L. Tube feeding dilemmas: can artificial nutrition and hydration be legally or ethically withheld or withdrawn? *J Advanced Nursing* 1997; 25: 217–222.

29. Kaw M, Sekas G. Long-term follow-up of consequences of percutaneous endoscopic gastrostomy in nursing home patients. *Dig Dis Sci* 1994; 39: 738–743.

30. Mazzini L, Corra T, Zaccala M *et al.* Percutaneous endoscopic gastrostomy and enteral nutrition in amylotrophic lateral sclerosis. *J Neurol* 1995; 242: 695–698.

Bile duct stones

9

D. Westaby

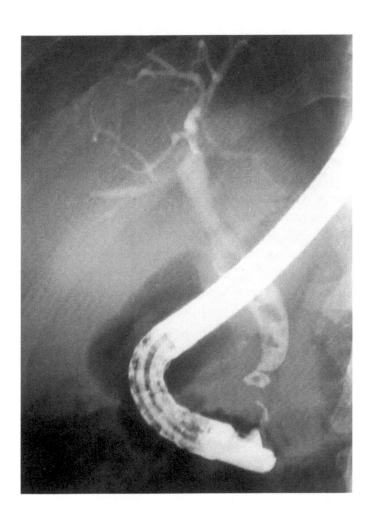

INTRODUCTION

Up until the early 1970s, the management of bile duct stones was entirely within the domain of surgery. In 1974, an endoscopic technique was described in which the sphincter of Oddi was cut to gain access to the common bile duct (CBD) [1,2]. This paved the way for endoscopic management of bile duct stones and stimulated a major industry producing equipment to facilitate this intervention. However, the role of the endoscopic management of bile duct stones has not been without controversy and has been further fuelled by the introduction of laparoscopic cholecystectomy (as well as laparoscopic common bile duct clearance).

PRESENTATION

The classical features of bile duct stones are biliary colic, fever and jaundice (Charcot's triad). However, in clinical practice this triad is present in only the minority of patients with bile duct stones. Abdominal pain is the most common symptom and has the typical features of biliary colic. This term encompasses an epigastric pain which is often of abrupt onset and radiates into the back and right shoulder with a crescendo characteristic. The pain may last for several hours and be of such severity as to produce sweating and agitation, as well as nausea and vomiting.

Presentation can be at any age, but gallstone prevalence increases with age (Fig. 9.1) and problems tend to present in the older age groups, though not exclusively so.

Jaundice is a variable accompaniment of bile duct stones. This is usually preceded by abdominal pain, although the interval between the two may be several days. A patient with bile duct stones may experience sequential episodes of pain, only some of these being accompanied by jaundice. In contrast to malignant bile duct obstruction the level of jaundice associated with bile duct stones characteristically tends to fluctuate.

Fever is only present in a minority of cases but is an extremely important symptom indicating biliary sepsis and associated septicaemia. The presence of biliary sepsis is an important adverse prognostic factor.

A small minority of patients with bile duct stones are discovered incidentally during imaging for gall bladder disease. Other ductular stones are discovered at the time of

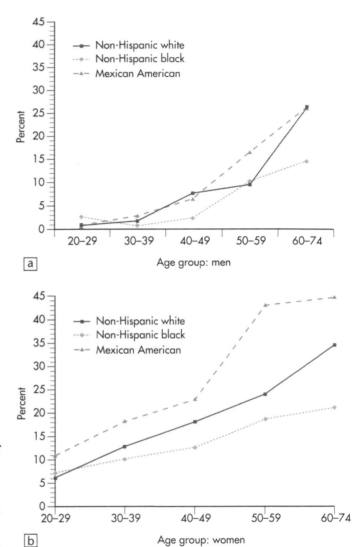

Figure 9.1. Rising prevalence of gallstones with age.

cholangiography as part of cholecystectomy. Abnormal liver function tests in an otherwise asymptomatic patient may on occasions lead to a diagnosis of bile duct stones.

DIAGNOSIS

Physical examination

If the patient is examined between episodes there may be no abnormal physical findings. During a symptomatic episode the patient may be jaundiced with a fever and associated tachycardia. There may be tenderness in the right upper quadrant varying from mild to extremely severe with rebound. In a minority of patients with bile duct stones and obstruction, the gall bladder may be palpable. More widespread abdominal tenderness extending from the epigastrium to the left upper quadrant, associated with distension, may indicate associated bile duct stone-related pancreatitis.

Laboratory tests

The full blood count is usually normal in the presence of uncomplicated bile duct stones. An elevated neutrophil count as well as raised inflammatory markers (erythrocyte sedimentation rate, ESR and C-reactive protein, CRP) are frequent accompaniments of cholangitis, the biochemical abnormalities reflecting the degree of bile duct obstruction. The hyperbilirubinaemia tends to be mild and often transient. Very high concentrations of bilirubin (>200 µmol/l) almost always reflect complete ductular obstruction. The serum alkaline phosphatase and gamma glutamyl transpeptidase are almost always elevated in relationship to the degree of hyperbilirubinaemia. Transaminase levels are usually mildly elevated, but with complete ductal obstruction may rise to 10 to 15 times the normal value. The serum amylase levels are often mildly elevated in the presence of acute bile duct obstruction, even in the absence of clinical evidence of gallstone-related pancreatitis.

The prothrombin time may be prolonged in the presence of protracted bile duct obstruction, reflecting decreased absorption of vitamin K. In the absence of established parenchymal liver disease the prolonged prothrombin time should respond to parenteral vitamin K.

Transabdominal ultrasound

Transabdominal ultrasound scanning is the initial imaging technique of choice for the investigation of possible bile duct stones, and in most cases the only imaging technique required. In the presence of jaundice the ultrasound is required to differentiate between extrahepatic biliary obstruction and hepatocellular causes. Bile duct obstruction is characterized by dilatation of intrahepatic biliary radicles. The distended biliary tree is best visualized in the longitudinal axis where the dilated ducts are seen to run parallel to the portal venous radicles, giving the appearance of a double channel. Acoustic enhancement beyond the dilated ducts is commonly observed. False-negative examinations may occur in early acute obstruction before the ducts have fully dilated. In such circumstances a repeat ultrasound scan one or two days later may identify dilated biliary radicles. It is easier to identify bile duct obstruction than to define the cause. The level of obstruction is identified by first defining the proximal CBD lying parallel and anterolateral to the portal vein. The duct is then followed distally to identify a change in duct calibre. The level at which this occurs can be identified in the majority of cases, but the cause of the obstruction will only be clearly shown in about one-half of the patients studied. Biliary stones are visualized as echogenic foci with a characteristic shadow seen distally; they may be found at any level in the biliary tree, but in general the more proximal they are lodged, the easier they are to identify. Unfortunately, the majority of stones causing obstruction are to be found in the distal CBD.

Ultrasound scanning will identify stones, if present, within the gall bladder in the vast majority of cases, although microcalculi may be missed. Biliary sludge is a term used to describe the layering of gall bladder bile with an echogenic zone separating out beneath echo-free bile. This has been shown to consist of precipitates of mucus, calcium bilirubinate and cholesterol crystals [3]. It is most frequently observed when there is biliary stasis. The description of sludge should not be confused with microcalculi, and while it may be a precursor of gallstones it should not be used as a marker that these are present.

In a patient presenting with jaundice, a finding of stones within the gall bladder is poorly predictive as to the cause of the obstruction. Asymptomatic gallstones are common (up to 15%) in patients in the cancer age group (65 years and older). Conversely, in 5–10% of patients with bile duct stones, calculi cannot be identified within the gall bladder.

Other imaging techniques (Fig. 9.2)

In a small proportion of patients, transabdominal ultrasound may leave sufficient doubt as to the diagnosis of bile duct stones to warrant alternative imaging before endoscopic retrograde cholangiopancreatography (ERCP). The choice of technique is influenced by local availability and expertise. Spiral computed tomography can be used to identify the common bile duct in the majority of cases. The definition can be enhanced by intravenous cholangiography using the newer (and safer) contrast agents such as meglumine iotroxate [4].

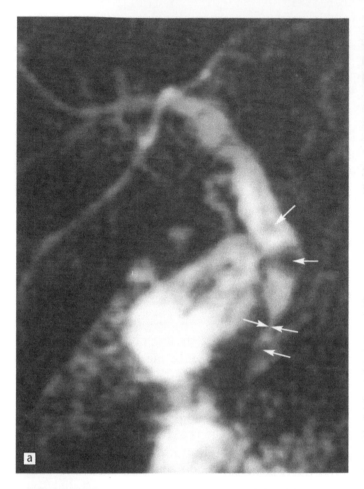

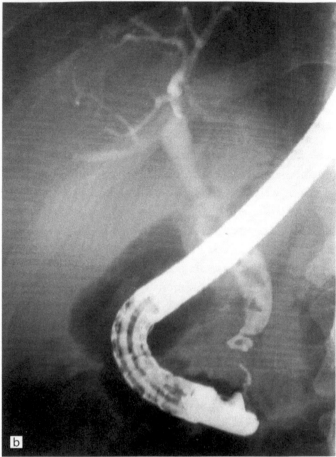

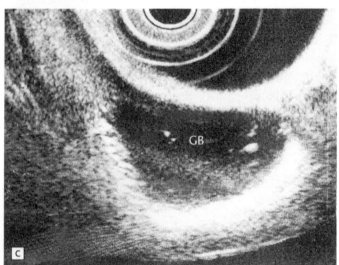

Figure 9.2. (a) An MRC in a patient with cystic fibrosis presenting with pain and jaundice. The cholangiogram shows evidence of a distal common bile duct stricture in close proximity to a small stone as well as a large stone in the mid-common bile duct (arrows). (b) An ERCP in the same patient showing identical biliary pathology as documented on the MRC. (c) Endoscopic ultrasound scan with the probe within duodenum (mid-upper margin of the figure) clearly demonstrating the gall bladder (GB) with multiple small stones within.

Magnetic resonance cholangiography (MRC)

MRC is an alternative non-invasive method for defining the biliary tree, and uses a fast spin-echo technique that can depict both the normal as well as the obstructed bile ducts. Recent studies evaluating MRC suggest similar diagnostic accuracy to endoscopic retrograde cholangiography (ERC) [5].

Endoscopic ultrasound (EUS)

Endoscopic ultrasound has enabled high-resolution imaging

of the common bile duct, gall bladder and pancreas. Recent comparisons with ERCP have shown EUS to be as sensitive for the detection of bile duct stones [6]. This imaging technique is particularly valuable for the detection of microcalculi which may easily be missed by transabdominal ultrasound as well as by ERC.

Endoscopic retrograde cholangiography (ERC)

ERC remains the 'gold standard' against which other imaging techniques are compared for the detection of bile duct stones. ERC also offers the opportunity of therapeutic intervention if ductal stones are identified. However, diagnostic ERC has a well-documented complication rate, with pancreatitis occurring in 1–2% of cases, although this is usually mild with less severe sequelae as compared with therapeutic intervention (see below). However, this complication rate compares very poorly with that of the non-invasive imaging techniques, as well as EUS described above. There is therefore an increasing emphasis upon identifying bile duct stones before ERC, and therefore reserving the latter as a therapeutic technique (see below).

Multifactorial approach to the detection of bile duct stones

In the patient presenting with jaundice, fever and dilated ducts on ultrasonography, early ERC would be a non-controversial intervention of choice to document the bile duct stones and to carry out endoscopic therapy. However, the introduction of laparoscopic techniques has led to a marked increase in the numbers of cholecystectomies being carried out, and hence a recurring need to assess whether bile duct stones are present. In the majority of cases the presence of bile duct stones would dictate preoperative ERC and duct clearance. With increasing expertise in laparoscopic bile duct exploration the preoperative detection of bile duct stones is also used as a guide to planning the operation.

A number of studies have investigated possible independent parameters predicting the presence or absence of bile duct stones [7–9]. Clinical, biochemical and ultrasonographic parameters have been evaluated, though no one single factor was able to predict CBD stones with both high sensitivity and specificity. Multivariate analysis has been used to identify independent predictors which, when used in combination, could provide a much higher sensitivity and specificity for the detection of bile duct stones. In one such study, four independent predictors were identified, namely age >55 years, elevated bilirubin (over

30 µmol/l), dilated CBD (>6 mm on ultrasonography), and suspected or detected bile duct stone on ultrasonography [10]. The probability of finding a CBD stone using this model ranged from 18% (no predictors present) to 94% (all four predictors present). Despite these encouraging figures, in clinical practice this model has proved of less value, with a much lower probability of finding a CBD stone with all parameters present. However, the negative predictive value when all the predictive factors were absent was validated, thus providing for a confident selection of a group of patients in whom precholecystectomy ERC is unnecessary.

Standard liver function tests have been disappointing in their predictive value as to the presence of CBD stones. In many cases this will reflect the passage of a calculus in the period following clinical presentation to the time of ERCP or cholecystectomy. Attempts have been made to monitor liver function tests in the period between presentation and contrast imaging of the bile duct [11]. This confirmed that a sustained elevation of liver function tests during this period is associated with a very high probability of finding a persisting bile duct stone. The converse was true in that a fall in liver function tests was associated with an absence of duct stones. To date, this information has not been incorporated into a wider predictive model.

In summary, standard clinical, biochemical and ultrasonographic findings have proved disappointing for predicting the presence of CBD stones, although a small group of patients with no predictive parameters present can be confidently excluded from any further biliary imaging. The remaining majority of patients with one or more risk factors present have on the whole been investigated by ERC. However, with the current trend towards avoiding unnecessary ERC (and its complications), other imaging techniques are being employed to confirm or exclude the presence of CBD stones. The techniques of spiral computed tomography (CT), MRC and EUS require additional expertise and incur extra cost. However, each of these techniques may provide additional predictive value and further reduce the need for ERC.

EVIDENCE-BASED MANAGEMENT OF BILE-DUCT STONES

Endoscopic and surgical approaches

The increasing popularity of endoscopic sphincterotomy

for the management of bile duct stones has been based upon a high success rate, as well as a complication rate considerably less than that seen with surgical bile duct exploration. This was particularly so with an elderly age group with co-morbid disease in whom surgical CBD exploration has been associated with an extremely high morbidity and mortality [12,13]. However, these comparisons (almost always historical) tend to overstate the complication rate associated with surgical CBD exploration. In a younger age group (<65 years of age) without co-morbid illness, the associated mortality rate would approximate to 1% – not dissimilar to that seen with endoscopic intervention. While most observers would support the contention that endoscopic intervention was considerably safer (than surgical CBD exploration) in the elderly age group, this has not gained support from one available controlled trial which showed no significant advantage for the endoscopic technique [14].

The era of laparoscopic cholecystectomy has introduced new variables into the equation as to the optimum management of CBD stones. In the early years after the technique's introduction, there were very few surgeons who would attempt bile duct clearance at the time of cholecystectomy. This therefore placed considerable emphasis on ERC and sphincterotomy for the management of patients with bile duct stones. With increasing experience, more operators are clearing the CBD either via the cystic duct, or by choledochotomy. However, such laparoscopic surgery requires considerable operating theatre time and has a high failure rate as well as an increased risk of complications. In such instances the endoscopist still has an important role to salvage the failures and manage some of the complications. To date, a single controlled trial has been reported comparing ERC and bile duct clearance followed by laparoscopic cholecystectomy, as compared with laparoscopic cholecystectomy and CBD exploration in a single procedure [15]. There were no significant differences between the outcome and complication rate of these two approaches, while the in-hospital time was somewhat shorter for patients undergoing laparoscopic CBD exploration. Despite this evidence in favour of laparoscopic CBD clearance, the majority of operators restrict the laparoscopic operation to cholecystectomy and cholangiography via the cystic duct. In such circumstances the investigational process described above is utilized to identify patients with CBD stones before the cholecystectomy and the ERC and sphincterotomy planned to be carried out within a few days of the operation. This therefore represents endoscopic decision-making being dictated by personal surgical preference. It is likely that a further move towards laparoscopic bile duct exploration and clearance will occur over the next few years.

ERCP and sphincterotomy

The endoscopic management of bile duct stones has been associated with a high success rate in duct clearance. In large series endoscopic sphincterotomy was successfully achieved in 90–95% of cases [16,17]. The failure to achieve sphincterotomy is almost always related to difficult gastroduodenal or biliary anatomy. In a further 5–10% of patients in whom the sphincterotomy is successful there will be a failure to clear the CBD of stones. The failure to clear the CBD following a successful sphincterotomy is usually the consequence of impacted or excessively large stones, but failure may also occur in the presence of a biliary stricture or other anatomical abnormality. A prerequisite of endoscopic intervention for bile duct stones is the establishment of adequate biliary drainage at the end of the procedure. This can be adequately achieved by the placement of either a nasobiliary tube or a pig-tail endoprosthesis. The use of the former has the advantage of easy access to further cholangiography, as well as flushing of the duct if small stones or fragments are present. Unfortunately, there is a major propensity for such tubes to become displaced. The insertion of pigtail endoprostheses has been associated with excellent biliary drainage with only a very small risk of displacement and has now become the most widely used technique [18].

Sphincter of Oddi balloon dilatation ('sphincteroplasty')

The complication rate associated with sphincterotomy (see below) has led to a search for alternative methods to gain access to the CBD. For the management of small stones there are reports of balloon and basket clearance of the duct in the presence of an intact sphincter [19]. This can be aided by the use of glyceryl trinitrate spray to relax the sphincter muscle. Because of the risks of stone impaction and papillary trauma, this technique should be restricted to small stones (2–3 mm). An alternative approach has been the use of balloon dilatation of the sphincter of Oddi using coaxially placed balloons expanding to 8 or 10 mm [20]. It was theorized that this technique might reduce the risks of haemorrhage and perforation that have been observed with sphincterotomy. At least some instances of sphincterotomy-induced pancreatitis have been attributed to thermal energy, and it was hoped that balloon dilatation might offer a safer alternative. There is evidence to show that sphincter of Oddi function returns to normal within a few weeks of balloon dilatation, and this might have important implications for the prevention of possible long-term complications of sphincterotomy (see below) [21].

In initial uncontrolled series, balloon dilatation of the sphincter of Oddi was shown to provide good access to the CBD and allow stone clearance in approximately 80% of cases, with a complication rate similar to that of sphincterotomy [20]. The efficacy was further confirmed in a large controlled trial comparing balloon dilatation with standard sphincterotomy [22]. Complication rates of both techniques were similar. The major disadvantage associated with balloon dilatation was the size of stone that could be safely removed from the bile duct. Standard sphincterotomy allowed stones in excess of 1 cm diameter to be extracted, but this was limited to 8–10 mm following balloon dilatation. There was therefore an increased requirement for lithotripsy in those undergoing balloon dilatation. Anecdotal concerns have been expressed about the risks of pancreatitis with sphincter of Oddi balloon dilatation, but this appears to be adequately refuted in the studies reported. While further controlled data would help fully to establish the role for sphincter of Oddi balloon dilatation, it might be suggested that this technique would be the ideal approach to the younger age group of patients with small bile duct stones who might otherwise be exposed to the potential complications of a long-term sphincterotomy (see below).

SPECIAL SITUATIONS

The difficult bile duct stone

In experienced hands the CBD will be cleared of stones in 80–85% of cases, without the need to resort to other techniques beyond sphincterotomy and basket or balloon extraction. However, in the residual 15–20% of patients additional techniques may be required. The difficult cases are usually secondary to large or impacted stones. Anatomical difficulties such as a papilla within a large diverticulum or a bile duct stricture may also present difficulties in stone extraction.

The presence of an impacted stone is frequently suggested by a bulbous papillary fold representing the stone within the intramural segment of the distal common bile duct. The downward distortion of the ampullary access may prevent cannulation by the standard technique. In such circumstances, a needle knife incision over the stone may allow retrieval and access to the CBD.

The size of stone that can be retrieved from the CBD is dependent upon the size of the sphincterotomy. This in turn is determined by the length of the intramural segment of the CBD. This is variable, but usually allows a cut up to 1.25–1.5 cm. However, any stone in excess of 1 cm in diameter may cause difficulties in retrieval. It is therefore essential that the size of stone within the CBD should be carefully assessed and matched to the size of the sphincterotomy before retrieval is attempted. It is wise to err on the side of caution and to avoid the risk of stone and basket impaction. When the stone is considered too large for the size of the sphincterotomy available, then a means of stone fragmentation should be considered.

Mechanical lithotripsy involves initial basket entrapment of the stone followed by crushing against the metal sleeve of the device. This is a crude procedure but in expert hands has facilitated bile duct clearance in up to 90% of cases treated [23]. Alternative means of stone fragmentation are much more difficult to use and are considerably more expensive. These include both laser and electrohydraulic stone fragmentation [24,25]. For these techniques to be both safe and effective they are optimally applied under direct cholangioscopic vision using the so-called 'mother and baby' endoscope. Alternative approaches avoiding cholangioscopy have involved positioning the laser or electrohydraulic probe using either a basket or balloon technique. This procedure has been further refined by laser devices that will only 'fire' when in direct contact with the stone, hence reducing the risk of CBD trauma [26].

Dissolution therapy
Chemical dissolution of bile duct stones has been attempted by instillation of mono-octanoin [27] and methyl-tert-butyl-ether (MTBE) [28]. These agents are specifically aimed at dissolving the cholesterol content of biliary stones.

However, most series reporting this technique have been disappointing with very low dissolution levels and high risk of complications including neurological side effects, elevation of liver enzymes as well as duodenitis.

Extracorporeal shock-wave lithotripsy (ESWL)

ESWL has also been used for the management of large CBD stones. Fragmentation may be directed either by ultrasound or radiological methods, and it may be necessary for an indwelling nasobiliary tube to allow contrast injection to delineate the stone. Repeated sessions may be required to achieve adequate fragmentation which will also be matched by the need for repeated ERC and duct clearance. Duct clearance rates of up to 90% have been achieved using this approach [29].

Endoprostheses

The insertion of a pig-tail endoprosthesis has been widely used for the immediate management of patients with difficult and in particular large bile duct stones (see above). This approach has also been adapted for the long-term management of stones in the elderly age group particularly with associated co-morbid disease. The aim of this approach was to reduce the procedural time as well as the degree of instrumentation required. Evidence from uncontrolled and controlled studies have confirmed the efficacy of pigtail stents in establishing the initial bile duct drainage. However, within a matter of 3–4 months almost 30% of patients can be expected to re-present with cholangitis following occlusion of the stent and accumulation of CBD debris [18]. As a consequence, this technique should – in almost all circumstances – be limited to the immediate bile duct drainage, after which definitive management should be undertaken.

Summary

In any centre undertaking endoscopic bile duct therapy an algorithm should be defined for the management of this small but significant group of patients with large bile duct stones. In the vast majority of centres the only additional technique that will be required is mechanical lithotripsy. In technically difficult situations such as those with multiple stones, the approach may be more safely undertaken as two or more procedures, leaving a pigtail endoprosthesis to maintain drainage. In the small number of failures from this approach, referral to a highly specialized centre may be indicated; alternatively, if the patient is otherwise well, surgical bile duct exploration remains an important alternative.

Anatomical difficulties

Diverticula

Access to the CBD may be impaired by a number of anatomical abnormalities. The most frequently encountered of these is a periampullary diverticulum which is present in approximately 12% of patients undergoing ERC, and which has a recognized statistical relationship with underlying bile duct stones. The papilla is usually found on the lateral lip of the diverticulum but may be more deeply situated, creating difficulties with selective cannulation and limiting the ability of subsequent sphincterotomy. Despite these potential problems, the presence of a diverticulum has only a modest effect upon the success rate of cannulation and sphincterotomy [29].

Gastrectomy

Previous gastric surgery may have a major effect upon the orientation of the papilla. This is particularly so in case of the Bilroth II anastomosis where the orientation of the papilla is entirely reversed. If a long afferent loop was created at the time of gastrectomy then it may not be possible to reach the papilla. The use of a colonoscope has been reported to reach the papilla in such circumstances [30].

In those cases in which cannulation of the papilla cannot be achieved, an alternative approach is to pass a guidewire percutaneously through into the duodenum; this can then be retrieved by the endoscopist. A sphincterotome can then be passed over this guidewire to allow sphincterotomy and bile duct access (combined technique).

Intrahepatic stones

Stones within the common hepatic and intrahepatic ducts may complicate any condition impeding bile drainage. In Asia, they are a serious consequence of the infective condition cholangiohepatitis or recurrent pyogenic cholangitis.

Clearance of the biliary tree – particularly when the stones are proximal to the common hepatic duct – may be extremely difficult using the endoscopic approach. Stone fragmentation using ESWL has been reported, with good results. An alternative approach has involved percutaneous hepatic cholangiography and lithotripsy of the intrahepatic stones [31]. This percutaneous technique has proved beneficial for large stones found proximal to a tight stricture.

PRACTICAL ASPECTS

Preliminaries

Before carrying out any endoscopic intervention for bile duct stones it is essential to have a full medical assessment available. This should extend beyond the biliary problem and include all co-morbid illnesses. All current and recent medication should be fully documented. The results of a prothrombin time and platelet count carried out in the previous 24 h should also be available.

Discussions aimed towards consent should be carried out at least 24 h before the procedure if at all possible. There should be a full discussion as to the aims and risks of the procedure and possible alternatives that may become necessary as a consequence of failure.

Venous access is obtained using an intravenous cannula. It is now standard practice for all patients undergoing intravenous sedation to receive continuous nasal oxygen at 2–4 l/min, as well as having a pulse oximeter in position. For patients with cardiopulmonary disease, continuous ECG monitoring should be used. Prophylactic antibiotics have been widely used, though recent evidence suggests that they are not necessary in the majority of patients [32]. However, antibiotics should be used in patients with preceding biliary sepsis and in all cases in which adequate bile duct drainage has not been obtained at the end of the procedure.

Standard sphincterotomy (Fig. 9.3)

The technical aspects of sphincterotomy are based upon the

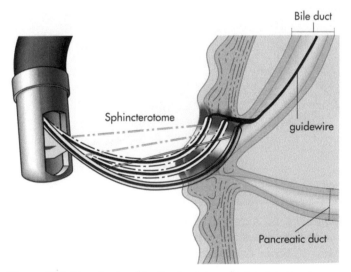

Figure 9.3. Standard sphincterotomy carried out over an insulated guidewire.

initial observation of the papilla, and particularly the length of the intramural segment. The diagnostic cholangiogram provides further important information as to the number, location and size of any ductal stones. The overinjection of contrast during this initial cholangiogram may mask the presence of small calculi and may also push proximal calculi into the intrahepatic ducts, causing subsequent difficulty in stone extraction. These problems may be overcome by taking sequential radiographs during the early filling phase.

There is a very extensive choice of equipment that has been developed for the purpose of sphincterotomy. The operator is advised to become experienced with a small selection of sphincterotomes sufficient to achieve bile duct access in the majority of situations encountered. The most commonly used sphincterotomes are pull-type bow string design. The main differences in the available designs are the length of the exposed cutting wire (20–30 mm), and the length of the leading cannula extending beyond the cutting wire, as well as the ability to be passed over a guidewire. With the availability of insulated guidewires it has now become possible to carry out sphincterotomy with a guidewire in position. This provides considerable stability for the procedure and avoids inadvertent loss of position in cases in which cannulation of the CBD has been difficult. The author would consider that the use of an *in-situ* guidewire is now the standard approach to sphincterotomy. This may be passed through the sphincterotome at the time of cannulation, or the sphincterotome can be passed over a wire that has been placed at the time of diagnostic cannulation (the author's preference).

A wide variety of electrosurgical units have been designed to generate the current necessary for sphincterotomy. These offer a pure cutting, pure coagulation and blended current modes. For the purposes of sphincterotomy, a waveform is restricted to either pure cut or blended current mode. The theoretical advantages and disadvantages of these different current modes has not been evaluated in formal trial. It has been suggested that pure cutting current reduces the risk of thermal damage to the pancreatic duct and hence lowers the risk of pancreatitis. However, the risks of papillary bleeding may be enhanced. In contrast, blended current may increase the risk of thermal injury but reduce the risk of bleeding. The author has a personal preference for the pure cutting current. There is a newly developed electrosurgical generator which automatically alternates between pure cutting and coagulation current as the procedure progresses. The theoretical advantages are the prevention of over-rapid cutting of the sphincter which might produce either bleeding or perforation.

Having obtained guidewire access to the CBD, the sphincterotome is advanced over this wire and a final fluoroscopic confirmation of position is obtained. The guidewire is carefully kept in position in the biliary tree throughout the procedure, which requires careful co-operation between the endoscopist and attending staff. The cutting wire of the sphincterotome is then positioned between the 11 o'clock and 1 o'clock positions on the papilla. No compromise should be sought as to this careful positioning so as to avoid inadvertent damage to the pancreatic duct. To optimize the cut, only a short length of wire should be in contact with the sphincter mucosa. This is achieved by inserting only a short length of the wire within the papilla, leaving at least two-thirds of the 20- or 30-mm wire within the duodenal lumen. The wire is kept in contact with the sphincter by gently bowing the sphincterotome as well as maintaining elevation on the bridge. This technique provides adequate diathermy density to achieve the cut, without risking excessive thermal damage to the pancreatic duct. As the cut progresses, further shortening of the wire by bowing is usually required and may extend to 35–50% of its original length. A recent technical development has been the insulation of the proximal half of the cutting wire which prevents placing too much of the cutting wire within the sphincter and also stops inadvertent shorting of the proximal end of the wire against the endoscope.

The length of the incision depends upon the length of the intramural segment and the size of the stone. There is no justification for carrying out a large sphincterotomy for small stones. However, such judgements may be extremely difficult to make, particularly for the inexperienced. Having defined the size of the intraductal stones the size of the sphincterotomy may be more formally assessed by the withdrawal of an inflated balloon or partially bowed sphincterotomy knife. In the case of large stones (>1.5 cm), lithotripsy should be considered rather than risk impacted stones and a trapped basket. In most circumstances a 1.5 cm sphincterotomy will be the largest required. Anatomical landmarks are essential guides for the larger sphincterotomy. The landmarks include the upper extent of the papilla itself, the bulging of the intramural bile duct, and the proximal transverse hooding fold. Using the extent of the papilla alone as the landmark is the safest of options, but may limit the extent of the cut in patients with larger stones. The presence of a bulging intramural segment secondary to an impacted stones allows a cut to be safely carried out along the full length.

Pre-cut sphincterotomy (Fig. 9.4)

Standard sphincterotomy is unsuccessful in 5–10% of cases. This is almost always related to difficult cannulation of the CBD, and may be the result of acute angulation of the distal CBD, an impacted stone, periampullary

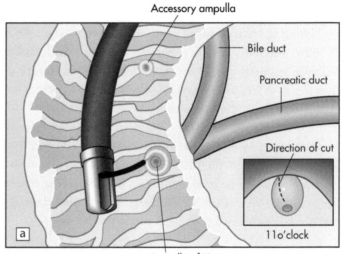

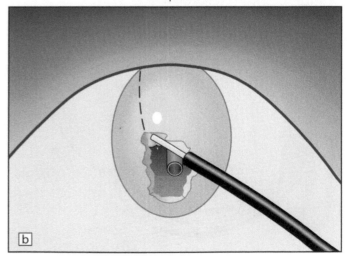

Figure 9.4. (a) A diagrammatic representation of pre-cut needle knife technique to gain access to the common bile duct. (b) Shows the direction of cut in an 11 o'clock position thus avoiding damage to the pancreatic duct.

diverticulum or previous gastroduodenal surgery. Two techniques of direct cutting have been developed to gain access to the CBD under such circumstances.

- The pre-cut sphincterotome. This is based upon the standard bowing wire technique described above. However, the leading catheter of the sphincterotomy is reduced to 1 or 2 mm; placing the tip of the sphincterotome within the papillary orifice will then bring the tip of the wire into contact with the roof of the papilla. The wire is then moved upwards in the direction 11–1 o'clock, applying cutting or blended current in small quanta and unroofing the papilla over about 5 mm to expose the CBD. This should then allow selective cannulation and standard sphincterotomy to be carried out. The technique may be technically difficult – particularly maintaining the correct orientation of the cut. The repeated application of current in a small area without adequate progression of the cut may produce local oedema and thermal trauma, both of which increase the risk of pancreatitis.
- The needle knife. This is the alternative approach to pre-cut sphincterotomy. The sphincterotome is of simple construction, with a 5-mm straight section of diathermy wire which is retractable within a Teflon catheter. The exposed wire is inserted into the papillary orifice, and the current applied to carry out the cut directed in the 11 to 1 o'clock position to expose the bile duct. The procedure needs very careful control to avoid inadvertent damage to the pancreatic duct or perforation of the duodenum. This can be best achieved by initial practice movements in the required direction before actually applying the cutting current. In the presence of a dilated papillary fold – and particularly when there is an impacted stone – the needle knife can be inserted directly into the intramural portion of the bile duct. The cut can then be extended upwards or downwards to achieve more open access.

Both the pre-cut sphincterotome and needle knife are techniques that can improve the success rate of CBD access in those patients in whom standard techniques have failed. However, they do require considerable expertise and have been associated with increased complication rates. Even in experienced hands they are restricted to cases in which therapeutic intervention is almost certainly indicated. Only highly experienced operators would consider using these techniques to gain access to the CBD for diagnostic purposes only. While there are no controlled studies comparing the two techniques described, most operators (including the author) would prefer the needle knife pre-cut as a technically easier technique with no clear evidence of a higher complication rate.

Balloon dilatation of the sphincter of Oddi (Fig. 9.5)

Balloon dilatation of the sphincter of Oddi can be considered the least demanding of the techniques to gain access to the CBD. The procedure is dependent upon initial guidewire cannulation of the CBD, allowing coaxial placement of a dilating balloon over the guidewire. Most modern dilating balloons have clear radio-opaque markers to delineate the proximal and distal extent, allowing accurate placement of the dilating segment across the sphincter of Oddi. The mid-point of the balloon should be approximated to the level of the sphincter; this will then prevent the migration of the balloon either proximally or intraduodenally when inflation occurs. Balloons of either 8 or 10 mm diameter have been used, depending upon the size of the stone to be extracted. It is the author's experience that the diameter of the balloon used will allow extraction of a stone 1–2 mm less in diameter. This therefore represents a major limitation in the size of stone that can be negotiated without the use of a lithotripsy technique. There has been no systematic attempt to use dilating balloons of a diameter greater than 10 mm based upon fears of complication, particularly that of pancreatitis. The presence of stones within the distal CBD, or impacted stones, presents the risk that balloon dilatation in contact with the stones might cause CBD rupture. This remains a theoretical risk, but in the author's experience has seldom precluded satisfactory dilatation of the sphincter without complication. In most circumstances the stones are moved proximally as the balloon is advanced over the guidewire. The time period over which the balloon is inflated within the sphincter has not been systemically studied. There has been some speculation that obstruction of the pancreatic sphincter during the balloon inflation is responsible for cases of post-procedural pancreatitis. As such, it may be wise to restrict the time period to no more than 30 s, though this could be repeated with a short period of deflation, thus allowing the pancreatic duct to drain.

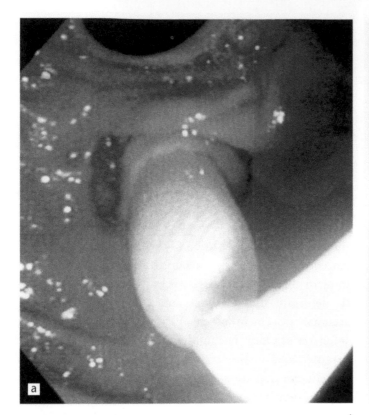

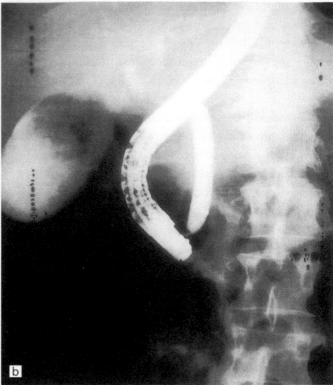

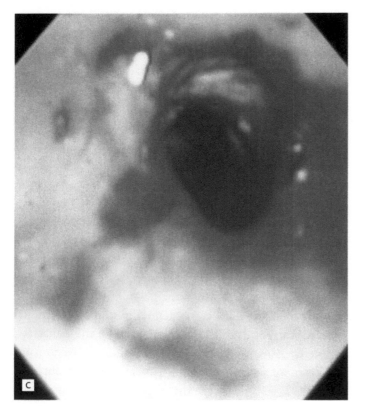

Figure 9.5. A 10 mm coaxial balloon has been placed over a guidewire and inflated across the sphincter of Oddi producing good access to the distal common bile duct.

Stone retrieval

Baskets (Fig. 9.6)

The standard approach to stone extraction following access to the bile duct (either by sphincterotomy or balloon dilatation) involves the use of a Dormia basket or stone extraction balloon. Using either or both of these techniques, the bile duct can be cleared of stones in 85–90% of cases. Baskets are available in several different sizes with four, six or eight wire strands of squared or spiral configuration. Newer designs incorporate nitenol as a so-called 'smart metal' with an enhanced ability to retain its shape despite distortion within the duct. The size and configuration of the basket to be used is dictated by the number and size of stones within the duct. The basket within its sheath is advanced beyond the stones and then opened to allow the basket to take shape. In cases in which the stone is impacted within the duct, a basket may be passed over a guidewire to facilitate access proximal to the stone. The basket is then withdrawn, the aim being to capture the stone within. Continual fine adjustments both of the basket and angulation of the endoscope may be necessary to achieve this entrapment. Only when the stone is clearly positioned within the distal end of the basket

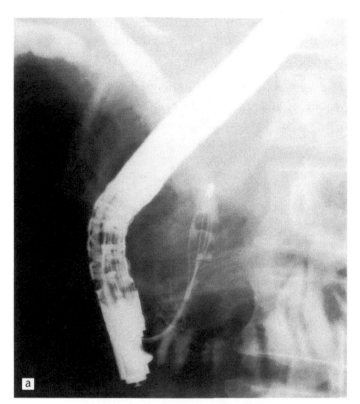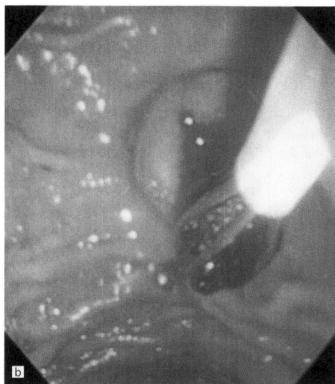

Figure 9.6. (a) Two stones trapped within a Dormia basket. (b) The stones are withdrawn into the duodenal lumen.

should closure be carried out and a slow withdrawal from the duct is maintained. If the size of the sphincterotomy has been carefully planned with regard to the size of the stone, withdrawal of the basket should not require excessive force. Any force that is applied should be in a distal (downward) direction, thereby avoiding damage to the roof of the papilla. If there are multiple stones, every attempt should be made to retrieve the most distal stone first thereby avoiding the risk of multiple stone impaction.

The use of the Dormia basket is the preferred method for the removal of the majority of stones encountered. It may however fail to capture small stones and has no role in the management of microcalculi.

Balloons (Fig. 9.7)
Balloon catheters for stone extraction are available in various sizes allowing a choice of catheter in relationship to the size of the bile duct. The balloon catheter can be advanced into the bile duct either with or without the prior placement of a guidewire. The advantages of a guidewire are the ability to gain repeated access to the duct, particularly in difficult complicated cases. The catheter is advanced beyond the stone and then inflated to a diameter

which fills the bile duct at that level. This is then slowly withdrawn with the stone passing through the sphincterotomy under the traction of the balloon catheter. One of the disadvantages of this technique is the ability of stones to roll proximally around the balloon and into the proximal duct. Repeated withdrawals of the balloon catheter under such circumstances may give a false impression that the duct is clear. It is important that a cholangiogram be obtained finally to confirm duct clearance before ending the procedure. The main advantage of the balloon catheter is its ability to sweep from the bile duct any small stones and fragments which would be missed by a standard basket technique.

The optimum approach to stone retrieval combines both the above approaches. Stones which are >0.5 cm in diameter should be retrieved using the basket technique leaving the balloon catheter for the management of smaller fragments or microcalculi. It is a useful manoeuvre to complete duct clearance with a basket and then to use a balloon for one or two bile duct sweeps to be absolutely sure that all fragments have been removed. It is also convenient to carry out a balloon occlusion cholangiogram at the end of the procedure so that contrast is injected into the bile duct as the inflated balloon is withdrawn. This is a sensitive way of excluding any residual stones.

Lithotripsy (Fig. 9.8)

The majority of bile duct stones >1.5 cm in diameter will require fragmentation before duct clearance. Stones of

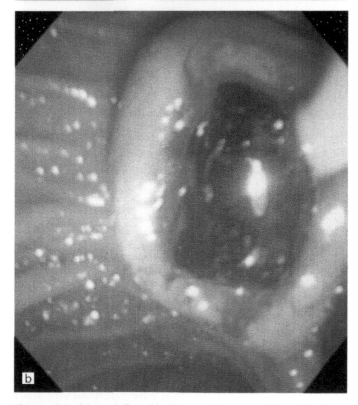

Figure 9.7. (a) An inflated balloon catheter positioned in the common hepatic duct with a stone distal to this. (b) This was subsequently withdrawn in to the duodenum.

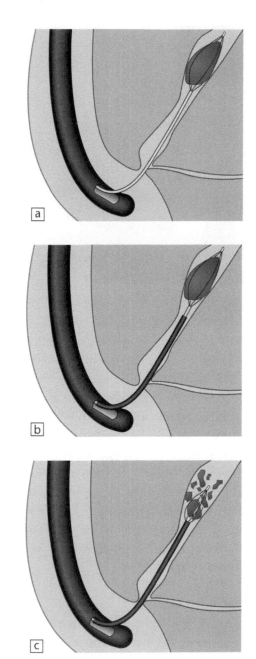

Figure 9.8. A diagrammatic representation of mechanical lithotripsy. This shows the through-the-scope technique. The stone is initially entrapped within the basket and a stiff metal outer sheath is then advanced to the level of the stone and using a winding device this is fragmented against the tip of the metal sheath.

smaller calibre may also need fragmentation in such circumstances as the presence of a bile duct stricture or a non-dilated CBD. On occasion, large stones that have formed within the duct may be removed without litho-tripsy as they are friable and will crumble when being withdrawn within a standard Dormia basket. They can then be easily cleared from the duct with a combination of standard balloon and basket techniques.

In the vast majority of centres carrying out this type of work the only available technique for stone fragmentation is that of mechanical lithotripsy. Only this technique will be discussed from the practical standpoint, although laser and electrohydraulic lithotripsy are mentioned in general terms above. There are two types of lithotripter in common use. The most popular of these is the through-the-endoscope lithotripter; the second approach is using an outside-the-endoscope technique in which lithotripsy takes place after the endoscope has been withdrawn.

Through-the-scope lithotripsy

The through-the-endoscope lithotripter is assembled from its four components, including the wire basket itself, a Teflon sheath, a flexible metal sheath, and a handle. The assembled unit is advanced through the endoscope with the Teflon sheath and basket within advanced ahead of the metal sheath. The Teflon catheter is then used to cannulate the CBD, after which the basket is advanced out of the Teflon sheath to take up its shape within the CBD. The basket is then manipulated within the CBD to entrap the stone. This is best achieved by rapid to-and-fro movement, with care being taken to fully entrap the stone and optimize the chances of subsequent fragmentation. The Teflon catheter is then withdrawn within the metal sheath such that the wires of the basket are in contact with the reinforced tip of the metal sheath. The winding device on the handle is then slowly turned until the stone is seen to fragment. This technique is best achieved with the endoscope in the short position so that the maximum tension can be applied via the basket wires to the stone. The final clearance of the duct is most conveniently achieved by using standard basket or balloon techniques, rather than persevering with the rather bulky lithotripter as the means of withdrawal.

Outside-the-scope lithotripsy

The outside-the-scope technique requires initial entrap-ment of the stone with a purpose-designed basket; this allows detachment of the wires at the basket's proximal end so that the endoscope can be withdrawn, as well as the outer Teflon sheath. A metallic coil spring sheath is then advanced over the basket wire using a coaxial approach, with gentle tension being maintained upon the basket wire itself. The metal sheath is visualized into position under X-ray screening, and when it is closely in apposition to the stone both the metal sheath and basket wires are secured in their independent positions on the crushing handle. Care should be taken to avoid advancing the metal sheath into the CBD, as subsequent crushing will lead to straightening of the sheath and potential damage to the CBD. Gentle sustained traction is then applied to the system using the crushing handle, until fragmentation occurs. It is then necessary to remove the lithotripter and to continue the endoscopic technique to clear the stone fragments by standard balloon or basket methods. The extra instru-mentation of the outside-the-scope technique has made it less popular than the through-the-scope lithotripter. However, it is an extremely valuable technique for the management of an impacted stone and basket after failed Dormia basket extraction. The practicalities are similar to those described above although in this setting the basket wires have to be cut at their proximal end to allow the Teflon sheath to be removed and the endoscope to be withdrawn. In most circumstances this will allow fragmen-tation of the impacted stone, although the wires in a standard Dormia basket may occasionally break and are a potential source of trauma.

SPECIAL CASES

Billroth II gastrectomy (Fig. 9.9)

Billroth II gastrectomy considerably increases the potential difficulties of managing bile duct stones. The afferent limb associated with this gastrectomy may be long and hence intubation to the level of the papilla may be either difficult or impossible. The endoscopic orientation of the papilla is reversed after this operation such that the bile duct is to be found in the 6 o'clock position. The sphincterotomy there-fore needs to be orientated in this direction. Specialized sphincterotomes have been designed for this purpose. The procedure can be achieved using either the side-viewing or end-viewing endoscope. However it is extremely important

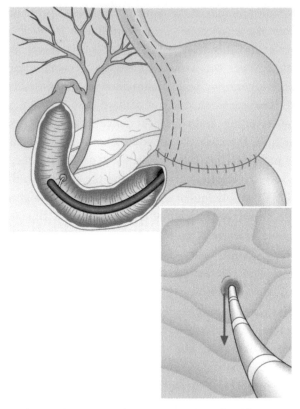

Figure 9.9. A diagrammatic representation of sphincterotomy in the presence of a Billroth II gastrectomy. In these circumstances orientation of the papilla is reversed requiring sphincterotomy in the direction of the 6 o'clock position. This is achieved by a specialized sphincterotome.

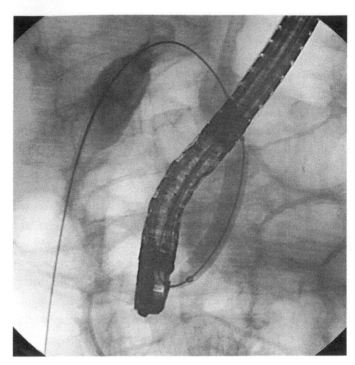

Figure 9.10. An unusual rendezvous procedure in a patient with both cholangitis and cholecystitis. Endoscopic access was initially prevented by the position of the papilla within a large diverticulum. The decision was made to drain both the gall bladder and biliary tree simultaneously and guidewire access to the common bile duct was via the gall bladder and cystic duct. Balloon dilatation of the sphincter of Oddi as part of the rendezvous procedure allowed the common bile duct to be clear.

to be fully conversant with the technique and the equipment used prior to attempting these cases. An alternative has been to use a needle knife papillotome to gain access to the CBD. This is most safely achieved by the prior placement of a 7 French straight endoprosthesis. An alternative approach to gain access to the CBD is by balloon dilatation of the sphincter of Oddi using a coaxial technique after the initial placement of a guidewire.

'Rendezvous' procedure (Fig. 9.10)

Failure to gain access to the bile duct occurs in approximately 5% of cases. This is most likely to occur in the presence of anatomical abnormalities such as diverticulae or previous gastrectomy. In such cases the combined procedure may provide a means of bile duct access. By the percutaneous route a guidewire is passed into the intrahepatic ducts and guided down into the duo-

denum. At this level the guidewire can be captured using either a snare or Dormia basket and then withdrawn perorally. The side-viewing endoscope is then passed over this guidewire (which needs to be of double length, 450–500 cm) until the papilla is visualized. It is then possible to pass a wire-guided sphincterotome through the endoscope and across the papilla. To facilitate this a certain amount of tension is maintained on both ends of the guidewire and it is therefore important to have an introducing catheter in place across the liver and to the level of the papilla to stop wire related laceration. This introducing catheter is slowly withdrawn as the sphincterotome is advanced into the common bile duct. The use of an insulated wire will allow the sphincterotomy to be carried out without the wire being withdrawn. An alternative approach would be the passage of a dilating balloon across the papilla to carry out balloon dilatation of the sphincter of Oddi.

Bile duct stone management in children

Bile duct stones are increasingly identified in children and adolescents. In many instances they are secondary to other disease processes such as haemolytic anaemia or cystic fibrosis. The practicalities of managing bile duct stones in children is not dissimilar from that of the adult population. In the large majority of cases this is best undertaken with general anaesthesia. Standard adult equipment can be utilized in the vast majority of children encountered. For the management of bile duct stones the 10 mm diameter endoscope with a 2.8 mm channel will provide all the therapeutic options required. Although this endoscope has been used in children down to the perinatal period, the author would have concerns about the risk of perforation. Specialized paediatric ERCP endoscopes have been developed and at a diameter of 7 mm provide considerably more room for manouvre. However ERCP in infants should be strictly within the realms of experts in the field.

Management of patients with an increased risk of haemorrhage

Assessment of the prothrombin time and platelet count is an essential prerequisite of bile duct stone management. In patients with cholestasis the prothrombin time may be prolonged secondary to vitamin K deficiency and this should respond within a few hours following intravenous supplements. In patients with established chronic liver disease there may be a defect in synthetic function which will not respond to vitamin K. In such circumstances fresh-frozen plasma may be required to cover the procedure although the author would only request this if the INR was more than 1.5 seconds. A further problem seen in patients with established chronic liver disease is the potential for variceal bleeding at the time of sphincterotomy or balloon dilatation of the sphincter of Oddi. There is evidence that varices may be found at the level of the papilla and may surround the distal common bile duct. As these vessels are usually not visible within the duodenum, there are few precautions that can be built into the procedure. It is the author's experience that major bleeding is very rarely a problem in such circumstances but balloon dilatation of the sphincter of Oddi may represent a safer alternative to sphincterotomy. Care should be taken not to traumatize the common bile duct in patients with portal hypertension, as choledochal varices found intramurally within the common bile duct may be ruptured and cause major bleeding.

Patients with established renal failure are at increased risk of bleeding during invasive procedures and this has been attributed largely to poor platelet function. It is our practice in patients with established renal impairment to give arginine vasopressin (DD-AVP) in a dosage of 0.04 μg/kg as a single bolus approximately 4 hours before the procedure. Formal haematological advice should be sought in patients with conditions such as haemophilia or von Willebrand's disease.

It is not an uncommon situation to find patients with bile duct stones who are also on anticoagulation for an associated medical condition. It is important to have a defined protocol for dealing with such patients. In the presence of gallstone pancreatitis or cholangitis it may be necessary to reverse the anticoagulation as an emergency using a combination of fresh-frozen plasma and vitamin K. For those patients in whom the anticoagulation is considered essential (such as those with prosthetic heart valves), titrated doses of heparin can be used intravenously to sustain anticoagulation over the minimum period required to achieve the procedure and confirm that there are no overt complications. Full anticoagulation can then be re-established initially with heparin and then with oral anticoagulants. An elective procedure should be planned based upon the observed necessity for continuous coagulation. In many cases this can be stopped over a period of a few days without excess risk of thrombo-embolic phenomena. Wherever possible, advice should be obtained from the physicians who initiated the anticoagulation. When continuous anticoagulation is considered necessary we would stop the oral anti-coagulants with two clear days prior to the procedure. On those two days the patient would receive a single sub-cutaneous injection of a low molecular weight heparin. On the evening before the procedure intravenous heparin would be started in full doses which would then be stopped approximately 2 hours before the procedure. The prothrombin time would be assessed the day before the procedure and on the morning of the procedure with the hope that the INR would be 1.5 s or less. Full doses of heparin would be restarted after the procedure when it is fully established that there are no complications. Oral anticoagulation could then be re-started the same evening.

COMPLICATIONS

Complications of endoscopic intervention for bile duct stones can be divided into early and late, the commonly used dividing point being 30 days post procedure. The literature addressing the problems of complications is difficult to interpret because of varying definitions of adverse events. A more objective grading system of complications and their severity followed on from a consensus conference in 1990 [33]. For each complication three categories of mild, moderate and severe were defined (Table 9.1). This has allowed a more objective means of comparing complications between different series and trials.

Acute pancreatitis

Acute pancreatitis occurs in approximately 3–5% of patients following sphincterotomy. In the majority of cases this is mild and self limiting, only a few extra days in hospital are required. However, there are occasional severe cases which may lead to extensive pancreatic necrosis and associated complications including pseudocyst, abscess formation and overwhelming sepsis. The overall mortality attributable to sphincterotomy-induced pancreatitis is approximately 0.5%. An important risk factor for post- procedural pancreatitis is suspected sphincter of Oddi dysfunction which may be associated with a 20% risk of pancreatitis [34]. Other important risk factors include difficulty in cannulating the bile duct, the use of a pre-cut sphincterotome, the presence of cirrhosis and the use of the percutaneous endoscopic approach [34]. The experience of the endoscopist has also been shown to be a risk factor, although less than might have been predicted [34]. The recognition of these risk factors offers a means of reducing post-procedural pancreatitis. Care should be taken to avoid ampullary trauma during cannulation. Overfilling the pancreatic duct with contrast was a common cause of pancreatitis in the early days of ERCP but is now so well recognized that this is obsessively avoided. In experienced hands sphincterotomy in the presence of probable sphincter of Oddi dysfunction would be accompanied by a temporary pancreatic stent to maintain post-procedural pancreatic drainage. This approach has

Table 9.1. Definitions of complications for ERCP

	Mild	Moderate	Severe
Bleeding	Clinical (i.e. not just endoscopic) evidence of bleeding, haemoglobin drop < 3 g, and no need for transfusion	Transfusion (4 U or less), no angiographic intervention or surgery	Transfusion 5 U or more, or intervention (angiographic or surgical)
Perforation	Possible, or only very slight leak of fluid or contrast, treatable by fluids and suction for 3 days days or less	Any definite perforation treated medically for 4–10 days	Medical treatment for more than 10 days, or intervention (percutaneous or surgical)
Pancreatitis	Clinical pancreatitis, amylase at at least three times normal at more than 24 h after the procedure, requiring admission or prolongation of planned admission to 2–3 days	Pancreatitis requiring hospitalization of 4–10 days	Hospitalization for more than 10 days, or haemorrhagic pancreatitis, phlegmon, or pseudocyst, or intervention (percutaneous drainage or surgery)
Infection (cholangitis)	> 38°C 24–48 hr	Febrile or septic illness requiring more than 3 days of hospital treatment or endoscopic or percutaneous intervention	Septic shock or surgery
Basket impaction	Basket released spontaneously or by repeat endoscopy	Percutaneous intervention	Surgery

Note: any intensive care unit admission after a procedure grades the complication as severe. Other rarer complications can be graded by length of needed hospitalization. Adapted from [33].

markedly reduced the risk of pancreatitis following biliary manometry and bile duct sphincterotomy. Infection has also been recognized as a cause of pancreatitis and this is minimized by careful attention to standard disinfection practices.

Bleeding

A certain amount of haemorrhage is common following sphincterotomy, but haemorrhage of clinical significance (ie a reduction in haematocrit or need for transfusion) is unusual, occurring in approximately 1–3% of cases. However, when there is a major arterial bleed usually arising from the retroduodenal artery this may represent a major emergency associated with a significant mortality. While the majority of bleeding episodes occur during the periprocedural period, delayed haemorrhage may occur up to 2 weeks after the sphincterotomy. If bleeding is observed at the time of the procedure this can usually be managed by either electro-coagulation or local injection of adrenaline.

A number of risk factors have been suggested as predictors of bleeding. The longer the incision and the more rapidly that this is achieved, the more likely that bleeding will occur. There is however no evidence that using a pre-cut or needle knife is more likely to precipitate bleeding. As discussed above, certain conditions such as cirrhosis and renal failure are more likely to be associated with bleeding, and appropriate precautions should be taken. Aspirin and non-steroidal anti-inflammatory drugs are best stopped at least 3 days before the procedure because of their prolonged anti-platelet action.

Cholangitis

Cholangitis is most likely to occur in patients with a preceding infected biliary tree. The potential for bile duct infection is extremely high in patients with bile duct stones. However, clinically significant cholangitis is only observed in 1–3% of patients post sphincterotomy. In most circumstances this will be observed in patients in whom biliary drainage is incomplete. Prophylactic antibiotics are commonly used in biliary intervention but their efficacy is in doubt [32]. The risk of infection can be reduced by avoiding overfilling the biliary tree at the time of contrast injection, but most importantly by establishing good bile duct drainage at completion.

Retroperitoneal perforation (Fig. 9.11)

Retroperitoneal perforation occurs when the sphincterotomy extends beyond the intramural segment of the bile duct. It is likely that this is a much underdiagnosed complication, as the majority of instances produce few or no symptoms. The more severe perforations can produce a catastrophic clinical picture with very large volume fluid loss into the retroperitoneal space, which requires urgent correction so that renal function is not impaired. Clinically important perforation occurs in approximately 1% of sphincterotomies. The diagnosis can usually be made by a plain abdominal radiograph when the extravasation of air into the retroperitoneal space can be seen. This can be confirmed by CT scanning if the clinical condition warrants further investigation.

Basket impaction

Basket impaction occurs when there has been a failure to judge the relationship between the stone and the size of the sphincterotomy. In many cases repeated attempts to move the open basket forward into the CBD will lead to dis-

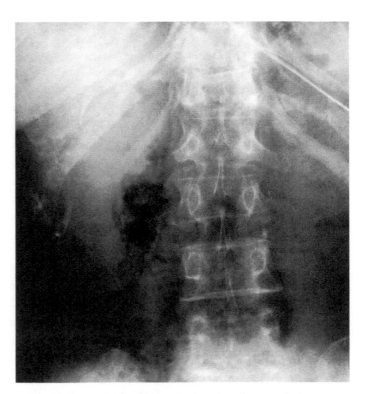

Figure 9.11. A plain radiograph showing the mottled appearance of retroperitoneal gas following perforation as a consequence of sphincterotomy.

impactation. When this is not possible, the wires of the basket should be cut and the endoscope and Teflon sheath of the basket removed. This will then allow the passage of a Sohendra lithotripter over the basket and the stone can then be crushed (see above).

Late complications

Reports of late complications have been somewhat variable but occur in approximately 5% of cases [35]. Recurrent stones within the bile duct are usually of the brown pigment variety, although occasionally cholesterol stones may be present. It is likely that the brown pigment stones are secondary to bacterial contamination of the CBD secondary to duodenal biliary reflux. Stone formation within the duct may also be secondary to papillary stenosis. This may occur in 1–2% of patients due to extensive fibrosis of the sphincterotomy cut.

Recurrent cholangitis following a previous sphincterotomy is usually an indication of a bile duct stone or reduced drainage because of stenosis.

CONTROVERSIAL ISSUES

Sphincterotomy as definitive treatment

There is controversy as to the need for cholecystectomy after sphincterotomy and bile duct clearance of stones. Evidence suggests that the risk of cholecystitis is under 20% over a 5-year period [36]. These relatively low values may justify leaving the gall bladder *in situ* in patients who are not a good risk for surgery.

Sphincterotomy in the young patient

There remains an unanswered concern as to the risks of sphincterotomy in young patients who are then exposed to duodenal bile duct reflux over a number of decades. Chronic bacterial contamination of the bile duct is now well recognized and this raises the possibility of chronic biliary damage [37]. There is also a concern as to the risk of cholangiocarcinoma. It is in such patients that balloon dilatation of the sphincter of Oddi may be a more appropriate alternative, as this will allow normal resolution of sphincter function.

ERCP and sphincterotomy preceding elective laparoscopic cholecystectomy

This issue has been referred to in the text and there is perhaps much less controversy than would have been recognized five years ago. The majority of surgeons carrying out laparoscopic cholecystetomy preferred to do so in the knowledge that the common bile duct was clear of stones prior to the procedure. However, indiscriminate ERCP in elective patients has never been a reasonable option because of the resources required and in particular for potential complications of the investigation. Pre-operative ERCP has therefore been based upon initial investigation that utilizes both standard liver function tests and imaging techniques, in particular trans-abdominal ultrasound scanning. As discussed above, extensive analyses have been carried out to identify those parameters most likely to predict accurately the presence or absence of bile duct stones. While limitations remain, a combination of liver function tests and ultrasound scanning will identify a small proportion of patients who would potentially benefit from pre-operative ERCP and bile duct clearance if stones are found. Operative cholangiography can then identify the small number of cases in which stones have not been predicted and these can then be managed endoscopically post-cholecystectomy; or, if the expertise is available, may be managed at the time of surgery itself. Currently it is only a minority of surgeons who prefer to carry out bile duct clearance at the time of cholecystectomy either by the transcystic or choledochotomy approach. This may reduce the hospital stay for patients involved although there is no evidence of reduced complications as compared to pre-operative endoscopic duct clearance. It therefore remains entirely a matter of local expertise as to how the patients are managed.

Sphincterotomy for acute gallstone cholangitis and pancreatitis

The endoscopic management of acute gallstone pancreatitis is discussed in detail in Chapter 12. There is however considerable overlap as to the indications for early endoscopic intervention for acute cholangitis and pancreatitis. It has been recognized for many years that emergency surgery in patients with severe gallstone cholangitis is associated with a high mortality rate of between 20 and 40%, depending on the degree of severity. There is now good evidence to show that emergency endoscopic decompression using sphincterotomy with or without nasobiliary drainage or pigtail endoprosthesis has a significantly lower morbidity or mortality as compared to surgical intervention [38,39]. To be of maximum benefit such endoscopic intervention should be timed within the first 24–36 hours after presentation, enabling only initial investigation and resuscitation to be implemented.

REFERENCES

1. Classen M, Demling L. Endoskopiche sphinkterotomie der Papilla Vateri und steinextraktion aus dem ductus choledochus. *Dtsch med Wachr* 1974; 99: 496–497.

2. Kwai K, Akaska Y, Murakami K *et al.* Endoscopic sphincterotomy of the ampulla of Vater. *Gastrointest Endosc* 1974; 20: 148–151.

3. Lee SP, Maher K, Nicholls JF. Origin and fate of biliary sludge. *Gastroenterology* 1988; 94: 170–176.

4. Stokberger SM, Wass L, Sherman S *et al.* Intravenous cholangiography with helical CT: Comparison with endoscopic retrograde cholangiography, *Radiology* 1994; 19: 657–680.

5. Soto JA, Banish MA, Yucel EK *et al.* Magnetic resonance cholangiography – comparison with endoscopic retrograde cholangio-pancreatography. *Gastroenterology* 1996; 110: 589–597.

6. Canto MF, Chak A, Stellato T, Sivak MV. Endoscopic ultrasonography versus cholangiography for the diagnosis of choledocholithiasis. *Gastrointest Endosc* 1998; 47: 439–448.

7. Santucci L, Natalini G, Sarpi L *et al.* Selective endoscopic retrograde cholangiography and pre-perative bile duct stone removal in patients scheduled for laparoscopic cholecystectomy: a prospective study, *Am J Gastroenterol* 1996; 91: 1326–1330.

8. Robertson GS, Jagger C, Johnson PR *et al.* Selection criteria for pre-operative endoscopic retograde cholangiopancreatography in the laparoscopic era, *Arch Surg* 1996; 131: 89–94.

9. Abboud PC, Malet PF, Berline JA *et al.* Predictor of common bile duct stones prior to cholecystectomy: a meta analysis. *Gastrointest Endosc* 1996: 450–452.

10. Barkun AN, Barkun JS, Fried GM. Useful predictors of bile duct stones in patients undergoing laparoscopic cholecystectomy. *Ann Surg* 1994; 220: 32–39.

11. Roston AD, Jackobson IM. Evaluation of the pattern of liver tests and yield of cholangiography in symptomatic choledocholithiasis: a prospective study. *Gastrointest Endosc* 1997; 45: 394–399.

12. Hatt RC, Butcher HR, Ballinger WF. Biliary tract operation: A view of 1000 patients. *Arch Surg* 1969; 98: 428–432.

13. Vellacott KD, Powell PH. Exploration of the common bile duct: a comparative study. *Br J Surg* 1979; 66: 389–394.

14. Tarqarona EM, Ayuso RM, Bordus JM *et al.* Randomised trial of endoscopic sphincterotomy with gall bladder left *in situ* versus open surgery for common bile duct calculi in high-risk patients. *Lancet* 1996; 347: 926–929.

15. Rhodes M, Sussman L, Cohen L, Lewis MP. Randomised trial of laparoscopic exploration of common bile duct versus post operative endoscopic retrograde cholangiography for common bile duct stones. *Lancet* 1998; 351: 159–161.

16. Vaira D, D'Anna L, Ainley C *et al.* Endoscopic sphincterotomy in 1000 consecutive patients, *Lancet* 1989; ii: 431–434.

17. Lambert ME, Betts Ch, Hill JD *et al.* Endoscopic sphincterotomy, the whole truth. *Br J Surg* 1991; 78: 473–476.

18. Chopra KB, Peters RA, O'Toole PA *et al.* Randomised study of endoscopic biliary endoprosthesis versus duct clearance for bile duct stones in high risk patients. *Lancet* 1996; ii: 791–793.

19. May GR, Cotton PB, Edmunds SEJ *et al.* Removal of stones from the bile duct at ERCP without sphincterotomy. *Gastrointest Endosc* 1993; 39: 749–752.

20. MacMathuna P, White P, Clarke E *et al.* Endoscopic sphincteroplasty: a novel and safe alternative to papillotomy in the management of bile duct stones. *Gut* 1994; 35: 127–129.

21. Sato H, Kodama T, Takaaki J *et al.* Endoscopic papillary balloon dilatation may preserve sphincter of Oddi function after common bile duct management: evaluation from the viewpoint of endoscopic manometry. *Gut* 1997; 41: 541–544.

22. Bergman JG, Rauws E, Fockens P *et al.* Randomised trial of endoscopic balloon dilatation versus endoscopic sphincterotomy for removal of bile duct stones. *Lancet* 1997; 349: 1124–1129.

23. Chung SCS, Leung JWC, Leong HT, Li AKC. Mechanical lithotripsy of large common bile duct stones using a basket. *Br J Surg* 1991; 78: 1448–1450.

24. Pouchon T, Gagnon P, Valette PJ *et al.* Pulsed dye laser lithotripsy of bile duct stones. *Gastroenterology* 1991; 100: 1730–1736.

25. Leung JW, Chung SC. Electrohydraulic lithotripsy with peroral choledochoscopy. *Br Med J* 1989; 299: 595–598.

26. Neuhaus H, Zillinger C, Born P *et al.* Randomised study of intracorporeal laser lithotripsy versus extracorporeal laser lithotripsy for difficult bile duct stones. *Gastrointest Endosc* 1998; 47: 327–334.

27. Palmer KR, Hoffman HF. Intraductal monoaction for direct dissolution of bile duct stones. Experience in 343 patients. *Gut* 1986; 27: 196–202.

28. Murray WR, Laferla G, Fullarton GM. Choledocholithiasis *in vivo* stone dissolution using methyl-tert-butyl ether. *Gut* 1988; 29: 143–145.

29. Chi Sin Cheng C. Do juxtapapillary diverticula of the duodenum interfere with cannulation? A prospective study. *Gastrointest Endosc* 1987; 33: 296–298.

30. Forbes A, Cotton PB. ERCP and sphincterotomy after Billroth II gastrectomy. *Gut* 1984; 25: 971–974.

31. Jan YY, Chen MF. Percutaneous trans-hepatic cholangioscopic lithotomy for hepatolithiasis: long-term results. *Gastrointest Endosc* 1995; 42: 1–5.

32. Van den Hazzel S, Speelman P, Danker J *et al.* Piperacillin to prevent cholangitis after endoscopic retrograde cholangiopancreatography. *Ann Intern Med* 1996; 125: 442–447.

33. Cotton PB, Lehman G, Vennes J *et al.* Endoscopic sphincterotomy complications and their management: An attempt at consensus. *Gastrointest Endosc* 1991; 37: 282–258.

34. Freeman ML, Nelson DB, Sherman S *et al.* Complications of endoscopic biliary sphincterotomy. *N Engl J Med* 1995; 225: 909–917.

35. Pereira-Lima JC, Jakobs R, Winter UH *et al.* Long term results of endoscopic papillotomy for choledocholithiasis. Multivariate analysis of prognostic factors for the recurrence of biliary symptoms. *Gastrointest Endosc* 1998; 48: 457–464.

36. Hammarströsm LE, Holmin T, Stridbeck H. Endoscopic treatment of bile duct calculi in patients with gall bladder *in situ*: long-term outcome and features predictive of recurrent symptoms. *Scand J Gastroenterol* 1996; 31: 294–301.

37. Sugiyama M, Atomi Y. Follow-up of more than 10 years after endoscopic sphincterotomy for choledocholithiasis. *Br J Surg* 1998; 86: 917–921.

38. Lai EC, Mok FP, Tan ES *et al.* Endoscopic biliary drainage for severe acute cholangitis. *N Engl J Med* 1992; 326: 1582–1586.

39. Sharma BC, Aqarwal DK, Bailjall SS *et al.* Endoscopic management of acute calculous cholangitis, *J Ganstroenterol Hepatol* 1997; 12: 874–876.

40. Everhart JE, Khare M, Hill M, Maurer KK. Prevalence and ethnic differences in gallbladder disease in the United States. *Gastroenterology* 1999; 117: 632–639.

10 *Biliary obstruction and leaks*

M. Lombard

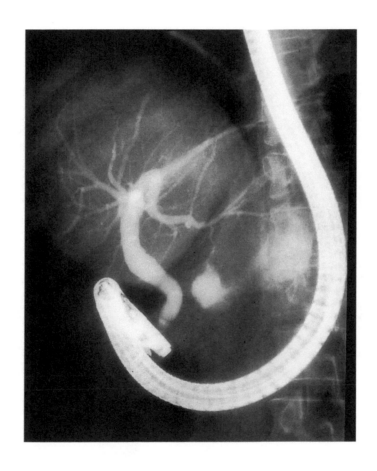

INTRODUCTION

Benign bile duct strictures present a major challenge because the consequences of making the wrong choices can cause long-term morbidity, especially when patients present at a young age. The presentation can mimic other causes of biliary disease or obstruction, and diagnosis and assessment is not always easy. Once the diagnosis has been established, there is some evidence to support the contention that outcome is dependent on the experience of the team managing the condition and, as in so many areas of advanced endoscopic therapy, a multidisciplinary team approach is essential.

PRESENTATION

The most common presentation for bile duct stricture of any cause is jaundice. If the presentation is temporally related to an identifiable event, e.g. trauma or occurring immediately following a cholecystectomy, the cause and nature of the problem may be very obvious. However, about 30% of bile duct strictures due to previous surgery do not manifest until more than 6 months after the event, 20% for 12 months, and at least 5% present later than 5 years [1]. Often, patients will present with recurrent pain in the right upper quadrant. Rigors with pyrexia or pain due to cholangitis is an uncommon presentation. Patients may have a variety of non-specific complaints for which biochemical tests may have been performed and, consequently, abnormal liver enzymes or raised bilirubin found. Bile duct leak or fistula is a rare presentation with pain, but has been described particularly in the early period following cholecystectomy when surgical clips may not have sealed the cystic duct remnant. If a peritoneal drain is *in situ*, the presence of bile should make the cause of pain more obvious.

Non-traumatic causes of benign biliary stricture such as primary sclerosing cholangitis (PSC) or cystic fibrosis have a very variable presentation. In some patients, a preceding history or diagnosis may be present; in the case of PSC, the history of ulcerative colitis or Crohn's disease frequently precedes the liver presentation. They may also be dis-

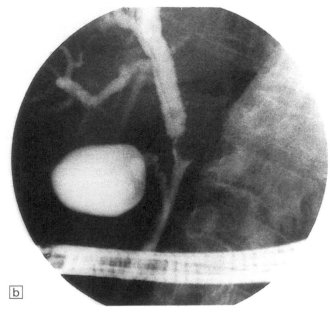

Figure 10.1. Bile duct stones can mimic strictures. (a) A cholangiogram from a patient with a stone in the bile duct. (b) A cholangiogram from a patient with a bile duct stricture due to cholangiocarcinoma.

covered during the course of investigation of abnormal liver enzymes. Similarly, chronic pancreatitis resulting in biliary stricture has a variable presentation but is less common than pancreatic carcinoma in causing biliary obstruction, especially in the older age groups.

Biliary-type pain in the absence of gallstones, or post cholecystectomy, may be due to dysfunction of the sphincter of Oddi, but this is uncommon and accounts for less than 5% patients with post-cholecystectomy pain.

Apart from biliary atresia which presents in the neonatal period, age of presentation is very variable. Although the peak incidence for PSC is in young adults, symptomatic presentation can be quite late. Bile duct stones (see Chapter 9) can mimic bile duct strictures both in their presentation and

their appearance on cholangiography (Fig. 10.1). These can occur in the very young when due to haemolytic syndromes, but otherwise tend to be more common in middle age.

DIAGNOSIS

Classification

Categorization of strictures can be on the basis of site (e.g. lower bile duct, hilar, intrahepatic) or aetiology (Table 10.1; Fig. 10.2). The site may influence choices for the immediate management, but identification of the nature and cause of the stricture will be essential in planning optimum long-term management.

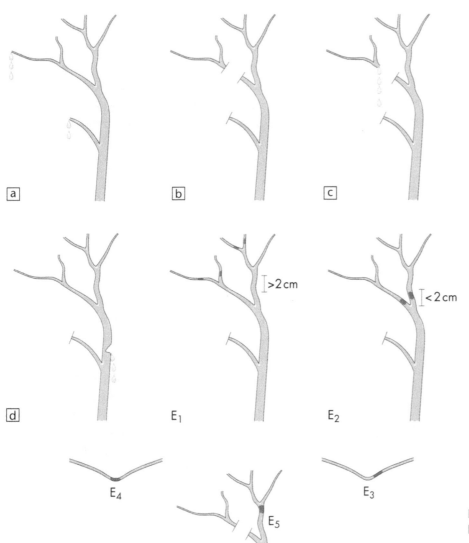

Figure 10.2. Proposed classification of bile duct surgical injury (illustration based on [2]).

Table 10.1. Classification and causes of benign bile duct stricture

Level of stricture	Cause
Intrahepatic	Primary sclerosing cholangitis
	Cystic fibrosis
	Recurrent ascending cholangitis (e.g. associated with parasites)
Upper CBD/CHD	Any of the above causes
	Ischaemia
	Traumatic (e.g. cholecystectomy)
	Inflammatory (e.g. with bile duct stones)
Lower CBD	Any of the above causes
	Chronic pancreatitis
	Papillary stenosis

CBD = Common bile duct; CHD = Common hepatic duct.

Assessment

The extent of assessment required is clearly dependent on the nature and history of the stricture – for strictures presenting early postoperatively, only limited assessment may be required, whereas for those presenting late or where the aetiology is uncertain, extensive investigation may be required.

Clinical examination

The patient is usually, though not invariably, jaundiced. Intense pruritus can be present. Evidence of weight loss or lymphadenopathy should raise suspicion that a stricture may not be benign. Concomitant signs of liver disease (e.g. spider naevi) may be present with sclerosing cholangitis. Splenomegaly, ascites or distension of abdominal veins are not associated with uncomplicated benign bile duct strictures.

Blood tests

Usually serum bilirubin and the 'biliary enzymes' (alkaline phosphatase and gamma-glutamyl transferase) are elevated as they would be in any case of bile duct problem. Occasionally, patients present with a flare or isolated rise in alanine or aspartate transaminase (ALT, AST). A low albumin or urea or low platelet count due to hypersplenism should alert to the possibility that other liver problems are present. A full hepatic investigation with autoantibodies, immunoglobulins, viral serology and special protein profiles such as caeruloplasmin, ferritin and alpha-1-antitrypsin may be indicated. If the patient has been jaundiced for any duration, vitamin K malabsorption may result in coagulopathy which should be corrected before any intervention is contemplated.

Tumour markers

These are not always helpful in differentiating benign from malignant bile duct strictures. There is more experience of their use in biliary strictures due to pancreatic cancer than cholangiocarcinoma. The most commonly used are serum markers CA19.9 and, latterly, CAM17.1. These are markers of mucin-producing adenocarcinomas (of pancreatic or biliary origin), but can also be raised in any cause of obstructive jaundice or ascites. CAM17.1 may be more specific in this regard. Nonetheless, marked elevations in the context of bile duct strictures are highly suggestive of a malignant process. Markers such as k-*ras* or *p53* in bile or pancreatic juice may be more sensitive, especially in the presence of hyperbilirubinaemia, but are no more specific for malignant disease (for review see [3]).

INVESTIGATION

Transabdominal ultrasound

Abdominal ultrasound (US) has achieved an important place in the investigation of patients with jaundice and abdominal pain of biliary origin because it is non-invasive, relatively inexpensive, widely available and versatile. Its senstivity for determining that the cause of jaundice is obstructive in nature is 80–89%, and its specificity should be 100% in expert hands. It may be less sensitive in the early phases and, if the clinical picture is suggestive, it should be repeated after a week or two. Dilated ducts are occasionally detected in non-jaundiced patients. For determining the cause of obstruction, ultrasound has a sensitivity of only 60% [4].

Computed tomography (CT) scan

Spiral CT with contrast is currently the best and most widely available non-invasive method of determining the cause and level of bile duct obstruction. It is especially useful in the context of lower common bile duct (CBD) strictures suspected to be pancreatic in origin, but has limitations for lesions less than 20 mm in size, and its senstivity is less than 50% for lesions of less than 10 mm.

Software developments have allowed advanced techniques such as image subtraction and three-dimensional reconstruction of anatomical structures, but these are not routinely employed in most institutions.

Magnetic resonance cholangiopancreatography (MRCP)

MRCP is possible because stationary fluids such as bile or pancreatic juice have a relatively long relaxation time following T2-weighted pulse sequences compared with surrounding tissue. Excellent biliary images can be obtained with a suitable magnet and the software to develop the image. Pancreatic duct images tend not to be as good, but undoubtedly will improve with technological advance.

Most MRCP data reflect non-invasive attempts to diagnose bile duct stones as ultrasound or CT scanning lack sensitivity in this respect, and diagnostic endoscopic retrograde cholangiopancreatography (ERCP) has a rate of morbidity which is becoming less acceptable. Early indications are that MRCP may be useful in differentiating benign from malignant bile duct strictures, though less discriminating for pancreatic strictures. Use of intravenous secretin improves the pancreatic image only in the absence of chronic pancreatitis. MRCP is more useful than ERCP for cystic lesions in the pancreas. MRCP has an especially important role in the context of failed ERCP or in the presence of a Billroth II gastrectomy.

Nuclear scan

Radioisotope scanning is used predominantly for assessing the excretory function of the liver, and to that extent can give valuable information regarding the functional integrity of the biliary tract. The information obtained by these scintiscans is dependent on hepatic function and also on the biophysical properties of the chemical vehicle of the radioisotope. Colloidal materials (e.g. sulphur, neoglycalbumin) are taken up by reticuloendothelial cells in the liver and provide information about hepatic architecture or its disruption; dyes such as iminodiacetic acid (IDA compounds) are taken up by hepatocytes, metabolized and excreted and therefore are used to delineate the biliary tract. Other compounds such as gallium citrate and selenomethionine may be preferentially taken up by particular cell types in the liver. The radioisotope is chosen for its short half-life and emission energy, ^{99m}Tc being the most commonly used with the -IDA compounds. Attention recently has concentrated on the rate of excretion of these compounds (dynamic -IDA scans) in determining the functional nature of mild biliary stenoses or in assessing papillary dyskinesia.

Endoluminal ultrasound (EUS)

This technique is becoming more widely available and compares very favourably with US, CT and MRCP for small lesions of the pancreas, where it may be superior [5]. It is a safe and efficient technique for the evaluation of the biliary tract and has a high sensitivity for stones. The lower bile duct can be visualized in about 90% of patients, and the upper part at the hilum in about 80%. EUS is not possible in the context of gastrectomy. The technique requires a high level of skill and dedication for investigators to become proficient, and is not yet widely available. Its accuracy in differentiating malignant from benign bile duct obstruction has not been fully evaluated.

Percutaneous transhepatic cholangiography (PTC)

In expert hands, thin-needle PTC can be achieved in more than 95% of patients. In large series, complications occurred in 3.4% of cases (of which sepsis and bile leakage accounted for the majority) and mortality occurred in 0.2% of cases [6]. Complication rates are higher when interventions such as dilatation or stenting are undertaken, and failure to pass through a stricture from above (though uncommon) can lead to potentially serious complications of peritoneal leakage and sepsis. Most centres use PTC as an adjunct to ERCP, but its use will also depend on local expertise. With the emergence of MRCP to identify the site of stricture before interventional measures are undertaken, PTC may become more desirable than ERCP for the management of hilar strictures because the risk of intrahepatic sepsis may be less.

Endoscopic retrograde cholangiopancreatography (ERCP)

ERCP has been the 'gold standard' for the assessment of bile duct strictures, and is likely to remain so in jaundiced patients because of the therapeutic options it allows. However, because of the potential for complications, especially pancreatitis, MRC and EUS have found an important role in the preliminary evaluation of such patients so that a rational plan of management can be developed.

Cytology and biopsy

Brush cytology can confirm malignant bile duct strictures in up to 75% cases, but in only 50% of pancreatic strictures [7]. In a practical sense, for the individual patient where the nature of the stricture is uncertain, a negative result is not wholly reassuring. The discriminating capability of brush cytology for PSC versus cholangiocarcinoma and for chronic pancreatitis versus pancreatic carcinoma is just over 80% for both sensitivity and specificity. Results can be improved by the enthusiastic participation of the cytologist in acquiring the samples and by combining several methods, i.e. brush cytology together with fine-needle aspiration and intrahepatic duct forceps biopsy.

Analysis of bile duct or pancreatic juice for k-*ras* mutations is not useful, as these are present in both chronic inflammatory conditions and malignancy. Analysis of other genetic mutations, e.g. *p53* may be more helpful. Interleukin (IL)-6 and tumour necrosis factor α (TNFα) are increased in cholangitis.

Which test should be used?

As previously stated, the extent of assessment will be guided by the presentation. An ultrasound scan should almost always be the first investigation used to diagnose bile duct obstruction. If the obstruction is in the lower bile duct and the patient is jaundiced, then ERCP with its options for tissue sampling and therapy would be the next appropriate investigation. If a hilar stricture is present, there is a case for undertaking spiral CT or MRCP followed by PTC to avoid introducing sepsis to undrained intrahepatic segments. However, these options are largely governed by availability of local expertise and facilities. Either ERCP or PTC can be used when PSC is suspected. EUS can be a very useful alternative to CT/MRCP and as a prelude to ERCP.

MANAGEMENT AND EVIDENCE

Endoscopic versus surgical

There are no directly comparable studies for surgical and endoscopic management of benign bile duct strictures. From published data on this, and comparable data for malignant strictures, it is reasonable to conclude that surgical management, where possible, produces the best long-term outcome for most patients. Endoscopic management has an important role to play in the initial assessment and management of jaundice, in the definitive management of those patients unsuitable for, or unsuccessfully managed by, surgery and also for a small number of conditions (e.g. PSC, cystic fibrosis) where surgery can jeopardize further treatment such as transplantation which may be required later. Endoscopic treatment can produce rapid relief of jaundice and pruritus with a lower short-term complication rate, but this has to be balanced against the requirement for long-term and repeated treatments.

In a series of 80 benign strictures managed endoscopically, one-third had already undergone surgery [8]. Satisfactory long-term results are possible because a proportion of patients do not require repeated insertion of stents and, if they do, metallic stents can be used after due consideration to the alternatives has been given [9,10].

ERCP and sphincterotomy

I do not routinely use sphincterotomy for insertion of stents, and in the case of benign stricture – where use of endoprosthesis may only be temporary – it may be even more important to maintain sphincter function. This has the immediate advantage of reducing the incidence of complications associated with the procedure, particularly haemorrhage and pancreatitis, but in the longer term also should reduce the likelihood of septic cholangitis which can occur in up to 10% patients on follow-up.

Sphincterotomy is useful in certain patients with biliary dyskinesia, including the neuropathic sphincter of Oddi which can occur following liver transplantation, but these are special cases (see below). Sphincterotomy may also be justifiable in the context of post-cholecystectomy leak from a cystic stump as an alternative to insertion of endoprosthesis, but again in younger patients I would try to preserve the sphincter.

ERCP: balloon dilatation (Fig. 10.3)

Balloon dilatation as an alternative to sphincterotomy is discussed in Chapter 9, and may be a useful alternative in sphincter of Oddi dyskinesia as some function is retained.

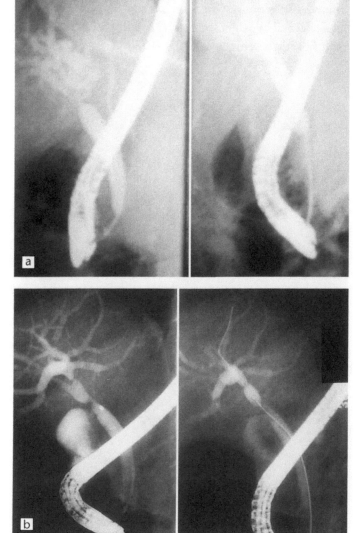

Figure 10.3. Balloon inflation of (a) a bile duct stricture and (b) an intrahepatic stricture.

For benign strictures above the ampulla, balloon dilatation may produce a fibrotic inflammatory reaction. If endoprostheses are inserted immediately, patency may in theory be maintained in the long term. Some authorities recommend the insertion of multiple stents in this situation to achieve as wide a diameter as possible.

There are no data to indicate that balloon dilatation is more effective than graduated cannula dilatation, but certainly a wider patency can be achieved. I use 8–10 mm Olbert dilators in the extrahepatic bile duct, and 4–6 mm balloons for intrahepatic strictures. Multiple repeat dilatations may be required. Dilatation of high strictures is more painful for the patient than balloon sphincteroplasty. It is useful to give an additional bolus of opioid analgesia immediately before dilatation and to talk the patient through the procedure. There are no data available to judge the duration of balloon insufflation, but empirically most operators use 1–2 min.

ERCP: stenting

There are several small series which demonstrate that an endoprosthesis left *in situ* across a benign stricture for 3–6 months can lead to improvement in symptoms, biochemistry and bile duct patency in at least 50% of patients long term. The aim should be to achieve as wide a patency as possible, and therefore multiple stents may be inserted [11]. This is a different rationale to placing stents into different segments of the liver, as might be the case for malignant disease. There is evidence that stents cause a fibroinflammatory reaction around the bile duct [12] which can make subsequent surgery difficult, and the aims of stenting at the outset – particularly for benign disease – should be clear.

Stent removal

The removal of endoprostheses is a straightforward process as long as they remain protruding from the papillary orifice into the duodenum. They can be held with a snare, basket or retrieval device, and pulled from the bile duct while the endoscope is being withdrawn. A screw retrieval device is available so that wire access can be maintained in the bile duct, but for benign strictures I prefer to obtain a clear cholangiogram following stent removal in order to assess whether or not it needs replacement.

Traumatic strictures and post-cholecystectomy strictures

Historically, cholecystectomy is the most common cause of benign bile duct strictures [13]. Before the introduction of laparoscopic techniques in the 1980s, the incidence of post-cholecystectomy bile duct injury was reported to be about 0.2–0.3%. In a large series of laparoscopic cholecystomy reported more recently, this figure was shown approximately to have doubled, even after the 'learning curve' had been surpassed [14], although there was ample evidence that the experience of the surgeon could also affect the incidence. Thus on average, a bile duct injury may be expected approximately once in every 300 cholecystectomies.

Factors associated with bile duct injury most commonly include a failure correctly to identify anatomical structures before clips, ligatures or cautery are applied. The reasons for such failure may include: misidentification of the common duct for the cystic duct when anatomy is normal; failure to appreciate aberrant anatomy [15]; difficulty in adequate visualization due to patient obesity, hepatomegaly or previous surgery resulting in adhesions; damage occurring during attempts to acquire urgent haemostasis; and distortion and limitation of the operating field when using laparoscopic instruments.

The bile duct, and particularly the subhilar hepatic duct, seems to be especially susceptible to ischaemic bile duct injury. The blood supply is derived from the right hepatic artery and the hepaticoduodenal artery, fine branches of which run along the bile duct fascia and can be easily injured. Resection or ligation of the hepatic artery can result in total bile duct ischaemia, and this may cause a very tight fibrotic stricture (Figs 10.4–10.7).

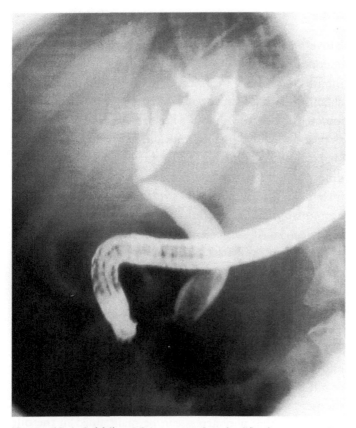

Figure 10.4. Subhilar stricture associated with placement of clip post cholecystectomy.

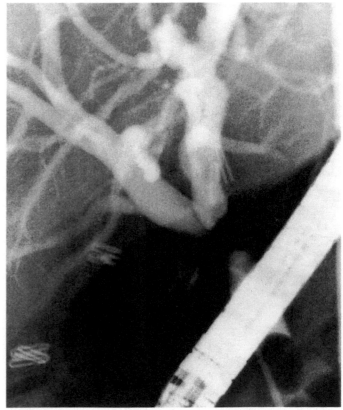

Figure 10.5. Type III stricture in a patient following difficult cholecystectomy. Note multiple clips around area of gall bladder and cystic duct. Endoprostheses were inserted as a temporary measure but this patient required surgical repair.

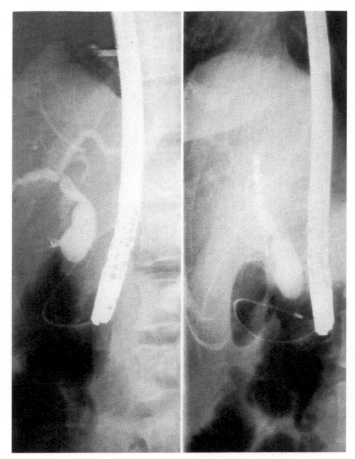

Figure 10.6. Hilar stricture presenting 12 years post-cholecystectomy. The patient was asymptomatic until this presentation with jaundice.

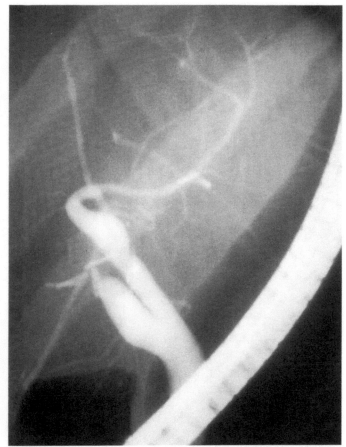

Figure 10.7. Total occlusion of the right intrahepatic duct following injury at cholecystectomy: patient presented with pruritis and abnormal biliary enzymes.

Post-cholecystectomy biliary leaks

Bile duct leak is usually a problem which arises after cholecystectomy, but occasionally can occur following liver biopsy if pressure in the biliary system is elevated for any reason (e.g. stones or stricture). There are a number of small series reported with biliary leak treated endoscopically. More than 90% of cases can be managed satisfactorily with an endoprosthesis or sphincterotomy [16].

The site of leak is most commonly the cystic duct remnant, but leaks from the main bile duct, aberrant right hepatic ducts, liver surface and gall bladder bed have also been reported (Figs. 10.8). It is my practice to preserve the sphincter in these patients (who are often young) and manage leaks by endoprosthesis alone. The stent is removed after 3 months. For leaks of the main pancreatic duct treated in this way, there has been some concern that a stenosis may develop at the site of the leak. Follow-up with liver enzymes and if necessary imino-iodoacetic acid (HIDA) scan may be indicated in these cases. Major bile duct injuries and complete transections should be managed surgically.

Orthotopic liver transplantation (OLT)

Bile duct complications have been reported in 13–40% of patients following OLT (Fig. 10.9). Currently, the majority (over 80%) of bile duct anastomoses for adult transplantation are end-to-end, but in most children and patients with PSC, and in some patients with previous biliary surgery, a choledochojejunostomy with Roux-en-Y anastomosis is required. In a recent survey in the USA of over 6000 transplant patients, 16% had bile duct complications [17]. In the same survey, just over 40% of patients investigated by ERCP or PTC had normal cholangiograms, and of the remainder 21% had stones, 28% strictures, 17% leaks and 11% papillary stenosis.

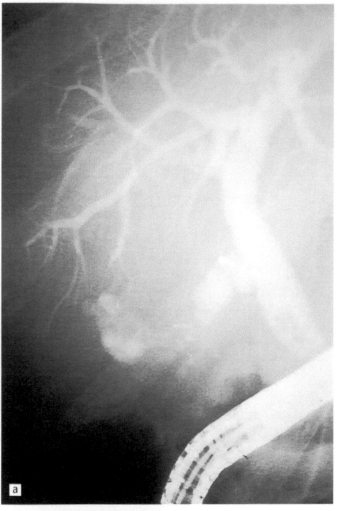

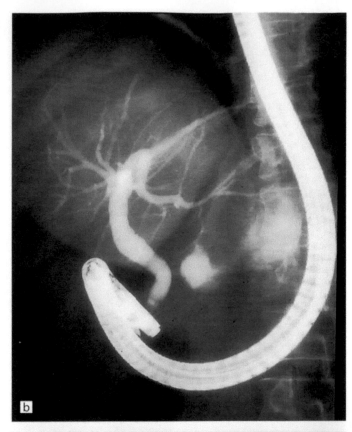

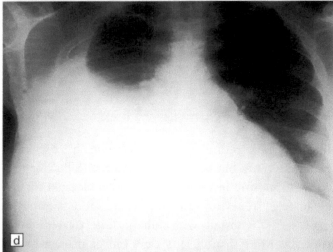

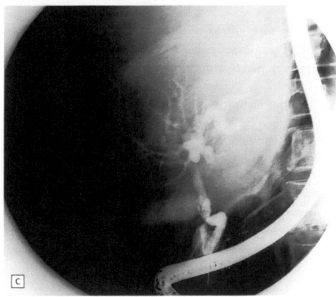

Figure 10.8. (a) Leak from cystic duct remnant and (b) gall bladder-bed post-cholecystectomy. (c) Peripheral biliary leak into pleural space and resulting in bile pleural effusion (d) following liver biopsy in a patient with biliary stenosis post-transplantation.

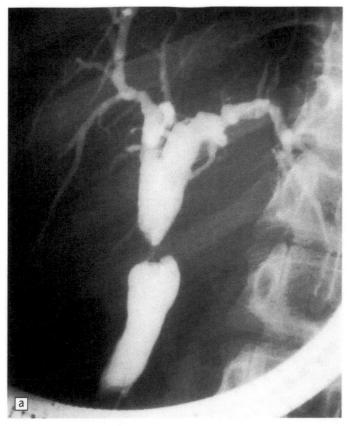

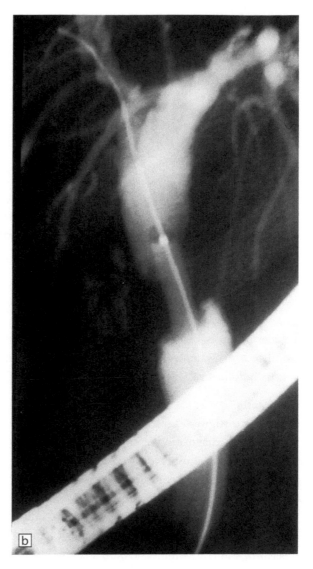

Figure 10.9. Anastomotic stricture following liver transplantation (a) and balloon dilatation of the same stricture (b). Note that the lower (recipient) common bile duct is also dilated.

Improved surgical technique and the use of perioperative stents may reduce the incidence of this complication. One-third of patients with biliary problems after OLT will require a re-transplant within 12 months, and therefore attempts at endoscopic treatment have become attractive. The complication rate for ERCP in patients with liver transplantation is higher than other groups at 17%, comprising cholangitis and pancreatitis predominantly.

Liver transplantation is an unusual cause of papillary stenosis which accounts for 20% biliary tract complications following transplant. This entity may be neuropathic in origin and has been successfully managed by sphincterotomy alone.

Papillary stenosis

Papillary stenosis can refer to a fibrotic stricture of the papillary orifice due to previous instrumentation, e.g. passage of a bougie during surgical exploration of the CBD or following a previous endoscopic sphincterotomy. Functional papillary stenosis can be due to an associated duodenal diverticulum, a penetrating duodenal ulcer, or to biliary dyskinesia. This latter entity is normally referred to as sphincter of Oddi dysfunction or dyskinesia.

Sphincter of Oddi dyskinesia may be responsible for pain in the right upper quadrant in 2–3% of patients after cholecystectomy. The patients are most commonly female, and aged between 30 and 50 years. Three groups have been identified, and a classification has been proposed based on the presence or absence of abnormal liver enzymes, dilated bile ducts, delayed drainage or kinetic measurements and the following clinical features:

1. Episodic pain with long pain-free intervals.
2. Constant daily pain, often described as an ache with intermittent severe episodes.
3. A subgroup of patients who are sensitive to opiates.

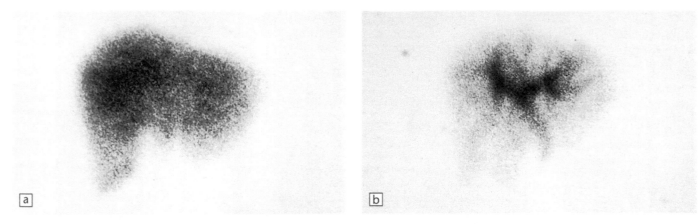

Figure 10.10. (a) HIDA scan from a patient with papillary stenosis (b) demonstrating delayed drainage after two hours.

Papillary stenosis or dyskinesia usually present with episodes of pain in the right upper quadrant similar to biliary colic. There is a similar entity of pancreatic sphincter dysfunction. Liver enzymes can be abnormal during an acute attack. Jaundice is unusual unless a true fibrotic stenosis is present – usually following a sphincterotomy.

Non-invasive tests

The morphine–neostigmine test was devised as a non-invasive method of diagnosing sphincter of Oddi dysfunction. Baseline blood samples are taken following intravenous saline and morphine. Reproduction of pain may occur in 30%, and a doubling of serum ALT activity signifies a positive test. Serial blood samples are taken at half-hourly intervals up to 3 hours. The test has the advantage of being simple to perform and relies on biochemical analysis, but it is not sufficiently sensitive or specific for routine use [18]. Radionuclide dynamic HIDA scanning is another non-invasive means of assessing sphincter of Oddi dysfunction, and may also distinguish those patients who may benefit from sphincterotomy [19] (Fig. 10.10).

Invasive tests

At ERCP, fibrotic stricture appears as a grossly dilated bile duct tapering to a point (Fig. 10.11), and drainage of contrast is delayed or absent. There are no specific radiographic findings in biliary dyskinesia, but local causes of obstruction can be excluded. Pain during injection is variable and dependent on the nature and amount of sedation given. Delayed emptying of contrast from the biliary tree for more than 45 min is unreliable and influenced by the shape of the ampulla and whether any oedema or spasm was induced by cannulation, particularly

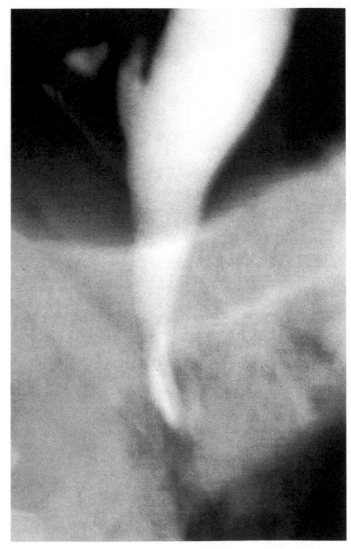

Figure 10.11. Dilated bile duct and tapering stricture in a patient with fibrotic papillary stenosis.

if this was difficult to achieve. Pancreatitis following cannulation or sphincterotomy is said to be more common in patients with biliary dyskinesia and sphincter of Oddi dysfunction.

Sphincter of Oddi manometry is the 'gold standard' for this diagnosis, but manometry is only possible in 70% of these patients. Pressures in excess of 35–40 mmHg are diagnostic, and in two series this was the discriminatory test for prediction of response to sphincterotomy [20]. Long-term follow-up data are limited. More recently, the entity of pancreatic sphincter dysfunction has also been studied, with similar results.

Primary sclerosing cholangitis (PSC) (Fig. 10.12)

PSC is a chronic inflammatory condition affecting medium- and larger-sized bile ducts, and results in ectasia, stricturing, irregularity, pseudodiverticula and dilatation. It is a variably progressive condition, resulting in liver failure in a minority of patients. Strictures below the bifurcation can cause obstruction with jaundice even in the absence of significant loss of hepatic function. In this situation a sudden clinical deterioration with jaundice is the usual presentation.

A variety of surgical techniques have evolved to manage PSC strictures, but many centres now try to avoid surgery in the right upper quadrant in these patients for fear of jeopardizing the success of OLT should that be required later. Data from uncontrolled series have shown beneficial results from a combination of stenting and dilatation. Endoprostheses are empirically placed for 6–12 months [21]. Sphincterotomy alone is not usually sufficient in these patients. Irrigation of the biliary tree with saline or steroids is not effective in preventing recurrence.

A common problem with PSC is discriminating dominant strictures from cholangiocarcinoma; this may occur in 8–20% of patients with PSC. Polypoid lesions within the bile ducts are nearly always malignant. Brush cytology is not helpful, having a sensitivity for cholangiocarcinoma of only 60% [22]; *p53* abnormalities in bile can be detected in 78% of cases. Serum CA19.9 appears to be of little value in the presence of jaundice. Some concern has been expressed with regard to managing dominant benign strictures endoscopically in such patients because of the possibility that temporizing in this way would preclude transplantation if carcinogenesis were to occur during the period when management was by

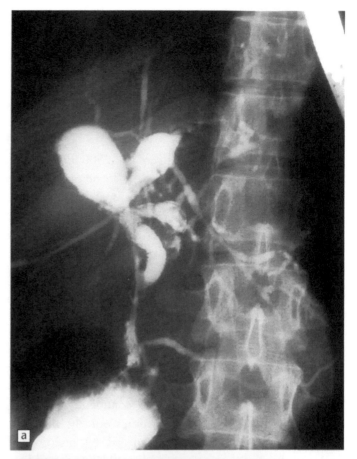
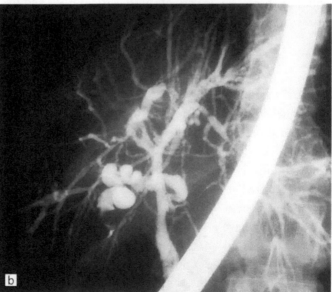

Figure 10.12. Tight subhilar strictures in a patient with PSC (a) before and (b) after 6 months treatment by balloon dilatation and stenting.

endoprosthesis. Such concerns may be tempered somewhat by a study which showed that up to 30% patients transplanted for PSC died within 8 years from OLT complications, while a more recent study showed that the risk of colorectal neoplasia in patients with PSC and concomitant ulcerative colitis was significantly increased following transplantation [23].

Cystic fibrosis

This genetic disorder, which affects 1 in 2500 live births in the UK, is due to a defect in the gene encoding a chloride transporter protein. It is best known for its effects on the respiratory tract and pancreatic insufficiency. With improved treatments, the survival for this condition has improved to a median of 30 years currently. A significant proportion of adults with this condition present with hepatobiliary disease; this can range from cirrhosis to rare occurrences of extrahepatic bile duct obstruction [24].

Particular care is warranted with these patients because of their respiratory problems, and this can be compromised further by the prone position required at ERCP and by the sedation used. The procedure should only be undertaken by experienced operators who can confidently cannulate and complete the required procedures quickly. Bile duct strictures, if present, can be managed by insertion of endoprostheses. Some patients with cystic fibrosis and liver disease may require OLT.

Miscellaneous strictures

Mirrizzi's syndrome
Gallstones impacted in Hartmann's pouch or in the cystic duct can cause mechanical or inflammatory obstruction of the bile duct. Two types have been described depending on whether a fistula has formed or not. Some of these cases are only recognized at the time of surgery [25]. Where a patient being investigated by ERCP for obstructive jaundice is discovered to have a Mirizzi syndrome, it is reasonable to undertake initial management by insertion of an endoprosthesis. Some endoscopists would also place an endoprosthesis into the gall bladder if possible in this situation. Most patients will ultimately warrant surgery.

Diverticula
Duodenal or periampullary diverticula are common, and can be found in about 10% of the population undergoing ERCP for a variety of reasons. An association with pigment gall bladder stones has been described. The intramural part of the CBD usually courses along the floor of large diverticulae, and it is conceivable that they could cause a partial functional obstruction. Bile duct dilatation without other cause is a frequent accompaniment. In view of the risks of sphincterotomy, dilated bile duct associated with duodenal diverticulum alone should not be regarded as sufficient justification for sphincterotomy.

Portal hypertensive cholangiopathy (Fig. 10.13)
Extrahepatic portal hypertension due to portal vein thrombosis is associated with paracholedochal varices. These can cause intermittent hyperbilirubinaemia (the pressure in the varices exceeds that in the bile duct), but this rarely produces clinical jaundice [26]. However, if these become thrombosed, a biliary stricture may ensue. Endoprosthesis is an effective treatment in this situation, and as OLT may not be possible due to cavernous

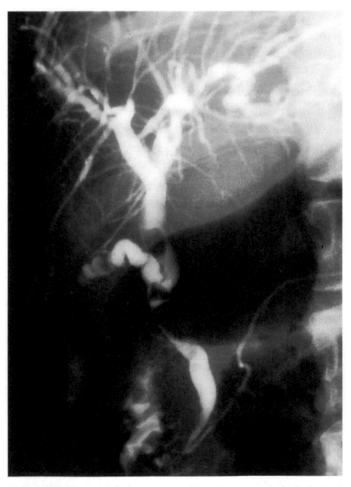

Figure 10.13. Partial duct obstruction due to paracholedochal varices in portal vein thrombosis. Note scalloped appearance of common bile duct.

transformation of the portal vein, the use of an expanding metal stent may be justifiable in this situation.

Duodenal ulceration

Occasionally, a deep penetrating ulcer can produce significant inflammatory reaction or oedema to result in partial bile duct obstruction. These lesions can be difficult to differentiate from invasive pancreatic carcinoma: biopsies may show necrosis or dysplasia, while a CT scan may show a mass related to the head of pancreas. Multiple biopsy sampling is usually required, and EUS may be helpful. Endoprostheses should be inserted while the ulcer is healing with proton pump inhibitors and reviewed with further biopsies 2–4 weeks later. Occasionally, surgery is required.

Chronic pancreatitis (Fig. 10.14, 10.15)

It can be extremely difficult to differentiate a stricture of the lower CBD due to carcinoma or to pancreatitis, though the former situation is probably more common. However, pancreatitis can be complicated by biliary stricture in approximately 10% of cases, and rates up to 30% have been reported – especially in the chronic calcific variety. Several series with small patient numbers have been reported in which such patients are managed endoscopically with endoprostheses. Improvements in jaundice, pain, cholangitis and liver biochemistry can be demonstrated. With long-term follow-up, symptoms usually recur once the endoprostheses are removed and this is not a viable long-term treatment option in these patients. Nonetheless, as a temporary measure, and to exclude carcinoma as a cause, ERCP plays an important role. Strictures, if associated with pseudocysts, usually resolve. Higher rates of stent migration also appear to be a particular problem in this group of patients.

Parasitic disease and infection

In certain parts of the world (or in patients returning from them), parasitic infestation is an important cause of biliary problems. *Echinococcus granulosus* infects the liver in 50–70% of affected patients, and 5–25% of these will get intrabiliary rupture with fistulae. Intrabiliary daughter cysts can be effectively cleared at ERCP following sphincterotomy, and the majority of fistulae will close with sphincterotomy alone or with temporary stenting [27].

Clonorchis (Chinese fluke) can cause intrahepatic stone formation with strictures (Fig. 10.16). A combination of

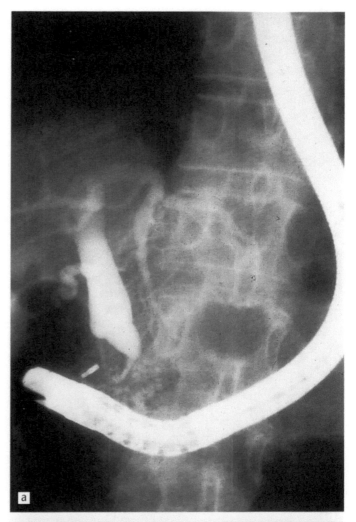

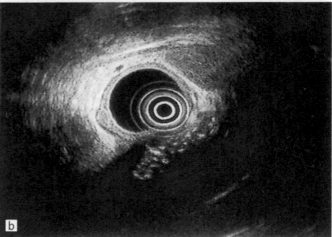

Figure 10.14. Calcific pancreatitis causing bile duct stricture (a). Note calcium flecks on accompanying EUS (b).

balloon dilatation, stenting, choledochoscopy and surgery may be necessary to restore bile duct patency for these and other causes (Fig. 10.17) [28].

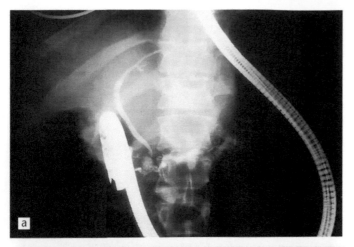

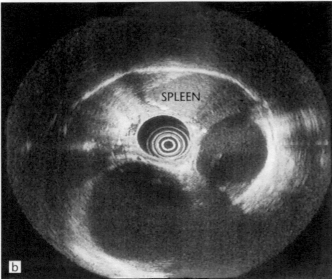

SPLEEN

Figure 10.15. Pancreatic pseudocyst producing distorted and compressed bile duct (a) which resorted to normal once the pseudocyst was decompressed. EUS of pseudocysts is shown at (b).

PRACTICAL ASPECTS

ERCP and access

Selective deep cannulation is required for management of bile duct strictures. There is no justification in confirming a stricture by injecting contrast (and introducing bacteria!) if the bile duct cannot be drained. Following cannulation, only a small amount of contrast should be introduced to delineate the level of stricture before a guidewire is passed across it to secure access for intervention. Once the guidewire or cannula has crossed the stricture, more contrast can be introduced if desired to demonstrate further the nature of the obstruction.

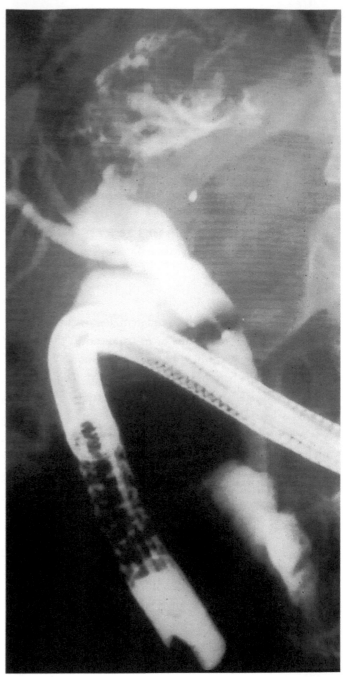

Figure 10.16. Multiple stone and stricture formation in a patient with intrahepatic parasitic infestation.

Standard 0.9 mm (0.035") guidewires with a floppy end and Teflon coating are usually used for therapeutic manoeuvres. Often, however, strictures are too tight or angulated to admit these, and thinner or hydrophilic wires may be required for initial access. Twisting, turning and 'jigging' the wire are all useful to get past difficult strictures, but cooperation between the endoscopist and wire assistant a rendezvous procedure with PTC may be useful (see Chapter 11).

Sphincterotomy techniques

A sphincterotomy, if desirable, should be undertaken in the standard way (see Chapter 9). For the purpose of inserting an endoprosthesis, a large sphincterotomy is unnecessary and may carry a higher complication rate. There may be some justification for stenting without a sphincterotomy as

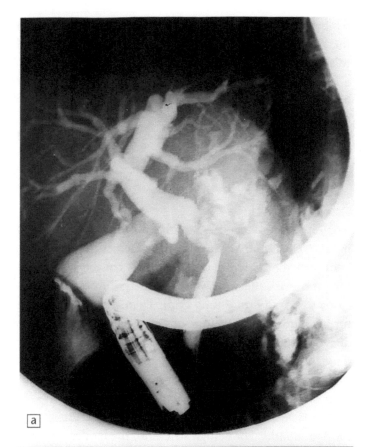

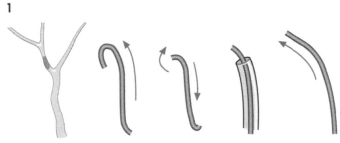

1

Form loop and gradually pull line to 'flick' tip into strictured duct. Stiffen line with cannula and advance in new direction.

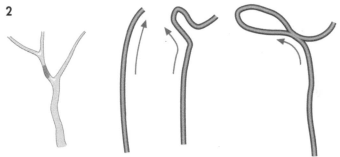

2

'Lodge' guidewire in patent duct and push to form loop into stricture so loop can pass through.

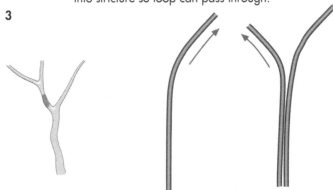

3

Place guidewire into first duct and second guidewire may 'course' more easily into second strictured duct.

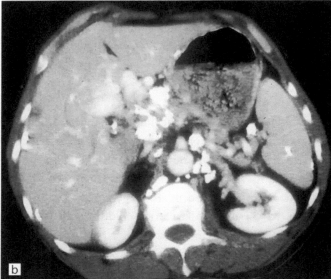

Figure 10.17. Extrahepatic bile duct compression (a) due to calcified tuberculous lymphadenopathy as shown on accompanying CT scan (b).

is essential (Fig. 10.18). Strictures may require dilatation following wire access before stents can be introduced. Where a stricture cannot be satisfactorily crossed at ERCP,

Figure 10.18. Guidewire tricks.

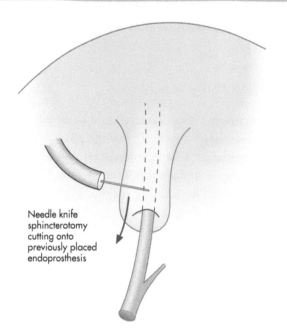

Figure 10.19. 'Cut-down' technique of sphincterotomy with pre-placed endoprosthesis.

Needle knife sphincterotomy cutting onto previously placed endoprosthesis

this reduces the potential for complications. I reserve its use for subsequent stent replacements when it can be undertaken in 'cut-down' fashion (Fig. 10.19).

Graduated dilatation

Benign strictures can be fibrous and very tight. Graduated dilatation can be difficult to achieve. After passage of a guidewire across a stricture, some assessment of its diameter can be made initially by passing the cannula through it over the guidewire. When even the 5 F cannula cannot be passed, it may be worthwhile switching to a 0.5 mm (0.021") wire and attempting passage of a tapered cannula which can be 'manufactured' by stretching a standard stenting cannula over heat. For very tight strictures it is worth considering managing these in stages rather than being too ambitious to achieve drainage at the first attempt – leaving a 5 F stent or cannula *in situ* is better than failing to place a standard-gauge stent. Where it is possible only to pass a wire, it can be helpful to leave this in place, withdrawing the endoscope over it and repeating the attempt 24 hours later.

Balloon dilatation

As discussed earlier, balloon dilatation can be useful to achieve a wide patency, but should be regarded as a temporary measure for benign strictures and a prelude to the insertion of an endoprosthesis. It is particularly useful to allow insertion of multiple side-by-side plastic stents.

Pain is common during dilatation of benign, particularly hilar, strictures. It may be useful to give an additional bolus of opiate analgesia before dilatation. Where repeated treatment episodes are needed some centres use general anaesthesia.

Endoprosthesis

Accurate measurement is essential. A simple method is to place the cannula with guidewire across the stricture. Withdraw the guidewire until it is just 1 cm above the stricture and mark the wire where it emerges from the endoscope (e.g. by a firm thumb grip). Then withdraw the wire further into the duodenum (visualize by screening or by direct vision through the transparent cannula in the duodenum) – the length of wire now withdrawn from the thumb mark to the endoscope corresponds to the length of stent required.

The stent is placed across the stricture and usually left for 3–6 months. For benign strictures, the best results may be obtained if as wide a stent as possible is left *in situ* for this time. Thus, attempts are commonly made to insert several such stents side-by-side across a stricture as in the series described by Davids [29].

Which stent should be used?
Plastic endoprostheses are the most widely used, and the least expensive stent for use in the biliary tract. Early experience indicated that stent occlusion would be a major limitation to the long-term management of benign strictures by this method of drainage alone. Occlusion is thought to be due to bacterial colonization from the duodenum with resultant build-up of proteinaceous debris. Strategies to reduce the incidence of this occurrence and prolong stent patency have included concomitant use of antibiotics, aspirin, ursodeoxycholic acid, use of ultraslick plastics or silver impregnation in the endoprostheses, or the omission of side holes. Recently, Teflon-coated stents with-. out side holes have been shown to have some advantage. Experimentally, placement of stents within the bile duct, wholly proximal to an intact sphincter (i.e. draining through the stricture but not through the sphincter) have been demonstrated to last longer – the practical difficulty

with their clinical use would be retrieving them if they were to require replacement.

The one consistent factor which determines the survival patency of endoprostheses is their internal diameter. Thus, 30 F stents last longer than 10 F, which in turn have been demonstrated to last longer than 7 F or 5 F stents. Small prospective studies have failed to demonstrate a difference between 11.5 F and 10 F stents, which are the standard sizes of larger plastic stents used. Stents with side holes clog up more quickly, as do pigtail stents when compared with straight stents. The standard stent used therefore remains a 10 F straight endoprosthesis.

Technical developments in the past decade have resulted in the introduction of a number of different designs of self-expanding metal stents. The advantage of these is that they can be introduced into the bile duct through standard instruments, but once deployed reach a patency of at least 10 mm; this greatly reduces the risk of occlusion due to build-up of biofilm and concretions. However, as these metal stents expand into the bile duct wall, they become epithelialized and are difficult – indeed mostly impossible – to remove. They are marketed particularly for malignant strictures where the major problem of tumour ingrowth and occlusion does not occur in most cases before the patient succumbs to the cancer.

Rarely, some benign bile duct strictures can have such a devastating effect on the patient's quality of life as to be considered 'malignant' in that sense. In some situations, OLT may be required for a bile duct stricture, though this is not always possible. In these situations, it may be justifiable to use permanent self-expanding metal stents for benign strictures, to temporize, or as definitive treatment. Even when used for non-malignant disease, in-growth occlusion due to bile duct epithelial hyperplasia can occur.

Nasobiliary drain

Occasionally, cannulation access and cholangiography can be difficult, particularly if a pre-cut sphincterotomy were required. Even if drainage can be achieved, further information may be required as to the nature of the bile duct problem and, in this circumstance, we have found nasobiliary drainage to be very useful. It allows further cholangiography, if necessary with concomitant CT scanning, while relieving the obstruction.

The technique follows standard insertion of a guidewire and passage of the nasobiliary draining catheter. Once placed across the stricture, the wire is withdrawn and the pigtail loop allowed to form. The endoscope is withdrawn over the nasobiliary drain, allowing generous loops to form in the duodenum and stomach. The exit of the nasobiliary drain via the mouth is converted to the nasal route by passing it retrogradely through a wide-bore nasogastric tube which is retrieved through the mouth (see Chapter 8, Fig. 8.4).

CHOICE OF TREATMENT

Endoscopic treatment is effective for the relief of jaundice and improvement in well-being and biochemistry in benign bile duct obstruction. However, it may not necessarily be the optimum treatment, and close collaboration with a hepatobiliary surgeon is essential. There are a number of specific issues which need to be resolved.

Controversial issues

Insertion of stents: to cut or not to cut?

The risk of death from sphincterotomy is 0.5–1%, of retroperitoneal perforation just less than 1%, of haemorrhage requiring transfusion or surgery 2%, and of pancreatitis perhaps 10% [30–32]. Many endoscopists do not use sphincterotomy routinely when inserting stents for this reason. However, in the context of benign strictures, if repeated endoscopic treatment is being considered (e.g. because of co-morbid factors in the patient), sphincterotomy may make further management easier and should be considered.

There is no evidence comparing the benefits and risks of endoprosthesis with and without sphincterotomy.

Endoscopic presurgical management: does jaundice matter?

Relief of jaundice preceding surgery is a controversial issue. Jaundice, and especially pruritus, can be intensely difficult symptoms for the patient to sustain. If surgical intervention is indicated for the long-term management of bile duct stricture, the question arises whether short-term drainage is worthwhile, given the risks of introducing infection. The nature of the bile duct stricture may also be delineated by EUS, spiral CT, MRCP or nuclear scan, and it is most important therefore that surgeon, endoscopist and radiologist work as a team for optimal management. When the nature of the stricture is uncertain, valuable histological or cytological information can be obtained at ERCP.

The earlier literature seemed to indicate that post-operative complications were more common in patients who were jaundiced at the time of surgery. However, several prospective studies have failed to demonstrate any significant difference in operative morbidity whether jaundice is first diminished by preoperative drainage or not [33]. Some surgeons find that placement of an endoprosthesis induces an unhelpful inflammatory reaction around the bile duct, whereas others find preplacement of a stent to be an advantage in cases of difficult dissection. This controversy underscores the importance of endoscopists, radiologists and surgeons having an intimate working relationship and mutual understanding.

Endoscopic versus surgical management

The only data directly comparing endoscopic against surgical management for biliary obstruction have been in the case of malignant strictures. The short-term advantages of endoscopic treatment (lower complication, shorter hospital stay) have to be balanced against the need for repeated stenting and risk of cholangitis with stent occlusion, if the patient survives. To a certain extent, the use of expandable stents has surmounted this problem, although some of the cost advantage against surgery is lost. In the case of benign stricture, the patient should clearly be expected to outlive stent patency and, as current expandable metal stents cause epithelial hyperplasia in the bile duct, they do not avoid the problem of stent occlusion completely. Data are available which demonstrate that patients managed endoscopically do well for some considerable time, but given that many are very young, a definitive surgical correction (if feasible) would seem to offer the best option at present for all but a few patients.

Prevention of bile duct complications: prelaparoscopic cholecystectomy ERCP

There have been several small studies looking at the efficacy of ERCP prelaparoscopic cholecystectomy. Tham *et al.* [34] examined 1847 patients and concluded that ERCP should be reserved for patients with recent jaundice or evidence of bile duct stones on ultrasound. The routine use of ERCP to discern the anatomy does not seem justified in view of the risks of pancreatitis. The issue of routine intraoperative cholangiography (IOC) in laparoscopic cholecystectomy has not been completely resolved. The arguments for are that normal and aberrant anatomy can be clearly identified, reducing the risks of bile duct injury, that stones in the bile duct will be identified and can be removed either laparoscopically or by conversion or by relying on subsequent ERCP to remove retained stones will fail in 5–10% of cases. The arguments against include a slight prolongation of operating time, the fact that small stones apparently will pass anyway, and that surgical exploration of the CBD adds to the risk of cholecystectomy. Where IOC is performed and the anatomy identified, bile duct stricture should be less common. When stones are found, the bile duct can be explored laparoscopically or by conversion to open cholecystectomy. Some surgeons prefer to leave stones for removal at early ERCP, in which case ligation of the cystic stump is usually accompanied by an adjacent drain until the stone is removed in case it obstructs the bile duct and causes a cystic stump leak. Alternatively – and particularly if the stone is thought to be impacted in the CBD – a fine drain can be inserted in the bile duct until the stone is removed.

Prevention of pancreatitis

The complication of pancreatitis occurs in 4% of patients undergoing diagnostic ERCP, and in a much higher proportion (up to 20%) in those undergoing therapeutic manoeuvres. The incidence is thought to increase with manipulation around the papillary orifice (i.e. difficult cannulation), multiple pancreatic cannulations and with sphincter of Oddi dysfunction. Many endoscopists assert that the rate is higher also in younger patients with normal-sized bile ducts, but this has been confirmed in only one of several studies [31].

Predicting those patients who will develop pancreatitis is not easy. An increase in serum trypsinogen-2 at 6 hours predicts most cases, but by that time most patients will begin developing abdominal pain necessitating their admission to hospital.

Somatostatin does not prevent post-ERCP pancreatitis, although in one study there was a significant difference in a placebo group following ERCP-sphincterotomy (18%) versus a somatostatin group (6%). Methyl prednisolone is not helpful.

REFERENCES

1. Pitt HA, Miyamoto T, Parapatis SK *et al.* Factors influencing outcome in patients with post-operative biliary strictures. *Am J Surg* 1982; 144: 14–21.

2. Strasberg S, Hertl M. Soper N. An analysis of the problem of biliary injury during laparoscopic cholecystectomy. *J Am Coll Surg* 1955; 80: 101–125.

3. Haycox A, Lombard M, Neoptolemos J, Walley T. Current practice and future perspectives in the detection and diagnosis of pancreatic cancer. *Aliment Therap Pharmacol* 1998; 12: 937–948.

4. Pasanen PA, Partanen KP, Pikkarainen PH *et al.* A comparison of ultrasound, computed tomography and endoscopic retrograde cholangiopancreatography in the differential diagnosis of benign and malignant jaundice and cholestasis. *Eur J Surg* 1993; 159: 23–29.

5. Snady H, Cooperman A, Siegel J. Endoscopic ultrasonography compared wth computed tomography with ERCP in patients with obstructive jaundice or small peri-pancreatic mass. *Gastrointest Endosc* 1992; 38: 27–34.

6. Harbin WP, Mueller PR, Ferrucci JT. Transhepatic cholangiography: complications and use patterns of the fine needle technique. *Radiology* 1980; 135: 15.

7. Mansfield JC, Griffin SM, Wadehra V, Matthewson K. A prospective evaluation of cytology from biliary strictures. *Gut* 1997; 40: 671–677.

8. Davids P, Tanka A, Rauws E *et al.* Benign biliary strictures: surgery or endoscopy? *Ann Surg* 1993; 217: 237–243.

9. Geenen DJ, Geenen JE, Hogan WJ *et al.* Endoscopic therapy for benign bile duct strictures. *Gastrointest Endosc* 1989; 35: 367–371.

10. O'Brien SM, Hatfield AR, Craig PI, Williams SP. A 5-year follow-up of self-expanding metal stents in the endoscopic management of patients with benign bile duct strictures. *Eur J Gastroenterol Hepatol* 1998; 10: 141–145.

11. Huibregtse K. *Endoscopic Biliary and Pancreatic Drainage.* Georg Thieme Verlag Stuttgart, New York: 1998.

12. Karsten T, Davids P, van Gulik T *et al.* Effects of biliary endoprothesis on the extrahepatic bile ducts in relation to subsequent operation on the biliary tract. *J Am Coll Surg* 1994; 178: 343–352.

13. Lillemoe KD. Benign post-operative bile duct strictures. *Baillières Clin Gastroenterol* 1997; 11: 749–779.

14. Wherry DC, Marohn MR, Malanoski MP *et al.* An external audit of laparoscopic cholecystectomy in the steady state performed in medical treatment facilities of the Department of Defence. *Ann Surg* 1996; 224: 145–154.

15. Charels K, Kloppel G. The bile duct system and its anatomical variations. *Endoscopy* 1989; 21: 300–311.

16. Davids P, Rauws E, Tytgat G, Huibregtse K. Post operative bile leakage: endoscopic management. *Gut* 1992; 33: 1118–1122.

17. Sossenheimer M. Slivka A, Carr-Locke D. Management of extrahepatic biliary disease after orthotopic liver transplantation: review of the literature and results of a multicentre study. *Endoscopy* 1996; 28: 565–571.

18. Roberts-Thomson IC, Pannall PR, Toouli J. Relationship between morphine responses and sphincter of Oddi motility in undefined biliary pain after cholecystectomy. *J Gastroenterol Hepatol* 1989; 4: 317–324.

19. Fullarton G, Allan A, Hilditch T, Murray W. Quantitative ^{99m}Tc-DISIDA scanning and endoscopic biliary manometry in sphincter of Oddi dysfunction. *Gut* 1988; 29: 1397–1401.

20. Bozkurt T, Orth KH, Butsch B, Lux G. Long-term clinical outcome of post-cholecystectomy patients with biliary-type pain: results of manometry, non-invasive techniques and endoscopic sphincterotomy. *Eur J Gastroenterol Hepatol* 1996; 84: 245–249.

21. Lee J, Schutz S, England R *et al.* Endoscopy therapy of sclerosing cholangitis. *Hepatology* 1995; 21: 661–667.

22. Ponsioen CY, Vrouenraets SME, van Millgen AWM *et al.* Value of brush cytology for dominant strictures in primary sclerosing cholangitis. *Endoscopy* 1999; 31: 305–309.

23. Luftus EV, Aguilar HJ, Sandborn W *et al.* Risk of colorectal neoplasia in patients with primary sclerosing cholangitis and ulcerative colitis following orthotopic liver transplantation. *J Hepatol* 1999; 30: 669–673.

24. Nagel RA, Westaby D, Javaid A *et al.* Liver disease and bile duct abnormalities in adults with cystic fibrosis (see comments). *Lancet* 1989; 2: 1422–1425.

25. Baer H, Matthews J, Schweiser W *et al.* Management of the Mirizzi syndrome and the surgical implications of cholecystocholedochal fistulae. *Br J Surg* 1990; 77: 743–745.

26. Malka G, Bhatia S, Bashir K *et al.* Cholangiopathy associated with portal hypertension: diagnostic evaluation and clinical implications. *Gastrointest Endosc* 1999; 49: 344–348.

27. Dumas R, Le Gall P, Hastier P *et al.* The role of endoscopic retrograde cholangiopancreatography in the management of hepatic hydatid disease. *Endoscopy* 1999; 31: 242–247.

28. Leung JW, Yu AS. Hepatolithiasis and biliary parasites. *Baillières Clin Gastroenterol* 1997; 11: 681–706.

29. Davids P, Ringers J, Rauws E *et al.* Bile duct injury after laparoscopic cholecystectomy: the value of endoscopic retrograde cholangiopancreatography. *Gut* 1993; 34: 1250–1254.

30. Sherman S, Lehman G. ERCP and endoscopic sphincterotomy-induced pancreatitis. *Pancreas* 1991; 6: 350–367.

31. Chen Y, Foliente R, Santoro M *et al.* Endoscopic sphincterotomy-induced pancreatitis: increased risk with nondilated bile ducts and sphincter of Oddi dysfunction. *Am J Gastroenterol* 1994; 89: 327–333.

32. Cotton P, Baillie J, Leung J *et al.* Correlations with post-ERCP pancreatitis. *Gastrointest Endosc* 1994; 40: P104.

33. Lai E, Mok F, Fan S *et al.* Preoperative endoscopic drainage for malignant obstructive jaundice. *Br J Surg* 1994; 81: 1195–1198.

34. Tham T, Lichtenstein D, Vandervoort J *et al.* Role of endoscopic retrograde cholangiopancreatography for suspected choledocholithiasis in patients undergoing laparoscopic cholecystectomy. *Gastrointest Endosc* 1998; 47: 50–56.

11

Malignant strictures of the biliary tree

M.L. Wilkinson

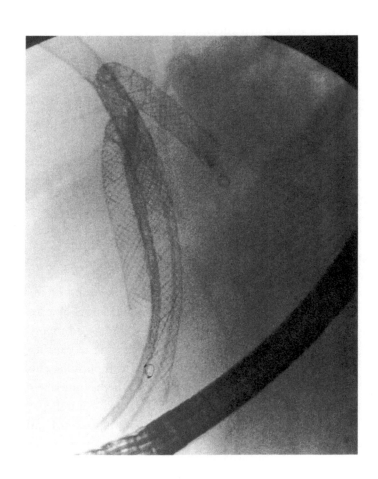

INTRODUCTION

There is no doubt that the advent of interventional endoscopy in the late 1970s revolutionized the management of malignant obstructive lesions affecting the biliary tree, from both a therapeutic as well as a diagnostic standpoint. Up until then the choice was limited to the dangerous and painful alternatives of surgery or percutaneous drainage, with or without the use of large plastic stents or drainage tubes. Assessment of operability was something of a hit-and-miss affair, with no computed tomography (CT) scanning, and ultrasound in its infancy, while there was little evidence of survival benefit even when therapy was technically feasible. There has been a huge leap forward in all of these areas since then, but such has been the impact of the endoscopic management of obstructive jaundice that it has become the standard against which other methods must be judged.

It would be wrong to trumpet the successes of endoscopy too loudly, however. Endoscopy has limitations, causes complications, and may not always be appropriate. The approach to malignant biliary obstruction is one that requires a close cooperation between gastroenterologist, radiologist, surgeon, pathologist and oncologist if the best results are to be achieved. Equally important is the input of community services and palliative care specialists towards the quality of life when therapeutic measures are inappropriate or exhausted. Such a multidisciplinary approach, now to be the norm in the UK since the Calman/Hine proposals [1], is expensive in terms of time, but before we leap ahead to develop further clever techniques by which to manage our patients the careful application of those advances already known in these diverse fields will bring dividends.

PRESENTATION

The most common malignant biliary strictures are extrahepatic (Table 11.1), usually leading to a presentation with progressive obstructive jaundice, but additional presenting complaints include: iron-deficiency anaemia, steatorrhoea, back or abdominal pain, gastric distension and/or vomiting from duodenal obstruction, an abdominal mass, thrombophlebitis migrans, diabetes mellitus, small-bowel infarction from superior mesenteric artery occlusion, acute cholecystitis as well as the familiar and non-specific general malaise or

Table 11.1. Malignant causes of biliary obstruction

Extrahepatic malignancies	Intrahepatic malignancies
Carcinoma of the pancreas	Hepatocellular carcinoma
Cholangiocarcinoma	Cholangiocarcinoma
Carcinoma of the ampulla of Vater	Cholangiocellular carcinoma
Carcinoma of the duodenum	Secondary carcinoma, especially breast
Carcinoid-like tumours	Sarcomas, haemangioendothelioma
Hilar lymph-node secondaries	Lymphoma
Carcinoma of the gall bladder	
Carcinoma of the stomach	
Lymphoma	

weight loss. The presentation of ampullary carcinoma also differs from the classical extrahepatic obstruction pattern. Many of these patients have a history of fluctuating cholestasis, often with cholangitis, indistinguishable from bile duct stones. Lack of gallstones on ultrasound in a person of appropriate age – usually the seventh decade onwards – is sometimes a clue.

Intrahepatic malignancies (Table 11.1) tend to present with biliary obstruction only when they are either strategically situated near the hilum, by which time other manifestations of malignancy are often present, or as a complication of primary sclerosing cholangitis (PSC) or one of the fibropolycystic diseases of the liver, when a worsening of existing cholestasis may herald development of a complicating cholangiocarcinoma.

Whether one labels hilar cholangiocarcinomas – 'Klatskin tumours' – intrahepatic or extrahepatic is arguable, and the presentation can mimic either, with a 'hepatitis-like' presentation being a particular catch (Fig. 11.1).

The assumption that a low bile duct-obstructing tumour was a pancreatic cancer until proven otherwise is no longer tenable, as it is now clear that far more than previously realized are cholangiocarcinomas. At present, this is frequently of no more than academic interest, but as chemotherapy regimes are increasingly shown to have benefit in particular tumour types, histological identification of the precise origin of a tumour will assume a greater importance (Fig. 11.2). Further molecular techniques to aid the process of histological diagnosis are under development.

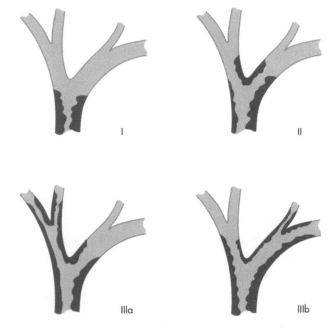

Figure 11.1. Diagrammatic Bismuth classification of malignant hilar strictures.

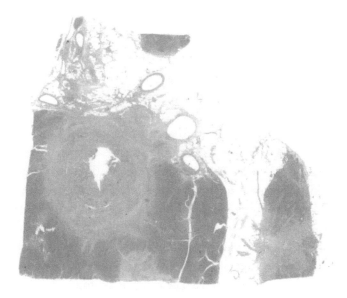

Figure 11.2. Histological specimen from a lower bile duct stricture thought endoscopically to be of pancreatic origin. The malignant process was demonstrated to be confined to the bile duct epithelium and did not invade the pancreas, that is a low CBD cholangiocarcinoma.

Initial clinical assessment

The management will depend critically on the state of the patient at the time therapy is planned, and therefore a careful assessment of general health and nutritional state,

Table 11.2. Initial clinical assessment

Age
Recent weight loss
Body mass index, skinfold thickness*
Haemoglobin
Coagulation status, platelet count
Albumin, prealbumin*
Urea and creatinine, urinary nitrogen*
Presence of ascites
Previous abdominal surgery, especially Billroth II or Roux-en-Y
Presence of chronic liver disease
Presence of encephalopathy
Bilirubin, liver enzymes
Presence of sepsis, C-reactive protein*
Tumour markers, CA 19-9, CEA, AFP, CA15-3*

* optional

the presence of concomitant or underlying diseases or metastases, as well as an appraisal of mental capacity and psychological preparedness should be carried out as early as possible (Table 11.2).

As well as a clinical assessment, blood tests may help somewhat in distinguishing malignant from benign biliary obstruction. The level of alkaline phosphatase tends to be greater in malignant obstruction, but this is a very poor specific finding, and should not carry much weight in the decision-making process.

Tumour markers

Tumour markers are not of great value at present in the biliary tree. Secondary tumours may be suspected with appropriate elevations of CEA. Pancreatic cancer is more likely with a raised level of CA 19-9 or CA 15-3, and bile duct cancer is more common with elevations of any of these or of alpha-fetoprotein. The distinction of cholangio-carcinoma from sclerosing cholangitis by tumour markers is not possible in an individual patient [2]. A very high alpha-fetoprotein level suggests hepatocellular carcinoma, as long as germ cell tumours have been ruled out. Clinical management should never be decided on tumour markers alone; corroborative evidence is necessary.

Radiological assessment

Ultrasound

Initial assessment of any case of obstructive jaundice will involve an early abdominal ultrasound examination [3]. Ultrasound is excellent at demonstrating dilated intrahepatic biliary radicles, but less effective at delineating the level or cause of the obstruction. The sensitivity for common bile duct (CBD) stones, for example, is only 50–60%. Occasionally, the appreciation of dilated intrahepatic biliary radicles is open to misinterpretation. A normal intrahepatic duct should not exceed 2 mm in diameter, or 40% of the diameter of the adjacent portal vein branch. The usual teaching that the biliary radicles lie anterior to portal vein branches is only correct about half of the time. In one-third, the bile ducts lie posterior, and in one-fifth they are sometimes anterior and sometimes posterior to the portal vein [4]. Doppler ultrasound, increasingly available on a routine basis, may help in difficult cases – particularly when confusing arterial branches exist.

In obstruction at the distal end of the CBD, the extra-hepatic biliary tree dilates before the intrahepatic, in some cases. The intrahepatic ducts may not dilate at all when they are constrained by fibrous tissue, as in cirrhosis, or by widespread intrahepatic malignancy. Similarly, the extra-hepatic ducts can be prevented from dilating by sclerosing cholangitis, by recurrent cholangitis (analogous to the Courvoisier rule in the gall bladder) or by choledochal varices or extensive extrahepatic malignancy. In general, the main bile duct is more dilated in the presence of malignant obstruction than with choledocholithiasis. If the ducts are not dilated on admission, they may become so after a few days. A repeat ultrasound examination is often revealing, especially if carried out by an operator with a special interest in hepatobiliary disorders.

Ultrasound examination may also be limited in looking at retroperitoneal structures, lymph nodes and pancreas especially. The pancreas can be examined very effectively by ultrasound, but it takes a highly skilled and dedicated operator to perform all the special manoeuvres to achieve this, such as filling the stomach with de-gassed water, and

scanning through it in the right posterior oblique position with the patient in the right lateral decubitus position when there is overlying gas or scanning in the transverse plane with the patient semi-erect and in the right posterior oblique (RPO) position.

Furthermore, not only gas (flatus) but also fat makes life difficult for the ultrasonologist. As the population in most Western countries continues to expand with annual rings of adipose tissue, so the problems for ultrasound increase. All this notwithstanding, its convenience, relative cost, lack of ionizing radiation, and the possibility of transporting it into the consulting room or to the bedside mean that ultrasound will remain the initial radiological tool for the time being.

In addition, training in the use of ultrasound by non-radiologists – already commonplace in Japan and certain parts of continental Europe [5] – will increasingly be available to gastroenterologists, and thereby enhance the specialized input to hepato-pancreato-biliary disorder. Certainly, having learned transcutaneous ultrasound examination accelerates the acquisition of the necessary skills for endoscopic ultrasound.

Computed axial tomography (CT)

CT scanning is the most useful single imaging technique for staging malignancies causing biliary obstruction, especially when used with intravenous contrast. The current generation of spiral scanners produce, when used appropriately, superb images with fine detail almost approximating to the mythical 'route map' which imaging techniques are supposed to give the surgeon. We are all aware, however, of the opposite side to this coin – poor-quality images from old or badly serviced scanners, produced with far too big gaps between slices, and without the aid of intravenous contrast. The interpretation of the images may also be insufficiently accurate. It is widely, but erroneously, believed that CT scanning is free of the operator dependence which is a cardinal drawback of ultrasound scanning. The truth is very different, and images of the pancreato-biliary tree are best interpreted by radiologists working in the context of a multidisciplinary team with surgeons and endoscopists.

CT scanning does have certain advantages compared with ultrasound which stem from the different technologies employed (Table 11.3). It is better able to produce good images of the retroperitoneal area, and it largely ignores the problems which occur due to gas or fat. CT may utilize the fat planes to delineate the various intra-abdominal organs. CT is superior to ultrasound in diagnosing the level of

Table 11.3. Comparison of computed tomography (CT) and ultrasound (US) for biliary obstruction

Advantages of US over CT	Advantages of CT over US
Cheaper	
Better in the slim patient	Better in the obese patient
More sensitive for gallstones	Intestinal gas minimal problem
Portable	Better in retroperitoneal area
Easier for guided biopsy	Good for assessment of viable liver mass
No ionizing radiation	Less operator-dependent
Simpler to assess blocked vessels*	Better at characterizing hepatic tumours
	More accurate staging

*With Doppler. CT angiography is also very useful.

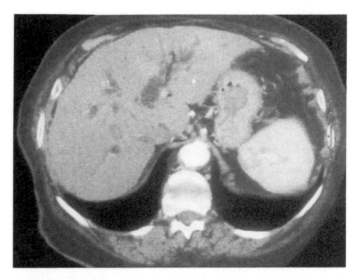

Figure 11.3. CT scan demonstrating asymmetrical dilation of the intrahepatic biliary tree suggesting hilar obstruction. Often no specific signs of a lesion can be demonstrated at the hilum and a malignant process is inferred from the pattern of dilatation.

obstruction, and its cause, with one important exception. Gallstones are not well seen on CT scans unless they are calcified [6]. Since calcification, even by CT criteria, is only present in 15–20% of gall bladder stones, and rather more ductal stones, to rely upon CT alone to make the primary diagnosis may be unwise. The proper investigation of possible malignant obstructive jaundice thus requires the combination of ultrasound and CT scans, ultrasound being performed first and CT once it is clear that a malignant process may be involved.

Magnetic resonance scanning

Until the arrival of magnetic resonance (MR) imaging, the non-invasive imaging techniques were no match for direct cholangiography in the demonstration of biliary obstruction and associated biliary and pancreatic duct lesions. Whereas ultrasound and CT are excellent initial screening tools and can provide much valuable staging data, they are essentially complementary to endoscopic retrograde cholangio-pancreatography (ERCP) or percutaneous transhepatic cholangiography (PTC) (Fig. 11.3). The introduction of magnetic resonance cholangiopancreatography (MRCP) (Fig. 11.3) has however provided new opportunities for pancreato-biliary imaging. Now, reasonably high-quality images of the biliary tree and, to a lesser extent, the pancreatic ducts, can be obtained, non-invasively, without the use of ionizing radiation and regardless of the presence or absence of obstruction or previous surgery. MRCP is increasingly available, and further improvements in image quality and speed of examination are certain.

The procedure is not devoid of problems, however. The expense is considerable, between 2% and 5% of patients cannot tolerate the noise and claustrophobia, certain sorts of metallic stents – principally Gianturco – may be moved by the magnetic force (an average pull of 7g towards the head) if they are not firmly embedded [7], and pacemakers contraindicate the test. The technical aspects of image production are quite difficult to perfect, although the original need to use a 20-s breath-hold is no longer necessary [8]. Not all MR scanners are suitable for MRCP, and the ultimate image quality remains at present inferior to that obtained by direct cholangiography [9].

MRCP is not useful where dynamic images are required. The sensitivity of MRCP in biliary obstruction exceeds 90% with a slightly lower figure – 80% – in bile duct stones [10]. These figures lie somewhere between the accuracy expected of direct cholangiography and the other indirect, cross-sectional techniques. MRCP is probably the method of choice where direct cholangiography is unsuccessful or where the images are incomplete or difficult to interpret. This may prove to be particularly useful where the intrahepatic ducts need to be visualized clearly, which can be difficult with ERCP, especially when there is widespread ductal abnormality, as in primary sclerosing cholangitis (PSC) or Caroli's disease, for example, both conditions predisposing to cholangiocarcinoma.

The final place of MRCP in the investigation of patients with malignant obstructive jaundice will become apparent with time and usage.

Choice of endoscopic or percutaneous management

Once an obstructed biliary tree is recognized, usually at US examination, an ERCP is routinely the next step. Should it be? I believe the answer is yes, but requires qualification. The chief advantage of performing ERCP first is to make the diagnosis secure. A recent study shows that ERCP increases the confidence in diagnosis in 35% of cases despite the use of all the other diagnostic tests already referred to [11]. Secondly, the ability of ERCP to treat definitively CBD stones means that it is logical to use it early, before the diagnosis is certain, to avoid complications such as cholangitis from untreated stones. Again, if there is a low bile duct obstruction from a tumour, ERCP is the logical first step since it is less invasive than the alternative percutaneous approach and is successful in about 90% of cases in palliating the obstruction, either by stent placement or, in the rarer ampullary carcinoma, sometimes by sphincterotomy.

The question of which procedure to do first if the obstruction is at the hilum is not so clear-cut, however. It is clear that successful endoscopic stenting of hilar tumours is less frequent than for low lesions, while PTC will nearly always lead to technically successful stenting, even if a second procedure is often necessary.

The argument against initial PTC remains the complication rate of the procedure ,which in one series was as high as 42%. These were not by any means all early or immediate complications, late drainage of infected collections constituting up to 25% [12]. Ascites and coagulopathy are contraindications, but nevertheless, infection (2–4%), bleeding (3%) and painful bile leaks (5–10%), into the peritoneum or pleural space, are the main serious complications. Haemobilia and pneumothorax are additional complications which can occur. However, the most frequent problem is pain; this can arise during the procedure, especially if balloon dilatation is required, or if analgesia is insufficient. Pain is also a significant problem in the post-procedure period, when bile drains are exiting via the lateral abdominal wall. Excessive pain may also be an indication of a bile leak. We must not forget, however, that for a few patients nothing compares with the discomfort and general unpleasantness of an ERCP.

Nevertheless, the choice of which approach to take must be individualized in respect of both patient and local facilities. It is very useful to have alternatives when things do not go as expected – hence the need for large centres – but also the need for an interested nucleus of specialists in a District General Hospital.

If initial ERCP fails completely, a second procedure can be scheduled, about 5 days later, to allow any papillary trauma to settle. Cannulation success in this context should exceed 50%. Failure at this stage should lead to PTC. If the duct is cannulated to the extent that contrast has passed the stricture, but either deep cannulation was not achieved or the stent could not be inserted, there is a significant risk of cholangitis and urgent PTC should be carried out providing that there are no absolute contraindications.

SURGERY AND MALIGNANT BILIARY OBSTRUCTION

The elation when a stent is successfully inserted at ERCP should be tempered by the knowledge that the best the endoscopist can ever achieve in malignant biliary obstruction is palliation. There is no problem when decisions about patients are taken in a multidisciplinary team, but endoscopists can forget that surgery may be curative and refer too few patients too late for sufficient to benefit. For the elderly, frail patient, endoscopic stenting can be a godsend, but both hilar cholangiocarcinomas and small pancreatic or periampullary tumours can be curatively resected. In anyone fit for surgery (itself an expanding group as anaesthetics and postoperative care have improved) with such a tumour, work-up for resection should be carried out. If patients are well hydrated, and coagulopathy is corrected, good anaesthetists and surgeons can perform major abdominal surgery safely. What many surgeons do not like operating upon is a bile duct which is inflamed and thickened from an indwelling endoscopic stent. Since it has been estimated that 25% of patients with pancreatic carcinoma will develop duodenal obstruction, it was suggested that, in patients fit for surgery, palliative choledochojejunostomy and gastrojejunostomy should be carried out rather than

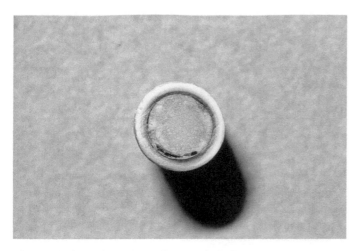

Figure 11.4. End-on view of an occluded plastic endoprosthesis. Debris comprising proteinaceous material and bacteria can cause total occlusion of 10-french stents in 2–6 months.

endoscopic stenting. Trials so far conducted to test this hypothesis have been inconclusive, stenting being safer and cheaper, but requiring more return visits for blocked stents [13] (Fig. 11.4).

TECHNIQUE OF THERAPEUTIC ERCP IN MALIGNANT BILIARY OBSTRUCTION

ERCP is carried out in the standard manner, with any extrinsic gastric compression being noted. Pyloric or duodenal stenosis may be present, and this may be impassable with a standard duodenoscope. A paediatric instrument can occasionally be helpful. Endoscopic balloon dilatation can also be accomplished for this indication, but there is a risk of perforation, which is difficult to quantify, as experience is limited. A further approach to duodenal obstruction is the insertion of an expandable metal stent, which will gently dilate the stricture, avoiding perforation and permitting cannulation and, if necessary, stent placement, through the mesh of the stent [14]. The stent cannot generally be removed, however. Probably the most straightforward way to deal with duodenal obstruction is to have a radiological colleague place a wire at PTC which can be manipulated retrogradely via the stenosis, grasped in the stomach by a basket, snare or forceps, and withdrawn through the duodenoscope which can often then be made to pass the obstruction by being 'railroaded' over the wire. Of course, once the radiologist is in position, if the obstruction is known to be malignant, a metal stent

can be inserted percutaneously rather than asking the endoscopist's help. These complex manoeuvres may perplex the surgeon, for whom a combined biliary and gastric bypass is a relatively straightforward procedure. If the patient is fit, surgery should be considered.

Once through into the second part of the duodenum, with a 'short scope', the papilla should be inspected for signs of infiltration or papillary tumours (Fig. 11.5). Attempts should then be made to cannulate the biliary tree selectively. If tumour is replacing the papilla, orientating the scope correctly and trying to advance the cannula through where the biliary orifice should be is sometimes successful in achieving biliary filling. If not, using a soft, hydrophilic-tipped guidewire may work, perhaps aided by a wire-guided sphincterotome to gain extra upwards angulation. Very low pancreatic lesions may make cannulation impossible, as may a distorted duodenal loop. Sometimes the papilla appears to be drawn upwards into an awkward position by a scirrhous-type tumour. Rarely, the papilla is widely patent, with thick, clear mucus exiting from the orifice caused by a mucus-secreting pancreatic tumour. If the papilla is replaced with an obvious papillary tumour, and the cholangiogram does not show a long stricture, initial therapy can be endoscopic sphincterotomy alone. A large tumour can also be snared in the manner of a colonoscopic polypectomy. Experimental treatments include laser therapy. These methods are useful for palliation, but all papillary tumours at the ampulla are potentially curable sugically, and careful consideration should be given before a solely palliative approach is taken (Fig. 11.6).

Needle-knife sphincterotomy

If cannulation is not achieved by standard and other methods, consideration should be given to the need for a needle-knife 'pre-cut' sphincterotomy. The latter is a very useful technique but associated with a well recognized complication rate, in particular bleeding and pancreatitis. It should rarely be used unless a therapeutic pay-off is likely (e.g. there is little justification for its use if the patient is not jaundiced). Nor should it be used by the relatively inexperienced endoscopist if alternative techniques or a more experienced operator are available locally. Nevertheless, it remains a valuable addition to the armamentarium of the endoscopist. The technique has been described as a downward, sweeping movement of the needle from

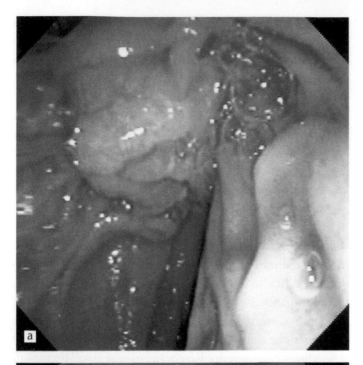

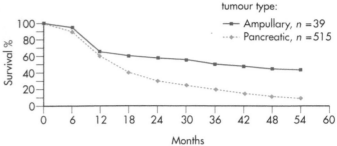

Figure 11.6. Survival curves of patients with carcinoma of ampulla of Vater and pancreas. Ampullary and bile duct tumours have a better prognosis and these diagnoses should be distinguished. Reproduced with permission from J. Neoptolemus, ESPAC.

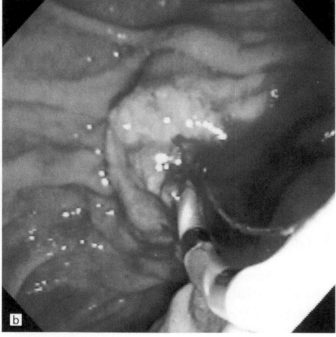

Figure 11.5. (a) Bulky papilla due to involvement by tumour. (b) Obstruction can be relieved by sphincterotomy with or without placement of endoprosthesis and biopsies should be taken from inside the cut edge.

longitudinal fold to papilla and also as an upwards cut, starting at the papillary orifice, using low power, cutting current, until biliary mucosa is revealed. The tendency is to cut too little and then try to insert a cannula into the cut

area. This often leads to a false passage or submucosal injection. It is better to make a somewhat larger cut and then probe the new orifice with a hydrophilic guidewire. Sometimes further progress is impossible due to bleeding, oedema or other factors. It is then tempting to call for radiological back-up, but if one can afford to wait, a second ERCP in a few days will usually be successful.

Cytology and histology

One of the advantages of an endoscopic approach to the bile duct is the ability to take cytological and histological samples for confirmation of malignancy and identification of tumour type. The overall yield in the best hands does not exceed 80%, however, and negative results are not reassuring [15]. The most common method used is brush cytology, in which a covered, disposable brush, within a catheter, is passed to the area of the stricture, and vigorously brushed through it, withdrawn, and the resultant cells smeared on one or more labelled glass slides and placed in preserving medium for transport to the cytology laboratory. As with other cytological techniques, a better yield is obtained if a cytologist is on hand to review the slides and to request further samples if necessary. This is not generally a cost-effective use of a cytologist's time.

Difficulties can arise in getting the brush to the desired area. These may be tackled in several ways. The brush catheter, without the brush, can be passed over a guidewire above the suspicious area, the wire withdrawn and the brush reinserted. The catheter is withdrawn just below the lesion and the brush is then withdrawn through the stricture far enough to get tissue, but not to lose position. The catheter can be reinserted over the brush and the latter withdrawn all the way to get specimens before reinserting the guidewire to commence stenting operations. One of the problems is that the brush wire is flimsy, kinks easily, and cannot be pushed through tough strictures. Employing the guidewire technique described above should overcome this problem, but much of the cellular material is lost on withdrawing the brush the length of the catheter. Getting the brush into position may be easier with double-lumen brush catheters, but I find these awkward to use, although their design is improving. Other ways of obtaining cytological samples are: bile aspiration (very poor yield); needle-aspiration; examination of stents on replacement, or, ingeniously, pioneered at the Royal London Hospital, the use of the Soehendra stent retriever literally screwed into the lesion, both to enable a wire to be passed and also to gain cytological samples from the screw threads. Unfortunately, the recent stipulations about non-reuse of disposable accessories [16] may make this last method too expensive.

Histopathology specimens are easy to obtain from ampullary lesions, although it should be noted that in-experienced pathologists may underestimate the malignancy of papillary lesions, which for practical purposes should always be considered to be at least locally invasive. Small endoscopic samples may not be representative of the whole lesion. Specimens from intraduct lesions are harder to get, but the manufacturers have devised some small forceps which tilt to one side in use to make samples easier to take. Clear benefit of these forceps compared with standard instruments is not yet available, but they are easier to use (Fig. 11.7). The main difficulty with getting any samples from biliary strictures is the desire to treat a stricture as soon as it has been demonstrated, for fear that any delay or additional manipulations may lead to a failed therapeutic manoeuvre. This is a real consideration, but the implications of a positive histological diagnosis are so profound that ways of achieving it should continue to be sought.

New techniques from molecular biology may soon be routinely available for examining biliary or pancreatic fluid or smear specimens, such as k-*ras* mutations, *p53* deletions or other molecular anomalies known to be associated with

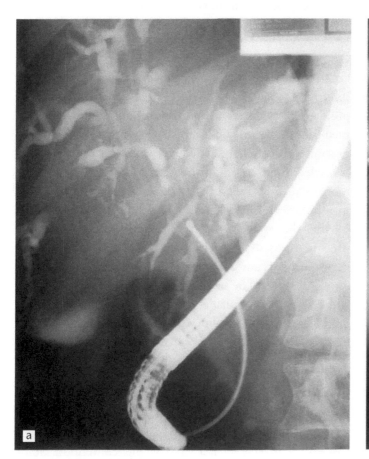
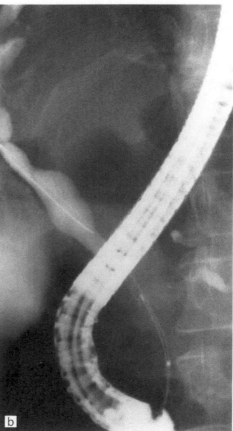

Figure 11.7. Samples of bile duct epithelium at the site of obstruction can be obtained by (a) brush cytology or (b) by 'blind' biopsy using a standard endoscopy forceps.

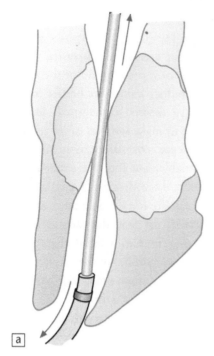

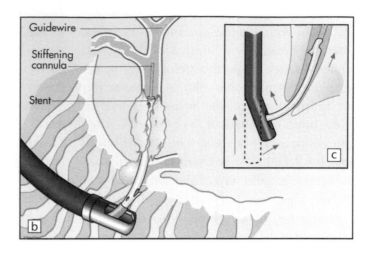

Figure 11.8. Illustration of technique for insertion of endoprosthesis. (a) The ampulla is cannulated in the usual fashion and a guidewire is passed through the occluding tumour. (b) After passing a stiffening tube over the guidewire, an endoprosthesis is pushed through the tumour over the stiffened guidewire. This is achieved by pushing a little at a time and elevating the stent into the bile duct by use of the bridge and upward angulation of the tip of the endoscope. (c) Once the stent is placed in satisfactory position, the guidewire and stiffening cannula are removed leaving the endoprosthesis to drain across the tumour.

malignancy in these organs. At present, any such test is at an experimental stage, but further developments are certain.

Stent insertion (Fig. 11.8)

After identifying the stricture, a guidewire is passed across it. Hydrophilic guidewires make the passage through tight strictures much easier, while nitinol-type kink-resistant wires are generally easier to handle. A wire with a hydrophilic tip of about 10 cm, but a stiff nitinol 'tail', seems to be an excellent compromise and removes the need to change to a stiffer wire for stent insertion, after crossing the stricture with a slippery wire. Unfortunately, the slippery tip cannot be recycled, unlike at least one make of nitinol wire. My practice is to use a reusable stiff wire where the stricture is not a difficult one, but a hydrophilic-tipped wire for tight or tortuous narrowings. Occasionally a fine, pure hydrophilic wire is still useful, but it must be changed to a stiff wire for stenting. Wires with radio-opaque or coloured markings help in monitoring wire position during catheter and other instrument placements, reducing the need for X-ray screening.

After the wire, the guide catheter or stent inner tube is inserted. Difficulty at this stage suggests that there may be problems with the stent, and the cautious endoscopist may predilate the stricture with either an angioplasty-type balloon or a push dilator of graduated type. I find that predilatation is needed less than 5% of the time, but others use it much more frequently. Balloon dilatation is invariably painful and may induce violent reactions in a lightly sedated patient.

After dilatation, if indicated, a plastic stent is selected. Most stents used for this purpose are the straight or slightly curved Amsterdam stents with barbs at each end to prevent stent migration. The standard calibre is 10 F, although 7, 8 and 12 F are also available. Stents of less than 10 F (actually 9.6 F) block with biofilm more rapidly, but, surprisingly, there is no evidence that 12 F stents last any longer than 10 F. Alternative stent patterns include the so-called Tannenbaum (Christmas tree) stent with a double row of narrow upper barbs and single lower row. This is alleged to last longer before becoming clogged, lacking as it does any side holes which is where the process often starts. Controlled studies do not support this contention. Some prefer this stent, but I dislike it, the chief reasons being its

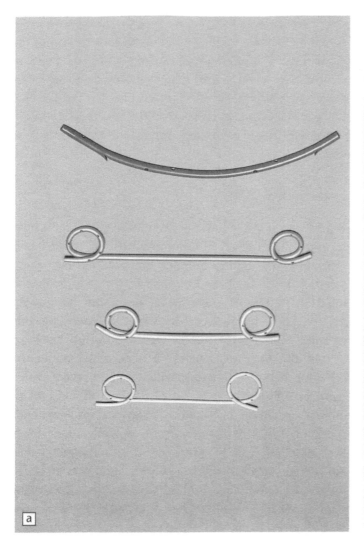

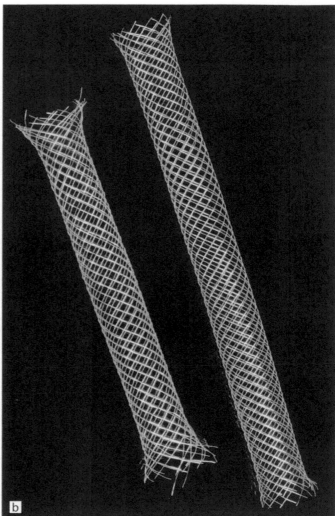

Figure 11.9. (a) A series of plastic stents incorporating both the straight and pigtail variety. (b) Two self-expanding stainless steel metal endoprosthesis in their release form.

greater stiffness and the propensity of the barbs to obscure vision. It is also considerably costlier than standard stents. There has been considerable attention to stent materials, both hydrophobic and hydrophilic coverings being tried. At present there is no clear advantage of one material over the others. Examples of endoprostheses are shown in Figure 11.9.

Picking the right length of stent can be done in several ways. The simplest, when images can be called up on the screening machine, is to measure from above the stricture to the spot in the duodenum where the lower barb will be on the screen, with a flexible ruler, and correct for the size of the endoscope. Others have calculated an average magnification in their room and marked a 'flexicurve' in appropriate centimetre marks to take this into account.

Another technique is to mark a metal-tipped cannula at the point where it exits the valve of the scope when the tip is at the top of the stricture and then mark it again when it is withdrawn into the duodenum, measuring the distance on the catheter. Catheters with radio-opaque centimetre marks in the distal portion can also be used, and the required length read off on the screening image.

Insertion of a plastic stent can either be very easy, or impossibly difficult. Whereas some strictures are inherently difficult, the endoscopist can make the task easier or harder for him/herself. A few principles should be followed:

- Keep the controls on the endoscope locked so that the scope is positioned below the ampulla looking up at it.
- Never allow too great a length of stent to get between scope and papilla, as this may result in control being

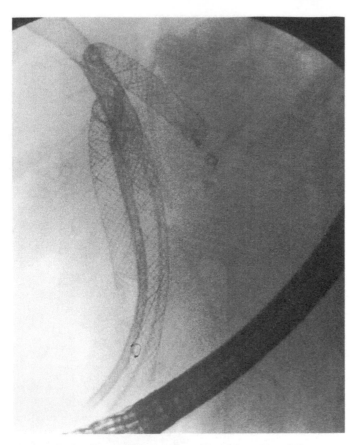

Figure 11.10. Stents may be placed in either side of the biliary tree when a Klatskin hilar stricture is present.

lost and the whole thing – scope included – being withdrawn and the process restarted.

• Stents can only be pushed, not pulled. Stent advancement should be by a four-step process – relax bridge, advance pusher sleeve, raise bridge, elevate scope tip.

• When obstructions are encountered, more force can be applied to the tip of the stent by withdrawing the scope slightly, or by rotating the scope shaft using the right hand.

The left thenar eminence tends to suffer during this period of stent insertion. The stiffer the stent, the more the force required. This is also when the bridge elevator tends to fail and should thus be used with care.

CONTROVERSIAL ISSUES

Pre-stent sphincterotomy

Initial sphincterotomy used to be employed routinely before stent placement, but there is no need for this in most cases. It does reduce the force required to insert a stent, but the complications of sphincterotomy are added to those of stent insertion, and a small sphincterotomy may make subsequent cannulation more difficult due to oedema or bleeding. Using solely wire-guided systems overcomes this last problem. If two stents are to be inserted, sphincterotomy may well be essential.

One stent or two?

If the lesion is in the lower or mid duct, or is a type 1 hilar lesion, a single stent is all that is required. When the lesion goes above the hilum, however, some authorities advise stenting of all undrained segments separately, with the insertion of two or more stents being the result (Fig. 11.10). There is much debate about the need for this technical tour de force, but few data to guide us. The logic behind inserting extra stents is impeccable: undrained segments become infected, therefore draining them avoids septic complications; draining all the liver should lead to quicker resolution of jaundice. However, draining one-third of the liver (assuming reasonable underlying liver function) will be sufficient to clear jaundice, and sepsis occurs in less than 10% of cases and it may be better to treat it as and when problems occur. Placing a second stent is often difficult, and may dislodge the first one. If one is going to use two stents, placing two wires first may help [13].

Stent blockage and changing

A further controversial area is whether stents should be changed routinely, when they are predicted to block, or only when jaundice or cholangitis herald that blockage has taken place. The policy adopted by a particular unit will be dictated by local factors, but the following points should be considered. Although all plastic stents block, with a median patency of around 5 months, the variation is very wide [17], and a policy of changing all stents at 3 months will result in several patients having extra visits to hospital for unnecessary stent changes, as well as some requiring emergency stent changes. Around 50% of plastic stents last longer than the patients in whom they are sited, who need no further instrumentation or re-appointment. On the other hand, a policy of emergency stent change only does require rapid and certain access to the stenting service, which may include the need for hospital in-patient beds. The latter can present major problems in modern health care systems. There is little more demoralizing than for a patient with known malignant disease and a short remaining lifespan to be sitting at home or in a District General Hospital with deepening jaundice waiting for a bed to become available. The more that independent beds protected from acute services are used, the better.

Stent-changing technique

To change stents is usually straightforward. The simplest method is to grasp the protruding stent in a Dormia basket, a snare or a stent-retrieval forceps and withdraw scope, stent and all, while holding the snare or forceps close to the biopsy-channel valve with the little finger of the left hand. This method has a number of disadvantages, however. The scope obviously must be reinserted, which is uncomfortable, and can be time-consuming. There may be difficulty in recannulating (unusual, as the stent will have widened the orifice, but the inevitable minor bleeding which accompanies stent removal may obscure the papilla) or in repassing the stricture. Other methods include passing a wire up the blocked stent – surprisingly, not usually a problem – and then inflating an angioplasty balloon within the stent sufficient to grip it and then withdrawing the balloon and stent while leaving the wire in place. Alternatively, the Soehendra-type stent retriever, referred to earlier, may be used. This can be screwed into the stent before withdrawing in a similar manner. These methods mean that wire position above the stricture is maintained, but under present regulations both the balloon and stent retriever are expensive and non-reusable – which makes these methods costly options. Furthermore, the stent retriever can split the stent, making removal difficult. Sometimes it is possible to grasp the end of the stent with a pair of forceps such that it can be withdrawn through the biopsy channel, but there is a possibility of dropping the stent within the channel or of damaging the plastic lining by this method. The removed stent can be sent for cytological examination.

Generally, stent changing is straightforward, but the need for repeated visits in patients who are otherwise fit, or have slowly growing tumours, can be trying and expensive. Consequently, better methods of preventing stent blockage are needed. One possible solution has been the development of metal stents.

Metal stents

The ingenious development of expandable metal mesh stents has meant that we are able to place palliative stents for far longer than before, since their larger size means biofilm-derived clogging takes longer to occlude the lumen, although tumour ingrowth through the mesh is a problem specific to this kind of stent. Application of metal stents is determined by these, as well as other properties. They are irremovable, except very soon after placement, and therefore are not generally appropriate for benign lesions. This means that histological confirmation of the diagnosis is essential. It also means that they are not usually suitable for a first stent, except where cancer is clearly present, as in, for example, disseminated breast or colorectal carcinoma with hilar metastases. 'Obvious' carcinomas of the pancreas on radiological grounds, even with 'highly suspicious' cytology, have a habit of becoming chronic pancreatitis with time.

Endoscopic metal stents come ready-mounted on catheter systems. These are slightly narrower than 10 F stents, are continuous, and are therefore easier to push past a stricture. Furthermore, once deployed, they slowly expand over a day or two to 1 cm in calibre, dilating the toughest strictures – even those that 12-atmosphere angioplasty balloons cannot deal with. The earlier need to pre-dilate or post-dilate strictures has passed. Initial types which required pressurizing the covering membrane with contrast are now obsolete, and insertion devices are simpler. The big disadvantage of metal stents is their cost, although if many repeat ERCPs are prevented, the money may be well-spent [18]. Indeed, one Dutch study claimed that metal biliary stents were cost-effective, but such judgements depend on local procedure costs, which were rather high in the study in question [19]. For metal stents to be used, it must be possible for the endoscopy centre to pass costs on to purchasers of health care. Further developments in design and delivery of stents are under way.

A simple rule of thumb about when to use plastic and when metal stents is therefore: first stent, plastic – second and subsequent stents, if positive histology and a predicted survival of 3 months, metal – if not, plastic.

'Rendezvous' procedures (Fig. 11.11)

If biliary cannulation or passing the stricture are unsuccessful, despite all appropriate manoeuvres, then PTC is performed

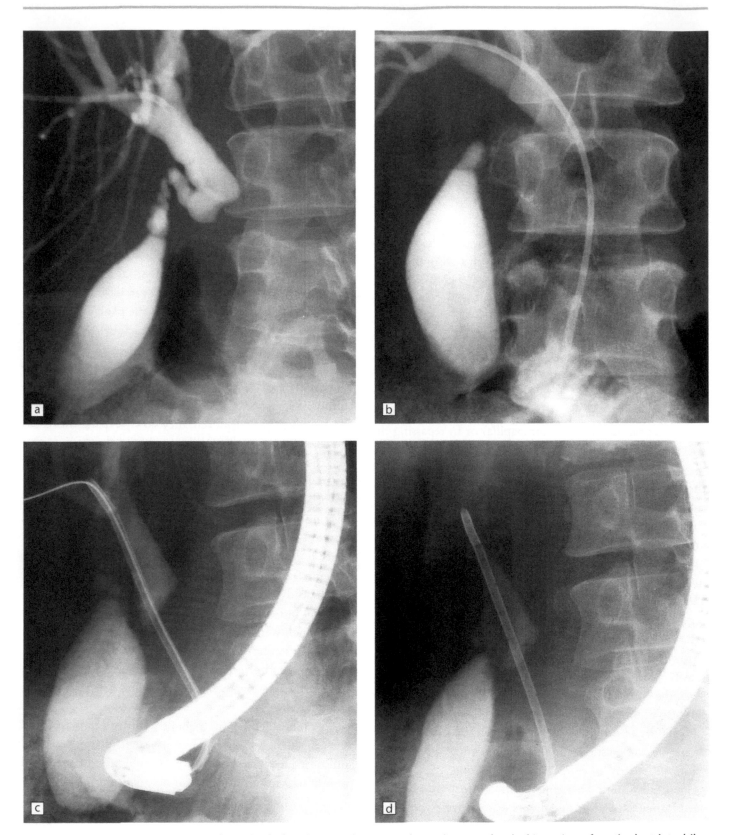

Figure 11.11. (a) Percutaneous transhepatic cholangiogram demonstrating stricture at level of insertion of cystic duct into bile duct. (b) A cannula is passed into the duodenum through which a guidewire can be passed and grasped by the endoscopist, rerouting the wire through the endoscope. (c) A stent is placed endoscopically across the wire 'tensioned' across the liver. (d) All wires and cannulae are removed to allow biliary drainage into the duodenum.

as soon as possible. A working catheter is left above the stricture, or sometimes passed through at the same session. The decision then is taken whether to insert a percutaneous stent or combine with the endoscopist to place an endoscopic plastic stent. If histology is positive, the best course is to place a percutaneous metal stent. Complications from these stents are few, once those from the initial puncture are discounted, because the diameter of the catheter is only 7 F. The only contraindication is price [20]. If percutaneous metal stents are unavailable or the diagnosis of malignancy is in doubt, the best approach is for the radiologist to advance a long (400 cm or more) wire into the duodenum. With the papilla and liver protected from 'cheesewiring' by a catheter, the wire is grasped by the endoscopist with a snare or basket, slowly withdrawn through the endoscope's biopsy channel, and a plastic stent inserted over the wire as already described. The fact that the wire is held at both ends means that greater mechanical force can be exerted and even very tight strictures can be stented. This mechanical advantage can lead to the stent being advanced too far. Careful observation of the stent should prevent this, and it is helpful if the stent and pusher catheter are different colours. One way of improving visibility when inserting a stent is to make sure that the light source is switched to react to average rather than peak illumination. A large white stent causes a brilliant reflection which reduces the light output from the light source automatically and can result in a very dark image.

Transplantation for malignant strictures

If one merely stated that transplantation had no place in the management of these tumours, one would probably not be far wide of the mark. The subject has, however, received a lot of attention over the years and needs considering. The problems with transplantation are mostly obvious. Unsuspected metastases grow rapidly in the immunosuppressed patient, and the slowly growing, rarely metastasizing Klatskin hilar tumour, for example, becomes a highly malignant tumour with multiple large secondaries following transplantation. Cholangiocarcinomas are still treated regularly, if inadvertently, by liver grafting in patients with sclerosing cholangitis. The results are dismal. Chemotherapy seems to have little to add. Hepatocellular carcinoma, on the other hand, has been successfully treated with transplantation on several occasions. The longest survivor of the Cambridge/King's College series had been treated for a large, but clinically silent hepatoma. It appears that single, preferably small, lesions which are situated in positions which preclude resection, usually at the hilum where they cause biliary obstruction, may be successfully transplanted, once strenuous attempts to rule out metastatic spread have proved negative. Although results are worse than with non-malignant disease, in a few, highly selected, cases it may be worthwhile. Obviously, transplantation has no role in low bile duct lesions.

REFERENCES

1. Calman K, Hine D. The Expert Advisory Group on cancer to the Chief Officers of England and Wales. *A Policy Framework for Commissioning Cancer Services.* Department of Health, 1995.

2. Ramage JK, Donaghy A, Farrant JM *et al.* Serum tumor markers for the diagnosis of cholangiocarcinoma in primary sclerosing cholangitis. *Gastroenterology* 1995; 108: 865–869.

3. Wilkinson M. The art of diagnostic imaging: the biliary tree. *J Hepatol* 1996; 25(suppl.): 5–19.

4. Bret PM, de Stempel JV, Atri M *et al.* Intrahepatic bile duct and portal vein anatomy revisited. *Radiology* 1988; 169: 405–407.

5. Martin DF. Ultrasound for gastroenterologists. *Gut* 1996; 38: 479–480.

6. Barakos JA, Rallo PW, Lapin SA *et al.* Cholelithiasis: evaluation with CT. *Radiology* 1987; 162: 415–418.

7. Taal BG, Muller SH, Boot H, Koops W. Potential risks and artifacts of magnetic resonance imaging of self-expandable esophageal stents. *Gastrointest Endosc* 1997; 46: 424–429.

8. Macauley SE, Schulte SJ, Sekijima JH *et al.* Evaluation of a non-breath-hold MR cholangiography technique. *Radiology* 1995; 196: 227–232.

9. Hintze RE, Adler A, Velzke W *et al.* Clinical significance of magnetic resonance cholangiopancreatography compared to endoscopic retrograde cholangiopancreatography. *Endoscopy* 1997; 29: 182–187.

10. Guibaud L, Bret PM, Reinhold C *et al.* Bile duct obstruction and choledocholithiasis: diagnosis with MR cholangiography. *Radiology* 1995; 197: 109–115

11. Topazian M, Kozarek R, Stoler R *et al.* Clinical utility of endoscopic retrograde cholangiopancreatography. *Gastrointest Endosc* 1997; 46: 393–399.

12. Adam A, Yeung E, Chettie N *et al.* Self-expandable stainless steel endoprostheses for the treatment of malignant bile duct obstruction. *Am J Roentgenol* 1990; 156: 321–325.

13. Cotton PB. ERCP – Therapeutic technique and ERCP and Therapy. In: Cotton PB, Williams CB (eds), *Practical Gastrointestinal Endoscopy*, 4th edn. Blackwell Science, Oxford, 1996, pp. 139–186.

14. Uno Y, Obara K, Kanazawa K *et al.* Stent implantation for malignant pyloric stenosis. *Gastrointest Endosc* 1997; 46: 552–555.

15. Pugliese V, Conio M, Nicolo G *et al.* Endoscopic retrograde forceps biopsy and brush cytology of biliary strictures: a prospective study. *Gastrointest Endosc* 1995; 42: 520–526.

16. Wilkinson ML, Simmons N, Bramble M *et al.* Report of the working party of the Endoscopy Committee of the British Society of Gastroenterology on the reuse of endoscopic accessories. *Gut* 1998; 42: 304–306.

17. Libby ED, Leung JW. Prevention of biliary stent clogging: a clinical review. *Am J Gastroenterol* 1996; 91: 1301–1308.

18. Lee JG, Leung JW. Biliary stents – plastic or metal? (editorial). *Gastrointest Endosc* 1998; 47: 90–91.

19. Davids PH, Groen AK, Rauws EA *et al.* Randomised trial of self-expanding metal stents versus polyethylene stents for distal malignant biliary obstruction. *Lancet* 1992; 340: 1488–1492.

20. Watkinson A, Wilkinson M, Adam A. Hepatobiliary intervention. In: Watkinson A, Adam A (eds), *Interventional Radiology – A Practical Guide*. Radcliffe Medical Press, Oxford, 1996, pp. 59–87.

12

Acute pancreatitis

J.P. Neoptolemos
With acknowledgement to J. Slavin

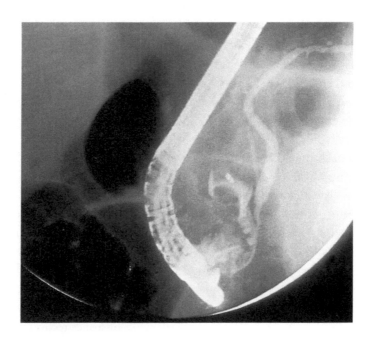

INTRODUCTION

There is an increasing role for endoscopic retrograde cholangiopancreatography (ERCP) and related endoscopic methods of management in the treatment of acute pancreatitis. While the role of such techniques has been evolving, knowledge of the natural history of this condition has developed dramatically, even during the past few years. This has led to new approaches to treatment such as prophylactic antibiotics and platelet activating factor antagonists. Radically new concepts such as the 'two-hit' hypothesis has placed disease processes such as multiorgan system failure and the systemic inflammatory response syndrome into a more rational context. The Atlanta classification has standardized nomenclature, not only between countries, but between specialties so that surgeon, gastroenterologist, internist, radiologist and endoscopist can better comprehend the same disease. The tremendous contribution that diagnostic and therapeutic endoscopy makes to the individual patient can be achieved only by its application within a multidisciplinary approach that is based on understanding a disease which, in many ways, remains enigmatic.

This chapter will review the evidence implicating gallstones in acute pancreatitis, and the current theories that account for this association. The diagnosis, assessment and management of patients with pancreatitis will be discussed. Finally, the role of ERCP and endoscopic sphincterotomy in biliary pancreatitis will be dealt with at some length.

AETIOLOGY

The incidence of acute pancreatitis is around 30–60 cases per 100 000 population per year, and this has risen in recent years [1]. Gallstones are the most common identifiable cause (Table 12.1). In an analysis of 5842 patients with acute pancreatitis from 26 studies, 2771 (47%) had gallstones [2]. Gallstone-associated pancreatitis, like gallstones, is more common in women. Although some series report an incidence as high as 65%, this variation is likely due to the use of different techniques for the detection of gallstones, the varying prevalence of gallstones, and the level of consumption and susceptibility to alcohol.

In 1901, Opie put forward his 'one channel' theory [3] proposing that impaction of a stone at the lower end of the main (common) bile duct (CBD) creates a single channel

Table 12.1. Causes of acute pancreatitis

Common causes	Other biliary causes
Gallstones	Sphincter dysfunction
Alcohol	Cholesterolosis
Idiopathic	Sclerosing cholangitis
ERCP	Sludge
Hypertriglyceridaemia	Parasitic infestation
Hypercalcaemia	Choledochal cyst
Steroids	Ampullary tumours
Trauma	Periampullary/intraluminal diverticulum
	Cholangiocarcinoma
	Pancreas divisum
	Biliary surgery
	Pancreatic duct abnormalities

of communication between the CBD and pancreatic ducts; this allows bile to reflux along the pancreatic duct, and this initiates acute pancreatitis (Fig. 12.1). Gallstone migration through the bile duct occurs in association with an attack of biliary pancreatitis, as stones can be retrieved from the faeces of individuals who are recuperating and the number of stones recovered is related to the severity of an attack [4]. It has also been suggested that oedema of the ampulla of Vater following passage of a stone may constitute a functional obstruction and that impaction is not a necessary prerequisite for an attack.

Between 3% and 8% of patients with symptomatic gallstones will develop acute pancreatitis and about 20% of those with microlithiasis [5]. Anatomical features which are consistent with Opie's theory are often found in individuals with gallstone acute pancreatitis, and include multiple small stones in association with a wider cystic duct, CBD, and a long common channel [6]. Hernandez and Lerch provided direct evidence for the existence of a functional common channel in individuals with gallstone acute pancreatitis [7]. Three groups of patients who had undergone cholecystectomy and CBD exploration with insertion of a T-tube were studied; those with gallstones alone, those

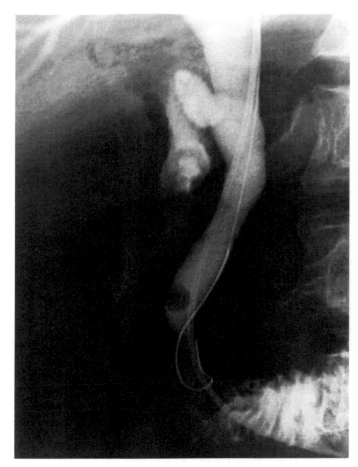

Figure 12.1. Impacted stone at papillary orifice causing acute pancreatitis.

the opossum have suggested that early decompression or relief of PD obstruction reduces the severity of an attack of acute pancreatitis [10]. These two observations provide a rational basis for the use of early pancreatic duct decompression in severe gallstone-associated pancreatitis.

PRESENTATION

An attack of pancreatitis usually begins with epigastric pain, often accompanied by profound nausea and vomiting. As inflammation spreads throughout the peritoneal cavity the pain spreads and gradually increases in intensity. Irritation of the retroperitoneum may cause back-ache. The tail of the pancreas overlies the left kidney, and inflammation in this area may lead to left loin pain. The patient may give a history of a previous attack of pancreatitis or of biliary disease. An attack may have been precipitated by a bout of heavy drinking; alternatively other aetiological factors may be identified (Table 12.1).

On examination the patient may have tachycardia, hypotension and be in distress. The initial presentation however may be indolent with minimal tenderness and constitutional upset, with signs of systemic upset developing only at a later stage. On abdominal examination there may be widespread abdominal tenderness with guarding, rebound and scanty or absent bowel sounds. Specific clinical signs that support a diagnosis of acute necrotizing pancreatitis include peri-umbilical (Cullen's sign) and flank bruising (Grey Turner's sign). A subset of patients with acute biliary pancreatitis usually of the severe variety will also have acute cholangitis. The features are jaundice, pyrexia and right upper quadrant pain and tenderness in addition to those of the underlying acute pancreatitis.

DIAGNOSIS

Blood tests

A diagnosis of pancreatitis is dependent on a typical history in the presence of a markedly elevated serum amylase. Provided that this is measured within 24 hours of the onset of symptoms, the sensitivity of a diagnostic level of three times the upper limit of normal is about 90%. If the diagnostic level is set at the upper limit of normal the sensitivity increases to 98%, but at the cost of reduced

with CBD stones, and those with acute biliary pancreatitis, which the authors took to indicate that stones had migrated into the duodenum. In the group of patients who had acute pancreatitis, amylase levels in the T-tube fluid after a test meal were much higher than in the other groups.

The mechanism by which reflux of bile up the pancreatic duct might cause pancreatitis is not entirely clear. However, infusion of bile salts into the pancreatic duct under physiological pressure has been shown to cause acute oedematous pancreatitis in the rat [8]. Low concentrations of certain bile salts can increase the autocatalytic activity of trypsinogen to over 50 times the normal rate, and it is possible that reflux of bile into the main pancreatic duct (PD) could activate trypsin locally and overcome the pancreatic trypsin inhibitor. Repeated bouts of PD obstruction in a rat model accentuate the severity of an attack of pancreatitis, suggesting that intermittent gallstone passage may contribute to the severity of human acute pancreatitis [9]. Further studies in

Table 12.2. Some other causes of a raised amylase level

Upper gastrointestinal perforation
Torsion of an intra-abdominal viscus
Mesenteric infarction
Retroperitoneal haemorrhage
Macro amylasaemia
Ectopic pregnancy
Salpingitis
Parotitis
Ectopic amylase-secreting tumours (ovary)

Table 12.3. Baseline investigations in acute pancreatitis

Full blood count
Plasma urea and electrolytes
Plasma glucose
Plasma bilirubin and liver enzymes
Plasma calcium
Arterial blood gases
Erect chest X-ray
Supine abdominal X-ray

specificity. Amylase levels gradually fall back towards normal over the following 5 days; thus delay in performing a test may lead to a false-negative level. Other conditions may occasionally cause a very elevated amylase level (Table 12.2).

Serum lipase levels are also raised in acute pancreatitis, and these remain elevated for a longer period of time than those of amylase. Thus the use of plasma lipase as an alternative to amylase has been suggested [11]. Although lipase is more specific for acute pancreatitis since it is not excreted by the salivary glands, it is still prone to false-positive results, for example following a perforated hollow viscus or mesenteric infarction. Overall the accuracy is not significantly greater than amylase, and it is technically more difficult to measure. In those cases where doubt remains contrast-enhanced computed tomography (CE-CT) of the pancreas will usually help to clinch the diagnosis. The amylase level is of no value in predicting the severity of an attack.

A number of other baseline investigations should be performed both to confirm the diagnosis of pancreatitis and assist with the assessment of severity (Table 12.3). An erect chest X-ray is mandatory to exclude a perforation as a cause of abdominal pain and an elevated amylase. A supine abdominal film may show gallstones, pancreatic calcification or the presence of a sentinel loop, but may also reveal obstruction or features more consistent with mesenteric infarction.

The identification of gallstones as an aetiological factor in acute pancreatitis is of increasing importance since early ERCP with or without endoscopic sphincterotomy (ES) is indicated in certain patients. In the convalescent stage it is important to identify those patients in whom early cholecystectomy will prevent a further attack. In the presence of lipaemic serum (which may cause a falsely low reading of the amylase) or in the absence of an obvious aetiology, fasting lipids need to be measured as hypertriglyceridaemia is a cause of acute pancreatitis in up to 5% of cases [11].

Radiology

Ultrasound (US) has an accuracy of 95% in identifying gallstones, and is now widely used for this purpose. Unfortunately, patients with acute pancreatitis usually have dilated gas-filled loops of bowel that obscure the gall bladder, and this reduces the accuracy of US to between 60% and 80%. If performed in the convalescent phase when bowel distension has resolved, then detection rates improve (Table 12.4). Ultrasound is poor at identifying CBD stones, with reported detection rates varying between 10% and 50% [12].

Contrast enhanced CT (CE-CT) during an acute attack will detect only 30–50% of gallstones, and is particularly poor at detecting bile duct stones [13]. Because of this, biochemical predictors of gallstones remain important for diagnostic purposes, even in the present day. The sensitivity of ultrasound can be enhanced 10–20% by the measurement of serum alanine or aspartate transaminase within 48 hours of an attack, with levels raised two-fold above normal suggesting a biliary aetiology. A bilirubin concentration >40 µmol/l has a sensitivity of 80% in predicting the presence of CBD stones [14].

Table 12.4. Detection of gallstones in acute pancreatitis

Site of stones	Method	Timing	Sensitivity (%)
Gall bladder			
	ALT >60 i.u./l	<24 h	70–80
	US	<72 h	60–80
	CT*	<72 h	30–50
	ERCP*	<72 h	90–95
	US	>96 h	90–95
	EUS#	>96 h	95
CBD			
	Bilirubin >40 μmol	<24 h	70–80
	US	<72 h	10–55
	CT*	<72 h	10–20
	ERCP*	<72 h	95
	EUS#	>96 h	95

*Similarly at >96 h; #No data on earlier time points.
ALT = alanine aminotransferase; CBD = common bile duct; CT = computed tomography; ERCP = endoscopic retrograde cholangiopancreatography; EUS = endoluminal ultrasound; US = ultrasound.

The role of magnetic resonance cholangiopancreatography (MRCP) or of endoscopic ultrasound (EUS) in the assessment of the CBD in acute pancreatitis is as yet undefined. Recent studies however have confirmed that the accuracy of both techniques in identifying CBD stones approaches that of ERCP [15,16]. Currently, ERCP remains the most accurate method of identifying CBD stones in the acute phase, although EUS may be particularly good at detecting microlithiaisis (stones <5 mm) in the gall bladder and CBD, at least in the convalescent phase. We would suggest that EUS, where available, should replace ERCP for the detection of gall bladder microlithiasis or CBD stones, especially in the convalescent phase. There is an associated morbidity and mortality for ERCP, even in the absence of acute pancreatitis, so that its use should be restricted for therapeutic indications or for the diagnosis of cases with an uncertain aetiology when non-invasive methods (US, CE-CT, MRI, MRCP and EUS) have been unhelpful or are not available (Table 12.4). Although CE-CT is poor at identifying CBD stones, it is an essential tool for demonstrating the extent of pancreatic necrosis and the presence of peripancreatic inflammation and collections [17].

Assessment: predicting a severe attack

The majority of cases of acute pancreatitis are mild, but

Table 12.5. Methods used to stratify acute pancreatitis into mild and severe cases, sensitivity predicting a severe attack

	Sensitivity (%)
Clinical assessment (general clinician)	50
Clinical assessment (expert clinician)	80
Ranson score (at 48 h)	80
Glasgow (Imrie) score	80
Peritoneal lavage	90
Alcoholic pancreatitis	–
APACHE-II (at <24 h)	76
APACHE-II (at 48 h)	80
Contrast-enhanced CT	80

about 25% can be graded as severe because of local or systemic complications [18]. In this group, about 50% will develop a progressively more severe clinical picture with haemodynamic instability and multiple organ failure leading to death in 20–30% of cases. Initial clinical assessment (except by genuine experts) has been shown to be rather poor at identifying which patients will suffer a severe attack. Thus, a number of clinical scoring systems have been developed in an attempt to identify those patients likely to suffer a severe attack (Table 12.5). In this way individuals who require intensive monitoring and support can be identified, and as new treatments are introduced they can be employed in appropriate patient groups.

The initial Ranson system used to predict the severity of an attack of pancreatitis was first described in 1974 and was based on a study of 200 patients. Unfortunately only 14 of these had gallstones, and dissatisfaction with this system led to the development of a further modified Ranson score specifically for use in biliary pancreatitis [19]. Based on the work of Ranson, the Glasgow group developed and validated a similar system. This scoring system was modified in 1981 and then again in 1984 (Table 12.6) [20–22]. The robustness, ease of use and accuracy of these clinical scoring systems has been repeatedly confirmed, and they are now in widespread use for clinical trials and should be in routine use.

The Acute Physiology and Chronic Health Enquiry Score (APACHE) was described in 1981 and was based on the premise that severity of an illness could be measured by quantifying the degree of abnormality of multiple physiological parameters. To this is added an assessment of the patient's premorbid health status. A much simpler APACHE-II system was introduced in 1985. When compared with

Table 12.6. The Glasgow (or Imrie) system for predicting severity in acute pancreatitis. Three or more factors present within the first 48 h predicts a severe attack

Prognostic factors	1981	1984
Age (years)	–	>55
Serum transaminases	>200 IU/l	–
White cell count	$>15 \times 10^9$/l	$>15 \times 10^9$/l
Blood glucose	>10 mmol/l	>10 mmol/l
Serum urea	>16 mmol/l	>16 mmol/l
PaO$_2$	<7.5 kPa	<7.5 kPa
Serum calcium	<2.0 mmol/l	<2.0 mmol/l
Serum albumin	<32 g/l	<32 g/l
Serum lactate dehydrogenase	>600 IU/l	>600 IU/l

the original Ranson score and a modified version of the Imrie score, an APACHE-II score of >8 was found to be an accurate indicator of a severe attack at admission, and at 24 and 48 hours. This is in contrast to the Ranson and Imrie systems which can only be used at 48 hours. Further continued use of the APACHE-II score during the course of an illness provides a good measure of disease progress [23]. Because of its relative complexity, the APACHE-II has not been universally adopted although it is invaluable for clinical trials assessing early methods of intervention. CE-CT performed soon after admission can also be used to predict the severity of an attack of pancreatitis [17]. Clinical scoring systems are however as good as CT at predicting outcome and identifying those patients who will develop organ failure. Thus, CT should be reserved for patients with severe acute pancreatitis, usually at the end of the first week of a continuing severe attack. It is important to be aware that the maximum accuracy of all the systems for predicting severity is at 48 hours following the onset of an attack. The most accurate system during the first 24 hours is APACHE-II, but this will mean that about 25% of severe cases will be misclassified as mild. Thus, clinical assessment by an expert remains extremely important, even if a scoring system is rigorously used.

In order to define the nomenclature used to describe acute pancreatitis and its local complications a consensus conference was held in Atlanta during 1992 [18]:

- Severe acute pancreatitis is associated with organ failure and/or local complications such as necrosis, abscess or pseudocyst (predicted by three or more Ranson/Glasgow criteria, eight or more APACHE-II points).

- Mild acute pancreatitis is associated with minimal organ dysfunction and an uneventful recovery; it lacks the features of severe acute pancreatitis.

Specific terms were also defined:

- Acute fluid collections are commonly seen in association with early acute pancreatitis and often lack a defined wall. They are distinct from pseudocysts which evolve more slowly and are not usually seen in the first few weeks. Acute fluid collections contain pancreatic enzyme-rich fluid, and are lined by a wall consisting of granulation or fibrous tissue. Most acute fluid collections resolve spontaneously, but a few mature into pseudocysts. They do not usually require drainage [18].

- An acute pancreatic abscess is a circumscribed collection of pus and usually arises at a late stage (≥6 weeks). Abscesses can usually be treated by percutaneous aspiration [18]. The mortality is low. In contrast, the mortality seen with infected pancreatic necrosis can be as high as 50%.

MANAGEMENT AND EVIDENCE

General measures

The initial management of acute pancreatitis is similar, whatever the cause. Fluid losses are often large and a central line and urinary catheter may assist in the estimation of the volume required. A large-bore intravenous line is inserted and fluids are given to replace losses. Nasogastric suction will help to empty the stomach and reduce nausea and vomiting. Irrespective of the scoring system used, measurement of an arterial blood gas is mandatory. Oxygen should be given for the first 48 hours by mask, and pulse oximetry should be instituted routinely for a similar period. If hypoxia is present an arterial line is inserted to allow regular arterial blood gas estimation. Blood pressure, temperature, pulse, urine output, central venous pressure and oxygen saturation are monitored regularly. Initial management of a patient with acute pancreatitis is thus supportive. Patients with a predicted severe attack should initially be managed on a high-dependency unit or intensive therapy unit. Further, any patients who subsequently develop features suggestive of a severe attack should be rapidly transferred to such an environment.

Infection and inflammation

Patients with severe pancreatitis usually develop a systemic inflammatory response syndrome (SIRS), characterized by widespread leucocyte activation. Multiple organ failure secondary to an overactive SIRS response is the most common cause of death in the first week [24]. Treatment in each individual needs to be directed towards the particular system that is affected. For example, lung failure may require oxygen supplementation and eventually positive-pressure ventilation. Inotropic support may be required to maintain blood pressure and organ perfusion. Renal failure that does not respond to fluid replacement may necessitate dialysis. The management of such patients can be complex, is often protracted and involves several disciplines.

Studies have demonstrated that administration of systemic antibiotics early in the course of an attack may reduce the incidence of septic complications, particularly infection involving areas of pancreatic necrosis [25,26]. Thus a patient with severe acute pancreatitis should be started on an intravenous broad-spectrum antibiotic at the time of diagnosis, probably either imipenem or cefuroxime. A recent placebo-controlled, randomized, multicentre study has shown that lexipafant – a potent antagonist of platelet activating factor (PAF) which is a mediator of SIRS – significantly reduces organ failure scores and mortality in severe acute pancreatitis, but only if administered within the first 48 h of the onset of symptoms [27].

In that study, all but one of the late deaths in both groups occurred in patients who had multiorgan failure within the first week [27]. This is consistent with the two-hit hypothesis of severe acute pancreatitis. Patients with an overactive SIRS will succumb to multiorgan failure, even if they survive the initial phase of acute pancreatitis (the first hit) if exposed to a second hit such as sepsis (at any time) or the trauma associated with laparotomy. This second hit may be relatively minor. Thus, in patients with severe acute pancreatitis it is pivotal to focus on preventing infection, dealing with infection in the least interventional manner (including endoscopic and radiological means of treatment), and avoiding laparotomy if possible [24].

Nutrition

Most patients with mild pancreatitis improve rapidly and may eat within 2–7 days; they thus require little in the way of nutritional support. In contrast, patients with severe pancreatitis may be unwell for a considerable length of time. They often have a prolonged SIRS response or persisting sepsis and remain in a catabolic state. There is only one prospective randomized trial of total parenteral nutrition (TPN) in patients with acute pancreatitis. A total of 54 patients were randomized to conventional therapy alone or conventional therapy plus parenteral nutrition [28]. No difference in clinical outcome was apparent, but increased rates of sepsis – particularly catheter sepsis – were seen in those patients being fed parenterally. As most of the patients in this trial had a mild attack of pancreatitis it is difficult to comment on the role of TPN in severe acute pancreatitis [28]. Recent studies have shown that early re-establishment of enteral versus parenteral nutrition reduces morbidity in patients with sepsis/SIRS, and a number of trials are currently assessing the value of early enteral nutrition in severe acute pancreatitis [29]. In any event, patients who are shown to have a severe attack extending beyond the first few days will require nutritional support, which should be instituted sooner rather than later.

Pancreatic necrosis

The degree of pancreatic necrosis is best assessed by CE-CT and may increase during the first two weeks. Lesser degrees of necrosis, for example up to 30%, are a common feature of clinically mild acute pancreatitis. Extensive necrosis (>50%) is associated usually with the need to intervene surgically [17]. Both necrosis and fluid in and around the pancreas can give similar appearances on CT scanning. Thus, solid pancreatic necrosis may be misrepresented as a pseudocyst. Moreover, a large pseudocyst may have a large solid (necrotic tissue) component. Abdominal US can define these components but often the pancreas cannot be fully visualized. MRI, when available, can be helpful. If non-surgical methods of pseudocyst drainage are considered, EUS may also be useful as the primary imaging modality.

Pancreatography observed at ERCP will distinguish peripheral from central pancreatic necrosis, as in the case of the latter there will be main PD disruption. Interestingly, the degree of pancreatic necrosis is associated with the site of disruption in that disruption of the PD in the tail of the gland is associated with limited necrosis, whereas that in the head of the gland is associated with almost complete necrosis. If there is any doubt about the presence of PD disruption from non-invasive investigations then ERP may be utilized for diagnostic reasons [30]. PD disruption may occur as early as 72 h, but is more often seen in the second week of the attack. In mild pancreatitis, minor irregularities of the PD may be seen sometimes in conjunction with peripheral minor duct disruption.

Pseudocysts

Pseudocysts should not be confused with infected pancreatic necrosis, which must be treated by necrosectomy because of the large solid and semi-solid component. The literature is surprisingly confused on the topic of endoscopic treatment of pseudocysts in patients with acute pancreatitis, first because there is no distinction from pseudocysts in chronic pancreatitis (or a mixing of the two types), and second because of selected patients (derived from endoscopic series without reference to the originating disease-specific population) [31]. In chronic pancreatitis there is usually a mature thick fibrous wall to the pseudocyst which may be accompanied by one or more strictures of the PD. In addition, the pseudocyst may be one of many features of the disease such as, calcifications in the parenchyma, stones in the PD, pancreatic ascites, an inflammatory mass of the head of the pancreas, obstructive jaundice, duodenal obstruction, diabetes mellitus, severe exocrine insufficiency, severe pain (unrelated to the pseudocyst), alcohol addiction, opiate addiction and catastrophic social circumstances. Outcome measures following pseudocyst drainage in chronic pancreatitis would thus be quite different from those in acute pancreatitis [31]. In acute pancreatitis pseudocysts will arise in about 15–18% of patients, but only 30–50% of these (i.e. 5–9% of the total disease population) will develop pseudocysts requiring treatment. By definition, pseudocysts can only be diagnosed 6 weeks after the onset of the attack [18]. Pseudocysts larger than 6 cm in diameter will not usually resolve and should be treated. Failure to do so may lead to pseudocyst rupture, haemorrhage into the cyst leading to a large pseudoaneurysm or, if the wall is not so thick, rupture with continuing haemorrhage into the peritoneal cavity. Pseudocysts may become infected, resulting in an abscess (note definition). Pseudocysts with a significant solid component may be drained endoscopically (or radiologically), but there is a risk of infection of the solid component or of early recurrence, and an open technique should probably be considered [31]. Very large

Table 12.7. Criteria for the endoscopic drainage of a pseudocyst in acute pancreatitis

Unresolving, >6 cm in diameter
>6 weeks after the onset of symptoms
Clearly defined wall
Lack of a significant solid component
Not containing blood
Transmural route: clear bulge into the stomach or the duodenum
Transpancreatic route: communication with duct

acute fluid collections which compromise respiratory effort because of a splinting effect on the diaphragm may occasionally need to be drained, but this should be done externally because of the absence of a fibrous wall. The criteria for draining a pseudocyst in acute pancreatitis endoscopically are shown in Table 12.7 [32].

Surgery

The role of surgery in acute pancreatitis is still controversial. The absolute indication for surgical intervention is clear evidence of infected pancreatic necrosis (CT-guided fine-needle aspiration with subsequent microscopy and culture) [31]. Patients with extensive pancreatic necrosis that remains uninfected may be treated with supportive measures and will sometimes recover. Surgery is preferred however if symptoms are prolonged, or for extensive pancreatic necrosis with a worsening clinical picture. Surgical intervention is occasionally required for specific complications such as massive haemorrhage, bowel obstruction and fistulae. Pancreatic abscess in isolation is best managed by percutaneous radiological drainage. Unresolving symptomatic pseudocysts are usually best treated by surgery, but there is an increasing role for endoscopic approaches.

TECHNIQUES

Endosocopic retrograde cholangiography (ERCP)

ERCP should not be undertaken in patients with acute pancreatitis unless there is an intention to treat, i.e. to perform an endoscopic sphincterotomy (ES) and remove stones if present (Fig. 12.2). The technique of sphincterotomy has been dealt with at length in Chapter 9. A few specific points will be made here as regards the use of this technique in patients with acute pancreatitis. Avoidance of infection is paramount, and to this end strictly sterilized instruments are used and prophylactic antibiotics are given.

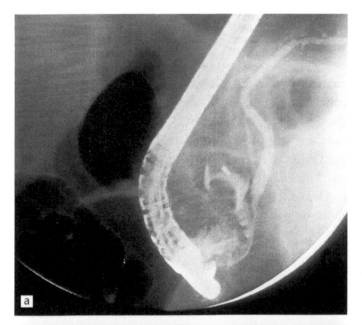

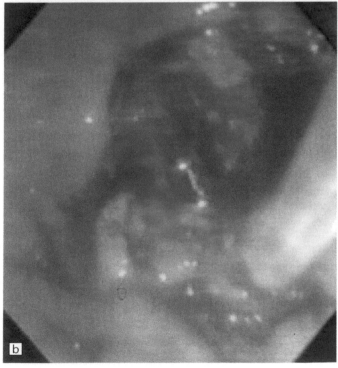

Figure 12.2. Sphincterotomy onto impacted stone.

Patients with acute pancreatitis already have a degree of lung injury and extra care therefore should be taken to avoid aspiration and sedation-induced hypoxia. The procedure may be performed in the radiology suite, but for intubated patients screening radiology can be used on the intensive care unit (ICU) itself. Because of oedema and distortion of the duodenum and ampulla, ERCP often becomes difficult after the first 72 hours, and cannulation of the CBD may be extremely difficult. Performance by an experienced ERCP operator is mandatory. Careful manipulation of the papilla is essential, and selective cannulation should be attempted using guidewires to identify the target duct before contrast is introduced. Incorrect cannulation of the PD may result in conversion of a sterile into an infected pancreatic necrosis. Conversely, cannulation of the biliary duct may increase and even cause cholangitis. The minimum amount of contrast should be injected to obtain the desired diagnostic or positional information.

Endoscopic drainage of pseudocysts

A side-viewing duodenoscope is still preferred for draining pseudocysts that bulge into the stomach or duodenum. If need be, radial EUS may be used immediately beforehand to be certain of the anatomy and pathology, especially if there has been a delay since the external imaging methods or the cyst wall is not bulging. Linear array EUS is invaluable, if available, in directing the puncture under ultrasound guidance.

In the absence of EUS, some operators inject contrast via a varices needle under fluoroscopic control through the bulging wall of a cyst: diffusion of contrast occurs in the cyst, whereas if the wall is too thick (>1 cm) or the content is more solid, concentration of contrast is seen. Puncture should be undertaken with a fine diathermy needle at the site of maximum bulge, sufficient to permit the introduction of a guidewire over which a wide-bore pigtail catheter is introduced into the cavity. The Huibregtse-type needle knife (Wilson Cooke Corp., USA) is ideal for this purpose as it allows withdrawal of the diathermy wire to be followed by introduction of a guidewire through the same cannula which has passed into the cyst upon its puncture. If necessary the tract may be dilated with a balloon catheter. Screening radiology is important to show correct positioning of the pigtail catheter. With good drainage the pseudocyst will collapse over a few days and be eliminated by fibrous healing and contracture over several weeks. The catheter will be discharged spontaneously, but occasionally will need to be removed endoscopically (see chronic pseudocysts, Chapter 13).

Sometimes the cyst, especially when under pressure, will decompress immediately (and explosively!) upon puncture and placement of a stent may be impossible. If possible, however, the pseudocyst contents should be aspirated to ensure that a pseudocyst has not become a pseudoaneurysm. The content of the pseudocyst should also be sent for culture in case it has become infected – in which case a course of specific antibiotics should be prescribed.

A wide diathermy cut into the pseudocyst increases the risk of major haemorrhage since the stomach is highly vascular, with an extensive submucosal plexus arising from the greater and lesser curves. Venous pressure will also be increased if there is splenic vein thrombosis – which is not uncommon in severe acute pancreatitis. The duodenum also has an extensive submucosal plexus arising from the anterior and posterior pancreaticoduodenal arcades situated in the pancreaticoduodenal grooves. Thus, in the duodenum bulging pseudocysts should be entered strictly in the mid-tangential axis. Some bleeding is to be expected on entering the pseudocyst. Occasionally, if an important vessel such as the left gastroepiploic artery or vein or one of their main branches is damaged, there may be massive bleeding. For these reasons also, EUS is an invaluable facility to have when undertaking these procedures. Emergency laparotomy is essential in this situation. Thus such invasive procedures should only be undertaken in expert multidisciplinary institutions.

CONTROVERSIAL ISSUES AND DECISION MAKING

The role of surgical biliary drainage in acute pancreatitis

Before the introduction of ERCP, two prospective randomized studies investigated the effect of surgical biliary decompression at the time of urgent cholecystectomy on the outcome of acute gallstone pancreatitis. In the first, 65 patients were randomized to transduodenal sphincteroplasty and decompression within 72 hours of admission, or delayed surgery until the patient was in remission [34]. Of 36 patients undergoing urgent surgery, complications occurred in 11% with one death (3%), compared with 11% and 7% respectively in the patients that had surgery while in remission. These differences were not statistically significant. In the urgent surgery group CBD stones were found in 75% compared with 28% in the delayed surgery group.

A second trial randomized 165 patients to undergo surgery within 48 h, or delayed surgery beyond this time [35]. Overall, 30% of patients in the urgent surgery group had complications and 15% died, compared with 5% with complications and 2.4% who died in the delayed surgery group. These poor results persuaded many in the surgical community that early operative intervention in acute biliary pancreatitis was unwise. Unfortunately, the trial was flawed as the group subjected to early surgery contained more severe cases due to incorrect use of the Ranson system. Moreover, most patients underwent supraduodenal bile duct exploration which will drain the CBD, but not the pancreatic duct, and is not the functional equivalent of either a transduodenal sphincteroplasty or an endoscopic sphincterotomy.

The role of endoscopic biliary drainage in acute pancreatitis

The earliest report of benefit from endoscopic decompression during an attack of pancreatitis was received with great caution, as it was felt that ERCP, being a cause of pancreatitis, might increase the severity of an attack [36].

The first prospective randomized trial of ERCP in acute pancreatitis was performed in Leicester [22]. A total of 223 consecutive patients with acute pancreatitis were screened for gallstones by US and biochemical tests. Patients with evidence of gallstones were scored prospectively into severe and mild cases according to the modified Glasgow criteria, and then randomized to receive either conservative management with prohibition on the use of ERCP for at least 5 days, or urgent ERCP with or without ES (within 72 hours of admission). ES was only employed if CBD stones were seen on cholangiography. All patients received intravenous antibiotics for 5 days. In total, 146 patients were thought to have gallstones, 15 could not be randomized due to non-availability of ERCP or incomplete data, and 10 were subsequently excluded because of an alternative diagnosis. Thus, 121 patients of known severity were randomized to the urgent ERCP ± ES arm (34 mild, 25 severe) or to the conservative arm (34 mild, 28 severe).

The overall mortality rate was 2% in the urgent ERCP group and 8% in the conservative group ($P = 0.23$). The complication rates were 17% versus 34%, respectively ($P = 0.03$). In those prospectively stratified as being severe, the mortality rate (4%) and the morbidity rate (24%) were less if patients had undergone ERCP compared with the conservative group (mortality 18%, morbidity 65%, $P < 0.01$ for morbidity). Outcome was unaffected by treatment in the group predicted to have a mild attack (morbidity was 12% in both groups with no deaths). Intervention also reduced the length of hospital stay in those patients with a predicted severe attack, from a median of 17 days for those on conservative treatment to 9.5 days for those undergoing ERCP ± ES ($P < 0.01$).

A second study from Poland [37], which was published only in abstract form, selected similar patients to those of the Leicester study, but with a higher proportion of tertiary referrals and without prospective stratification for severity. In total, 250 patients underwent endoscopy within 24 hours of admission, although in some cases this was several days after the onset of pancreatitis. Those with a bulging ampulla were assumed to have a stone impacted at the ampulla of Vater and were treated by sphincterotomy ($n = 62$). The rest were randomized to sphincterotomy

($n = 94$) or conventional treatment ($n = 94$). The results showed a significant reduction in both complication rate (13% versus 34%, $P < 0.001$) and mortality (0.6% versus 11%, $P < 0.001$) for ES compared with conservative treatment, even in those patients in whom ES was delayed for more than 72 hours.

A similar study in Hong Kong randomized 195 patients with pancreatitis (from all causes) to receive ERCP ± ES within 24 hours ($n = 97$), or conservative treatment ($n = 98$), unless they had signs of cholangitis or sepsis [38]. Overall, there was a reduction in biliary sepsis in the urgent ERCP ± ES group compared with the conservative group (0% versus 12%, $P = 0.001$), but no significant reduction in other systemic or local complications. The authors concluded that ERCP ± ES was indicated, but may have underconstrued their data. Further, there are flaws in the methodology employed for this study; for example, nearly one-third of the conservatively treated group actually underwent ERCP ± ES, mostly within 72 hours of admission, and all patients underwent ERCP ± ES by the end of the study. Only 127 of the patients in the Hong Kong study actually proved to have gallstones as the cause of their pancreatitis. Analysis of data from these patients alone demonstrated that the results (for local and systemic

Table 12.8. Combined results of the Leicester [22] and Hong Kong [38] randomized clinical trials of ERCP and ES in patients with 'proven' acute gallstone pancreatitis

Severity of attack	Treatment	Location	No. of patients	Complications			
				Local	Systemic	Deaths	Total
Mild	ERCP/ES	Leicester	28	3	1	0	4
		Hong Kong	34	4	2	0	6
		Total	62	7 (11%)	3 (5%)	0	10 (16%)
	Conventional	Leicester	29	4	0	0	4
		Hong Kong	35	1	5 (4)[a]	0	6
		Total	64	5 (8%)	5 (8%)	0	10 (16%)
Severe	ERCP/ES	Leicester	22	3	1	0	4
		Hong Kong	30	3	3	1	4
		Total	52	6 (12%)[b]	4 8(%)[c]	1 (2%)[d]	8 (15%)[e]
	Conventional	Leicester	24	6	9	3	13
		Hong Kong	28	8	16 [8][a]	5	15
		Total	52	14 (27%)[b]	25 (48%)[c]	8 (15%)[d]	28 (54%)[e]

[a]Biliary sepsis; [b]$P < 0.05$; [c]$P < 0.01$; [d]$P < 0.05$; [e]$P < 0.01$.

Table 12.9. Results of the multicentre German trial of ERCP in acute biliary pancreatitis [39]

Clinical details		ERCP <72 h	Conservative
Patients	Randomized	126	112
	Ineligible	19	13
	Eligible	107	99
Predicted severity	Severe	26	20
	Undefined	16	16
	Mild	84	76
Respiratory failure		15	5
Renal failure		9	4
Jaundice		1	12
Acute cholangitis		17	13[a]
Sepsis		13	16
Deaths	'Related'	10	4
	'Unrelated'	4	3
	Total	14	7

[a]Eight patients underwent delayed ERCP/ES.
Patients with jaundice were excluded from the trial, and no details of local pancreatic complications are available.

complications, and mortality) were very similar to those of the Leicester study (Table 12.8).

The most recently published study reported a multicentre trial performed in Germany between 1989 and 1994 (Table 12.9) [39]. A total of 238 patients from 22 centres were randomized to undergo either ERCP ± ES within 72 hours, or conservative treatment alone. Since the premise of the study design was that patients with coexisting biliary obstruction had already been shown to benefit from early ES, patients with jaundice, a temperature >39°C or persisting biliary cramps were excluded as they all received ERCP ± ES. The study therefore aimed to ascertain the benefit of early sphincterotomy in acute pancreatitis in the absence of overt biliary obstruction, and concluded that it was of no benefit.

Unfortunately, the study was terminated early after the second planned interim unblinded review by an independent board of referees. At that time, 14 of 126 patients in the interventional group and seven of 112 (not significant) in the conservative group had died of pancreatitis. It is difficult to interpret the results of this trial since there are major problems in both study design and conduct. There were 22 participating hospitals, and thus recruitment rates from individual centres were very poor, being less than two cases per centre per year. No explanation is given as to why 17 patients in the treatment group developed acute cholangitis

(compared with 13 cases in the control group). No previous study of ERCP and ES in acute pancreatitis has produced similar figures. A partial explanation is provided by the observation that in the predicted severe group of 26 patients who underwent ERCP only 10 patients had ES (U. Folsch, personal communication). Prophylactic antibiotics were not routinely used; recent evidence shows a favourable influence on outcome in acute pancreatitis.

A recent meta-analysis which combines the results of all four studies (Table 12.10) supports the value of early intervention to decompress the biliary/pancreatic duct system in severe acute pancreatitis. The morbidity and mortality of acute pancreatitis in a predicted mild attack is low, and there is no evidence from individual clinical trials to suggests that ERCP + ES is beneficial in the absence of cholangitis or

Table 12.10. Meta-analysis combining results of the four randomized prospective controlled clinical trials in this area

Prognosis	Outcomes	Odds ratio	(95% CI)
Mild	**Morbidity**	0.66	(0.42–1.03)
Severe		0.27	(0.15–0.48)
All grades		0.51	(0.36–0.70)
Mild	**Mortality**	0.60	(0.16–2.30)
Severe		0.37	(0.16–0.85)
All grades		0.44	(0.23–0.87)

Table 12.11. Endoscopic sphincterotomy for gallstone acute pancreatitis in patients with gall bladder *in situ*

Reference	Year	No.	Recurrent attacks	Biliary complications	Follow-up (months)
Davidson et al. [43]	1988	19	0	0	39
Shemesh et al. [44]	1990	9	0	0	22
Hill et al. [45]	1991	14	0	N/A	38
Uomo et al. [46]	1994	19	1	6	30
Wellbourn et al. [47]	1995	48	0	2	27

N/A = Data not available.

obstructive jaundice. In contrast, patients with a predicted severe attack of pancreatitis who have ultrasound, biochemical or clinical evidence of biliary disease should undergo urgent ERCP ± ES. All are agreed that acute cholangitis or obstructive jaundice in acute pancreatitis warrants emergency ERCP: all other severe cases should have an ERCP on the next elective routine list.

There is increasing agreement that if ERCP is performed for a severe attack of pancreatitis due to gallstones, an ES should be performed irrespective of the presence of CBD stones at the time of ERCP for the following reasons:

- Small stones may only be revealed following ES.
- Stones are often regularly passed from the gall bladder into the CBD and may not be present at the time of ERCP.
- The resultant oedema of the papilla may itself be sufficient to cause reflux of bile into the PD, even in the absence of a stone.

Prevention of further attacks of acute pancreatitis due to gallstones

Most patients with a mild attack of pancreatitis settle rapidly. Without removal of the cause (gallstones) by cholecystectomy, the risk of a recurrent attack following a single attack is in the region of 30% [2] and the average delay before the second attack in one series was 108 days [40]. Morbidity and mortality may be increased in patients with acute biliary pancreatitis who undergo laparoscopic cholecystectomy within the first week of an attack [41]. As in open cholecystectomy, the best timing for laparoscopic cholecystectomy is once an attack of pancreatitis has resolved, but before discharge [2].

In patients with mild biliary pancreatitis the use of EUS immediately before laparoscopic cholecystectomy is ideal, as this allows identification of those patients who require ERCP and ES. A normal preoperative ERCP or EUS does not however guarantee that further stones will not have migrated into the CBD before surgery, particularly if there has been an appreciable delay between the two procedures. At laparoscopic surgery an operative cholangiogram should be performed and the duct explored laparoscopically or by open surgery if necessary. Alternatively, peroperative or postoperative endoscopic sphincterotomy can be performed. The approach is dependent upon local expertise, as all the methods are effective [42].

Endoscopic sphincterotomy without cholecystectomy is a useful way of preventing further attacks of acute pancreatitis in individuals who are unfit for surgery. Further attacks of acute pancreatitis are really quite uncommon (Table 12.11). If they are fit for surgery, patients who have already undergone an ES for severe disease or because of biliary obstruction in the presence of mild disease should have their gall bladder removed. The reason is that there is a 10–15% risk of significant gall bladder complications such as empyema of the gall bladder, acute cholecystitis and chronic cholecystitis after several years' follow-up, possibly because of increased rates of biliary infection [42].

REFERENCES

1. Sinclair MT, McCarthy A, McKay C *et al.* The increasing incidence and high mortality rate from acute pancreatitis in Scotland over the last ten years. *Gastroenterology* 1997; 112(4 Suppl.): A482 (abstract).

2. Howard JM. Gallstone pancreatitis. In: Howard JM, Jordan GL, Reber HA (eds), *Surgical Diseases of the Pancreas*. Lea & Febiger, Philadelphia, 1987, pp. 265–283.

3. Opie EL. The aetiology of acute haemorrhagic pancreatitis. *Bull Johns Hopkins Hosp* 1901; 12: 182–188.

4. Acosta JM, Ledesma CL. Gallstone migration as a cause of acute pancreatitis. *N Engl J Med* 1974; 290: 484–487.

5. Farinon AM, Sianesi M, Zanelle E. Physiopathological role of microlithiasis in gallstone pancreatitis. *Surg Gynecol Obstet* 1987; 164: 256–266.

6. McMahon MJ, Shefta JR. Physical characteristics of gallstones and the calibre of the cystic duct in patients with acute pancreatitis. *Br J Surg* 1980; 67: 6–9.

7. Hernandez CA, Lerch MM. Sphincter stenosis and gallstone migration through the biliary tract. *Lancet* 1993; 341: 1371–1373.

8. Arendt T, Broschewitz U. Bile induced oedematous pancreatitis in rats: non-parallel changes in pancreatic morphology and amylase release *in vitro*. *Gut* 1994; 35: 1127–1131.

9. Hirano T, Manabe T. A possible mechanism for gallstone pancreatitis: repeated short term pancreaticobiliary duct obstruction with exocrine stimulation in rats. *Proc Soc Exp Biol Med* 1993; 202: 246–252.

10. Runzi M, Saluja A, Lerch MM *et al*. Early ductal decompression prevents the progression of biliary pancreatitis: an experimental study in the opossum. *Gastroenterology* 1993; 105: 157–164.

11. Winslet MC, Hall C, London NJM, Neoptolemus JP. Relationship of diagnostic serum amylase levels to aetiology and severity of acute pancreatitis. *Gut* 1992; 33: 982–986.

12. Winslet M, Neoptolemos JP. The place of endoscopy in the management of gallstones. *Clin Gastroenterol* 1991; 5: 99–129.

13. London NJM, Neoptolemos JP, Lavelle J *et al*. Contrast enhanced abdominal computer tomography scanning and predicition of severity in acute pancreatitis. *Br J Surg* 1989; 76: 268–272.

14. Neoptolemos JP, London N, Bailey I *et al*. The role of clinical and biochemical criteria and endoscopic retrograde cholangiopancreatography in the urgent diagnosis of common bile duct stones in acute pancreatitis. *Surgery* 1987; 100: 732–742.

15. Lomato D, Pavone P, Laghi A *et al*. Magnetic resonance cholangiopancreatography in the diagnosis of biliopancreatic disease. *Am J Surg* 1997; 174: 22–26.

16. Amouyal P, Amouyal G, Levy P *et al*. Diagnosis of choledocholithiasis by endoscopic ultrasonography. *Gastroenterology* 1994; 106: 1062–1067.

17. Balthazar EJ, Robinson DL, Megibow ASJ, Randon JHC. Acute pancreatitis: value of CT in establishing diagnosis. *Radiology* 1990; 174: 331–336.

18. Bradley EL. A clinically based classification system for acute pancreatitis. *Arch Surg* 1993; 128: 586–590.

19. Ransom JHC. Etiologic and prognostic factors in human acute pancreatitis. A review. *Am J Gastroenterol* 1982; 77: 633–638.

20. Imrie CW, Benjamin IS, Ferguson JC *et al*. A single centre double blind trial of trasylol therapy in primary acute pancreatitis. *Br J Surg* 1978; 65: 337–341.

21. Blamey S, Imrie CW, O'Neill J *et al*. Prognostic factors in acute pancreatitis. *Gut* 1984; 25: 1340–1346.

22. Neoptolemos JP, Carr-Locke DL, London NJ *et al*. Controlled trial of urgent endoscopic retrograde cholangiopancreatography and endoscopic sphincterotomy versus conservative treatment for acute pancreatitis due to gall stones. *Lancet* 1988; ii: 979–983.

23. Larvin M, McMahon M. APACHE-II score for assessment and monitoring of acute pancreatitis. *Lancet* 1989; ii: 201–205.

24. Wilson PG, Manji M, Neoptolemos JP. Acute pancreatitis as a model of sepsis. *J Antimicrob Chemother* 1998; 41(Suppl.): 51–63.

25. Sainio V, Kemppainnen E, Puolakkainen P *et al*. Early antibiotic treatment in acute necrotising pancreatitis. *Lancet* 1995; 346: 663–667.

26. Pederzoli P, Bassi C, Vesentini S, Campedelli A. A randomised multi-centre trial of antibiotic prophylaxis of septic complications in acute necrotising pancreatitis with imipenem. *Surg Gynecol Obstet* 1993; 176: 480–483.

27. Kingsnorth AN. Early treatment with lexipafant, a platelet activating factor antagonist, reduces mortality in acute pancreatitis: a double blind, randomised, placebo controlled study. *Gastroenterology* 1997; 112: A453.

28. Sax HC, Warner BW, Talamini MA *et al.* Early total parenteral nutrition in acute pancreatitis: lack of beneficial effects. *Am J Surg* 1987; 153: 117–124.

29. Kudsk KA, Croce MA, Fabian TC *et al.* Enteral versus parenteral feeding: effects on septic morbidity after blunt and penetrating abdominal trauma. *Ann Surg* 1992; 215: 505–513.

30. Neoptolemos JP, Carr-Locke MA. ERCP in acute cholangitis and pancreatitis. In: Jacobson IM, ed. *ERCP: Diagnostic and Therapeutic Applications.* New York: Elsevier Science Publishing Co., Inc, New York, 1989, pp. 91–126.

31. Grace PA, Williamson RCN. Modern management of pancreatic pseudocysts. *Br J Surg* 1993; 80: 573–581.

32. Huibregtse K, Kwan CP. Pancreatic pseudocysts. In: Testoni EP, Tittobello A, (eds), *Endoscopy in pancreatic disease.* London: Mosby-Wolfe, 1997, pp. 107–112.

33. Uhl W, Schrag HJ, Wheatley AM, Büchler MW. The role of infection in acute pancreatitis. *Dig Surg* 1994; 11: 214–219.

34. Stone HH, Fabian TC, Dunlop WE. Gallstone pancreatitis: biliary tract pathology in relation to time of operation. *Ann Surg* 1981; 194: 305–310.

35. Kelly TR, Wagener DS. Gallstone pancreatitis: a prospective randomised trial of the timing of surgery. *Surgery* 1988; 104: 424–428.

36. Classen M, Ossenberg W, Wurbs D *et al.* Pancreatitis – an indication for endoscopic papillotomy? *Endoscopy* 1978; 10: 223(Abstract).

37. Nowak A, Nowkowska-Dulawa E, Marek TA, Rybicka J. Final results of the prospective, randomised, controlled study on endoscopic sphincterotomy versus conventional management in acute biliary pancreatitis. *Gastroenterology* 1995; 108: A380 (abstract).

38. Fan ST, Lai EC, Mok FP *et al.* Early treatment of acute biliary pancreatitis by endoscopic papillotomy. *N Engl J Med* 1993; 328: 228–32.

39. Folsch UR, Nitsche R, Ludtke R *et al.* Early ERCP and papillotomy compared with conservative treatment for biliary pancreatitis. *N Engl J Med* 1997; 336: 237–242.

40. Paloyan D, Simonowitz D, Skinner DB. The timing of biliary tract operations in patients with pancreatitis associated with gallstones. *Surg Gynecol Obstet* 1975; 141: 737–739.

41. Tan E, Stain SC, Tang G *et al.* Timing of laparoscopic cholecystectomy in gallstone pancreatitis. *Arch Surg* 1995; 130: 496–500.

42. Wilson PG, Ogunbiyu O, Neoptolemos J. The timing of endoscopic sphincterotomy in gallstone acute pancreatitis. *Eur J Gastroenterol Hepatol* 1997; 9: 137–144.

43. Davidson BR, Neoptolemos JP, Carr-Locke DL. Endoscopic sphincterotomy for common bile duct calculi in patients with the gall bladder *in situ* considered unfit for surgery. *Gut* 1988; 29: 114–120.

44. Shemesh E, Czerniak A, Schneabaum S, Nass S. Early endoscopic sphincterotomy in the management of acute gallstone pancreatitis in elderly patients. *J Am Geriat Soc* 1990; 38: 893–896.

45. Hill J, Martin DF, Tweedie DEF. Risks of leaving the gall bladder *in situ* after endoscopy for gall stones. *Br J Surg* 1991; 78: 554–557.

46. Uomo G, Manes G, Laccetti M, Rabitti PG. Endoscopic treatment of acute biliary pancreatitis in pregnancy. *J Clin Gastroenterol* 1994; 18: 1109–1110.

47. Wellbourn CRB, Beckley DE, Eyre-Brook IA. Endoscopic sphincterotomy without cholecystectomy for gallstone pancreatitis. *Gut* 1995; 37: 119–120.

13

Chronic pancreatitis

A.R.W. Hatfield

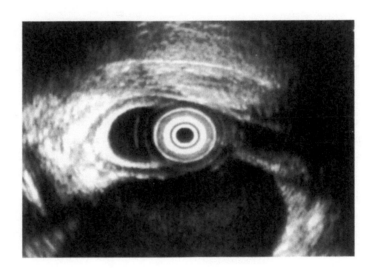

INTRODUCTION

Chronic pancreatitis accounts for at least 80% of the burden of pancreatic disease, affecting the population with a prevalence of 100–150 per 100 000 of the population per annum. This estimate reflects the fact that, although pancreatic cancer and acute pancreatitis have a higher incidence, the average duration of each is only one year whereas chronic pancreatitis is a debilitating illness which may last 20 to 30 years.

AETIOLOGY AND PATHOGENESIS

By far the most common cause of chronic pancreatitis is alcohol, accounting for 60% to 80% of cases. In developing countries, malnutition may be an important factor and 'tropical pancreatitis' is thought to be related to dietary factors. Conversely, high-protein diets have also been implicated in some cases. Approximately 1% of cases are due to hereditary pancreatitis, an autosomal dominant condition with an 80% penetrance in affected families. Systemic disease such as lupus, cystic fibrosis and hyperparathyroidism are all associated with chronic pancreatitis. The cause remains unclear in 20–30% of cases.

Gender predisposition for chronic pancreatitis is thought to be equal, but males present more commonly with alcoholic pancreatitis.

Obstruction of the pancreatic duct due to trauma, stenosis, adenoma, malignant stricture or papillary dyskinesia can lead to chronic pancreatitis. Pancreas divisum remains controversial as a cause – it occurs in 4–7% of the general population but only a tiny fraction of these present with pancreatitis. Nonetheless, it is found in between 7% and 50% of patients presenting with pancreatitis, and many clinicians believe it is implicated, though the mechanisms remain unclear and attempts at improving dorsal duct drainage have not been conclusively beneficial.

Chronic pancreatitis is usually a patchy and focal pathological process. Chronic alcohol administration is thought to lead to alteration in acinar cell lipid membranes, alteration in the ratios of different proteins secreted by those cells – most notably a disproportionate increase in trypsinogen compared with trypsin inhibitor, and an increase in the production of cholecystokinin (CCK) hormone.

Ductal cells secrete less bicarbonate, and this may help to precipitate protein plugs within the duct lumen. These form a nidus for calcification – the hallmark of chronic pancreatitis – but are also thought to perpetuate inflammation because of ductal obstruction. In this context, cytokine activation and oxidant stress are thought to play a role. Elevated pressures in the sphincter of Oddi have been demonstrated in chronic pancreatitis, but it is not certain whether this is cause or effect. Removal of debris from the duct sometimes produces relief, but reduction of pressure within the duct has less consistent results. New insights in the pathogenesis of pancreatitis have come from studies in hereditary pancreatitis where mutations in enzyme inhibitory proteins result in their unopposed action. Virtually all enzymes are secreted in an inactive proenzyme form and rely on a series of mediators to activate them – and often another series of mediators to limit their activity. Thus, trypsinogen is activated to trypsin by an activation peptide, a process which is usually initiated within the intestinal lumen by enterokinase. Mutations in the trypsin molecule have been found at hydrolytic sites involved in its degradation. Thus, in hereditary pancreatitis, if trypsin is inappropriately activated in the pancreas, its degradation and limitation of its deleterious action at this site may be impeded. Human trypsinogen has a propensity to auto-activate, and this may be more likely in the case of pancreatic hyposecretion or reduced flow rates due to ductal obstruction. As a general model for pancreatitis, this balancing act between increased or inappropriate enzyme activity and a dysfunction of the limiting or controlling mechanisms has been widely accepted.

PRESENTATION

Pain is the most common presentation of chronic pancreatitis, occurring in up to 95% of patients, but becoming a less prevalent symptom with increasing age of presentation. Presentation can be at any age but peaks in the early 20s and 50s are well recognized. Exocrine and endocrine insufficiency develop more rapidly in late-onset chronic pancreatitis and occasionally diarrhoea or diabetes mellitus are presenting features. Jaundice, due to fibrosis in the head of pancreas constricting the bile duct, is the presenting feature in 5–10% of patients. Very occasionally, patients present with haemorrhagic complications of portal vein thrombosis due to pancreatitis.

DIAGNOSIS

Chronic pancreatitis most commonly presents with pain, but this is often poorly characterized. The pain is usually epigastric, but can be more diffuse. It commonly radiates into the mid-back, being most frequently described as a dull ache which is persistent and relentless in about 30% of patients – half of whom may have a pseudocyst causing the pain. Usually these features, or unexplained abdominal pain, will require investigation in order to make a diagnosis. The other presentations of chronic pancreatitis discussed above often have more common causes which should be excluded. The gland is not easy to investigate because of its retroperitoneal location and its anatomic relationship with stomach and bowel, so that several modalities may have to be used to diagnose or exclude chronic pancreatitis.

Clinical and laboratory investigations

In general, laboratory blood tests are surprisingly normal in chronic pancreatitis. Serum pancreatic enzymes, trypsinogen, lipase and amylase, are usually normal except in acute exacerbations when they may be only slightly raised. Chronic severe pancreatitis is characterized by very low serum levels of enzyme.

Insulin and C-peptide concentrations are low in incipient endocrine insufficiency due to chronic pancreatitis, but are not sufficiently specific to be useful in this context. Similarly, pancreatic polypeptide, glucagon and somatostatin have been found experimentally to be depleted.

Pancreatic function tests

Unfortunately, most of these tests are not sensitive except in advanced disease when a diagnosis is usually obvious from the structural assessment of the pancreas. It has been estimated that 90% of the pancreas gland has to be destroyed or non-functioning before clinical insufficiency becomes manifest.

Duodenal intubation and sampling of juice for concentrations of bicarbonate, proteases, amylase and lipase is the best available pancreatic function test, though this is not widely used as it is time-consuming and not tolerated well by patients. Various modifications using secretagogues (secretin, ceruletide, CCK or Lundh test meal) have also been used. Non-invasive tests such as the pancreatolauryl test are less sensitive and specific, though easier to administer and better tolerated. They are based on the principle that presence of pancreatic enzyme in the duodenum will result in hydrolysis and subsequent absorption of a complex substrate taken orally. The proportion absorbed can be measured by analysis of breath, serum or urine depending on the substrate [C13/14, fluorescein or p-aminobenzoic acid (PABA), respectively] and is an indirect reflection of enzyme concentration.

The least invasive method – faecal fat estimation – is also the least sensitive. However, recently assays have been devised to measure chymotrypsin and elastase in faeces and these may be more helpful in less severe cases.

Radiological investigations

A number of radiological investigations are available for chronic pancreatitis:

- Pancreatic calcification occurs in all forms of chronic pancreatitis, but is more prevalent and occurs three times more rapidly in alcohol-related pancreatitis and can be seen on a plain abdominal X-ray lying across the midline. It is not a sensitive test.
- Ultrasound is limited by the overlying bowel gas, but in expert (and persistent!) hands real-time ultrasound can be as good as other imaging techniques. It is very operator-dependent, and this may explain discrepancies in various studies from Asia, Europe and North America. It has major advantages in terms of its ubiquity, safety and cost.
- Endoscopic ultrasound (EUS) is used widely in certain countries but not in others. EUS of the pancreas and biliary tree is a difficult technique to master, but is a very sensitive, non-invasive test for chronic pancreatitis and may be the best test available for the condition in its mild form. Therapeutically, it has an important role in the management of pseudocyst puncture.
- Computed tomography (CT) scanning is excellent at detecting abnormalities in severe pancreatitis, but much less so with less advanced disease. Spiral CT with contrast has improved its sensitivity further in this respect but it is very interpreter-dependent and, though widely available, remains a relatively expensive modality.
- Magnetic resonance cholangiopancreatography (MRCP) is developing rapidly. The current state of the

art is similar to that of CT scanning in terms of sensitivity – duct abnormalities are demonstrable in moderate to severe disease but not in less advanced or mild disease. Undoubtedly further improvements will make this an important modality, but the technology is expensive and the time involved in enhancing images can be a major constraint. At present there are not well-defined magnetic resonance criteria for detecting parenchymal abnormalities.

- Endoscopic retrograde cholangiopancreatography (ERCP) has been the 'gold-standard' imaging modality for chronic pancreatitis and has additional function as a therapeutic modality. However, experienced ERCP operators find it useful to plan therapeutic strategy with the additional, and preliminary, information given by other modalities discussed above.

Grades of severity and prognostic factors

There are well-defined prognostic scales for acute pancreatitis (see Chapter 12), but the course of chronic pancreatitis is more difficult to predict. A multicentre study [1] of more than 2000 patients indicated that age at presentation (older being worse), smoking, male gender, continued alcohol use and presence of cirrhosis were the most important factors influencing outcome. The standardized mortality ratio for this group was 3.5, with 10- and 20-year survival rates of 70% and 45%, respectively. There was a significant increase in the incidence of pancreatic cancer compared with the general population, but this accounted only for a small fraction of the mortality.

Differentiation from malignancy

One of the most difficult areas for diagnosis is the differentiation of pancreatic abnormalities due to pancreatitis or malignancy. As usual, where gross features are present, or invasion in the case of malignancy, the imaging modalities are more accurate. A range of options including cytology, juice aspiration, serum tumour markers detection of k-*ras* and *p53* mutations in pancreatic juice may be helpful in about half of the difficult cases. EUS-guided fine-needle aspiration holds considerable promise for focal lesions, but in the context of pancreatitis, histological interpretation is fraught with difficulty.

MANAGEMENT AND EVIDENCE

The study and management of chronic pancreatitis has been hampered by problems with classification. Symptoms, course of illness, morphology and aetiological factors have all been used to classify subgroups, but are not helpful in predicting the outcome for individual patients. It is well established that recurrent episodes of acute pancreatitis are a feature of chronic pancreatitis. However, chronic pancreatitis is characterized by progressive irreversible damage to the gland with loss of both exocrine and endocrine function. Usually, the acute episodes are treated as for acute pancreatitis with supportive measures and analgesia. The longer-term management of complications is considered here.

Conservative management

Conservative or medical management has evolved out of a realization that the natural history of pain in chronic pancreatitis is self-limiting, albeit that it takes a prolonged course with disabling morbidity in many patients. Thus, in several series, 60–80% of patients have diminution or absence of pain after 4 to 20 years, depending on the population studied. Thus, supportive care and analgesia is aimed at getting the patient through exacerbations and helping them to tolerate symptoms until the disease process wanes. In uncontrolled series, surgical or endoscopic drainage has resulted in more rapid pain relief, but this often recurs and there have not been any comparative studies. Narcotic analgesia is frequently required, though is not recommended as a first line, and dependence occurs in up to 20% of patients. Tricyclic antidepressants seem to have important pain-relieving properties in addition. Coeliac axis and thoracic sympathetic nerve blockers provide useful, albeit temporary, relief.

In addition to analgesia, the avoidance of alcohol is thought to be important, but there are no data on which to judge whether this helps to relieve pain. Other strategies have been to reduce pancreatic secretion with somatostatin analogues and to replenish antioxidant levels on the grounds that some of the damage is mediated by free radical chemistry.

Dietary supplementation of pancreatic enzymes is usually given once clinical exocrine insufficiency is manifest. Recent evidence suggests that, if these are given earlier, pain relief may be enhanced because free proteases in the duodenum destroy the CCK-releasing factor which is a major stimulus to pancreatic secretions.

Surgical management

The most common indication for surgical intervention in chronic pancreatitis is to relieve intractable pain. Other indications include the management of pancreatic pseudocysts or abscess, or the differentiation of pancreatic cancer from focal pancreatitis where other modalities fail. Ideally, pain relief should be achieved while preserving pancreatic endocrine and exocrine function. A variety of duct drainage operations and limited resections have been devised to this end, and can relieve pain in about 80% of patients, but mortality occurs in up to 5% of cases. Recurrence of pain is not uncommon and reoperation is less successful with a higher morbidity.

Endoscopic management

Although endoscopic therapy in the biliary tree has been established for over 25 years, pancreatic endotherapy has been developed, by and large, in specialist centres since 1990. There is a wide range of possible techniques available, and the remainder of this chapter attempts to put these in their clinical perspective.

PRACTICAL ASPECTS

Pseudocysts

The endoscopic drainage of pseudocysts represents one of the more commonly performed and therapeutically satisfactory procedures. The therapeutic concept is simple. A puncture or cut is made into an endoscopically obvious bulge within the gastric lumen and the cyst drained internally, with or without endoscopic stent placement to keep the lumen open between the stomach and cyst cavity. Early series achieved good results in terms of successfully draining cysts, but often with a considerable morbidity and occasional mortality [2,3]. Internal drainage is altogether more satisfactory than percutaneous external drainage as there is less chance of infection developing in the cyst cavity and the formation of pancreatic fistulae. The technical details of draining cysts have now been refined and the use

of high-quality, contrast-enhanced, spiral CT scanning and EUS allows safe procedures to be performed in appropriate patients.

The main complications in early series were mainly bleeding, as well as infection and retroperitoneal perforation, occurring in about 10–15% of patients [2–4]. Few series detail long-term follow-up, but probably about one-third of cases will have a cyst recurrence. In one series [4], despite a good initial 90% success in endoscopic drainage, 10 of 37 patients needed surgery for recurrent disease within a mean 32-month follow-up period. Pre-procedure CT scanning will show if the cyst is closely approximated to the gastric or duodenal wall, and show whether there are any variceal collaterals between the stomach and cyst wall. Unfortunately, it is common to find quite a thickening and gap between the stomach and cyst due to retroperitoneal inflammation even though the cyst produces an endoscopically visible bulge. If the cyst is more than 5–6 mm away from the gastric lumen, endoscopic puncture and drainage can fail. Commonly in chronic pancreatitis – but less so in cysts associated with acute disease – there will be portal vein compression or thrombosis, with portal collaterals coursing along the gastric wall; this represents a significant hazard to endoscopic therapy. These vessels are not visible from the lumen endoscopically, and the use of endoscopic ultrasound will determine both the distance between the gastric lumen and cyst and the presence of any significant blood vessels beneath the area of intended puncture in some detail. A conventional ultrasound endoscope cannot be used for therapy, and a suitable puncture site would have to be marked by clipping or dye injections submucosally before performing a procedure with an end-viewing or side-viewing instrument. The use of endoscopic ultrasound miniprobes facilitates the procedure, as a direct ultrasound scan can be performed down an ordinary endoscope at the chosen site of puncture.

The assessment and practical aspects of this technique are illustrated in Figures 13.1–13.13. Pseudocysts drain extremely quickly following this procedure, and invariably the cyst has completely decompressed within 24–48 hours. Loculated pseudocysts represent a challenge for any mode of drainage, and follow-up CT is mandatory to assess efficacy of therapy. Undrained loculi may still produce symptoms or become infected and may need separate, usually percutaneous, drainage.

Some centres have, because of the substantial complication rate of direct transmural endoscopic drainage,

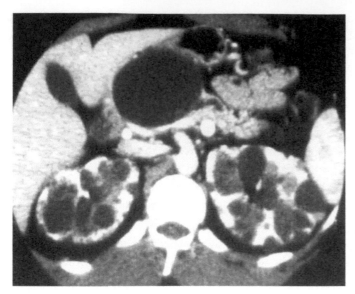

Figure 13.1. CT scan showing a pancreatic pseudocyst with a thin wall in close proximity to the posterior wall of the stomach. This is ideally situated for endoscopic puncture and drainage.

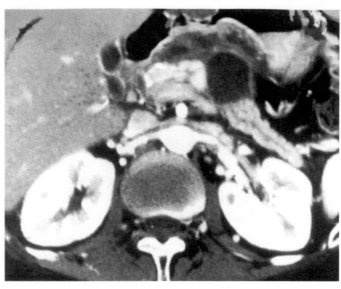

Figure 13.2. CT scan showing a significant amount of soft tissue thickening between the cyst and the gastric lumen. This would be unsuitable for endoscopic puncture and drainage.

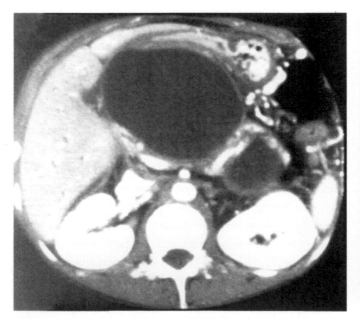

Figure 13.3. CT scan showing significant collateral portal varices between the cyst wall and the lumen of the stomach. Such blood vessels might pose a distinct hazard for endoscopic puncture.

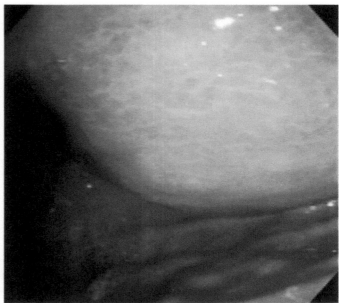

Figure 13.4. Endoscopic view showing a large bulge on the posterior wall of the stomach projecting into the lumen. The bulge is due to an underlying pseudocyst.

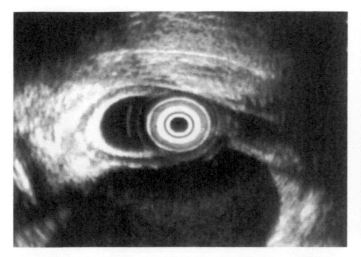

Figure 13.5. An endoscopic ultrasound scan (M20 Olympus instrument) showing a thin-walled cyst immediately adjacent to the gastric antrum. This would be ideal for endoscopic puncture.

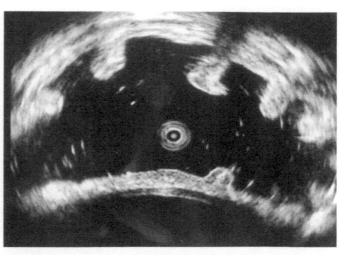

Figure 13.6. This endoscopic ultrasound scan has been obtained with an Olympus UM-3R miniprobe, which can be applied to the gastric wall at the site of intended puncture. It shows the rugal folds of the stomach and a thin-walled cyst adjacent to the posterior wall.

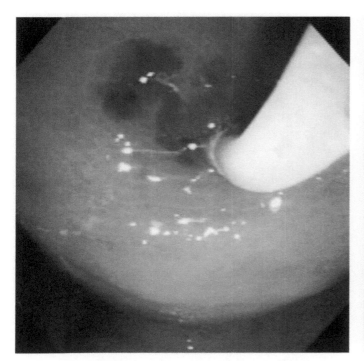

Figure 13.7. A wide-bore endoscopic needle, 1.5 cm long, capable of taking a 0.9 mm (0.035") guidewire, which is inserted through the gastric wall into the pseudocyst.

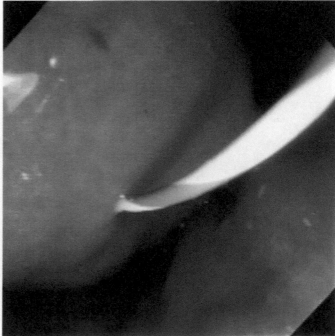

Figure 13.8. A guidewire has been passed down the needle into the pseudocyst and the needle withdrawn.

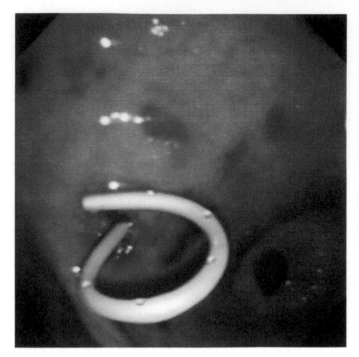

Figure 13.9. A 7FG double pigtail stent has been inserted over the guidewire into the pseudocyst and the proximal end is seen draining into the gastric lumen.

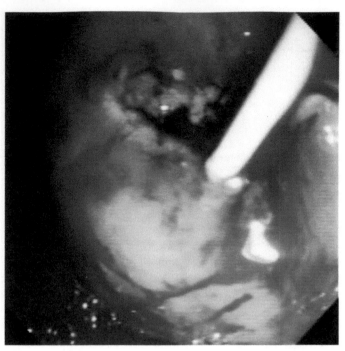

Figure 13.10. In order to achieve better drainage a small cut can be made in the wall of the stomach using an over-the-wire sphincterotome or a needle-knife. Care must be taken in case such a cut causes bleeding.

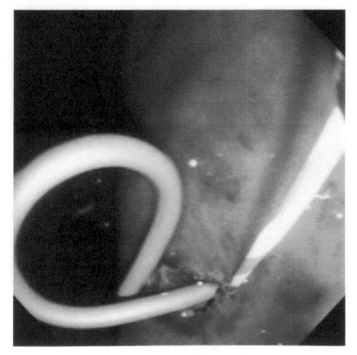

Figure 13.11. When draining very large pseudocysts, as well as making a small cut, two stents can be placed. The guidewire is reinserted into the cyst, through the small cut, alongside the first stent.

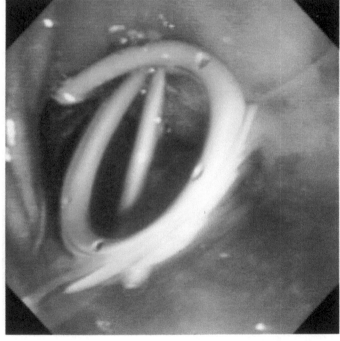

Figure 13.12. A second stent is now inserted alongside the first with pancreatic juice flowing freely into the lumen of the stomach.

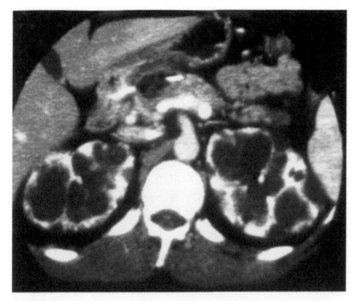

Figure 13.13. A CT scan four days after endoscopic cyst puncture and drainage. There is little fluid left in the pseudocyst and the stents are seen in situ.

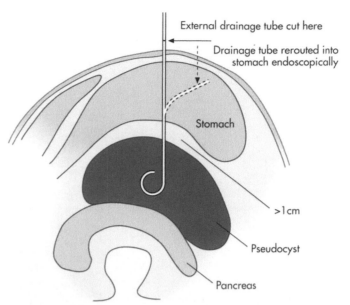

Figure 13.14. Diagram of percutaneous transgastric pseudocyst drainage and subsequent endoscopic rerouting.

advocated transpapillary drainage of cysts, where a free communication between the cyst and the duct exists [5–7]. This seems to occur in about 50% of patients with pseudocysts, which clearly would limit the application of this particular technique. Although bleeding and perforation are avoided, pancreatitis, inadequate drainage, subsequent cyst infection and the need for repeated endoscopic stent or drainage tube changes, are a disadvantage. The initial success of transpapillary drainage and the late failure rate seen similar to results of direct transmural puncture for drainage.

Follow-up management

In most instances, the pigtail stent(s) will be left in for 1–2 months before removal, provided that the cyst had completely decompressed. Removal of the internal stent is straightforward and need not be done under screening. Cyst recurrence after the stents are removed does occur, but few series have given long-term follow-up results to quantify this precisely. In general, cysts secondary to a duct disruption – which settles with subsequent restoration of continuity of pancreatic duct drainage – will drain very satisfactorily and not recur. Cysts filled from the distal pancreas behind ongoing duct obstructions are less likely to settle with simple internal drainage, and cyst recurrence or distal pancreatitis are not uncommon and may need surgical intervention in due course.

Management of deeper pseudocysts

Pseudocysts that are 1 cm or more from the lumen of the stomach can still be drained non-surgically without the use of external drainage catheters – which might introduce infection and increase the risk of pancreatic fistula formation. If a pigtail drain is inserted percutaneously into a pseudocyst under ultrasound guidance, and care is taken to route this transgastrically across the lumen of the stomach, the external catheter can then be rerouted internally, by endoscopic means. This is an extremely useful technique, not only for cysts that are too far from the stomach for endoscopic puncture, but also for endoscopists with limited experience in pancreatic endotherapy. The technique is demonstrated in Figures 13.14 and 13.15, which show the endoscopic appearances of rerouting the cut external drainage catheter into the lumen of the stomach. This achieves the same end result as if the drainage catheter had been placed endoscopically in the first instance.

There are some patients with a duct disruption and pseudocyst where internal pancreatic stenting or drainage via the main duct and papilla might be suitable.

Pancreatic duct leaks and disruptions and peripancreatic collections

Patients with disruption of the main pancreatic duct or side

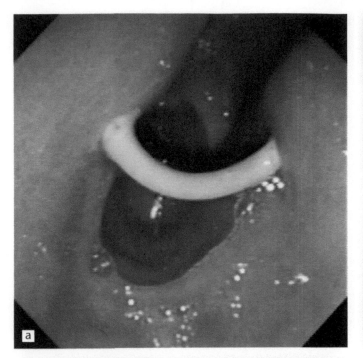

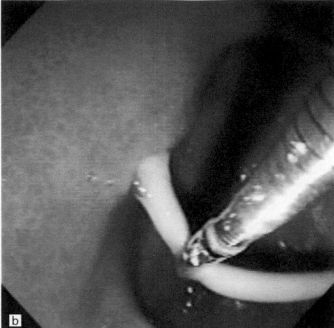

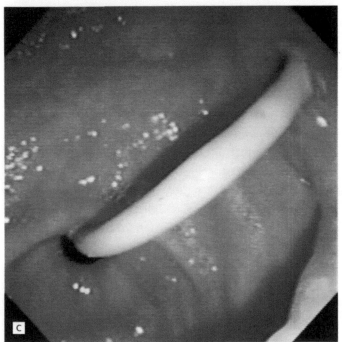

Figure 13.15. (a) Here the percutaneous drainage catheter can be seen entering and leaving the lumen of the stomach. (b) Once the drainage catheter has been cut at skin level it is straightforward to grasp the catheter with endoscopic forceps and pull the cut end into the lumen of the stomach. (c) The cut end of the stent pulled through and drainage well in the stomach lumen near the pylorus.

branches may not develop a formal pseudocyst, and CT scanning often reveals more widespread peripancreatic inflammation, with or without separate fluid collections around the pancreas. It may be clear from the CT scan that the pancreatic duct has become disrupted, but often the precise site of duct disruption and assessment of continuity of the pancreatic duct (which is of extreme importance) cannot be assessed until the ERCP is performed. There are two ways of draining the pancreatic duct and such collections: first, by the insertion of a pancreatic stent; and second, with a nasopancreatic drainage tube [8,9].

Where there is continuity of the pancreatic duct, a stent or drainage tube can be passed over a guidewire and should ideally be positioned across the area of disruption. However this is not always technically possible, and drainage to the proximal side of the leak is often all that can be achieved. Where there is complete duct disruption and no continuity with the body or tail of the pancreas, proximal drainage is clearly all that can be achieved.

The scanning and endoscopic appearances and the therapeutic manoeuvres involved are illustrated in Figures 13.16–13.20.

The technique of placing a stent or drainage tube into the pancreatic duct is essentially the same. It is not always necessary to perform a pancreatic sphincterotomy for this purpose and, if short-term drainage in acute disease is required, the pancreatic duct can be cannulated and a stent

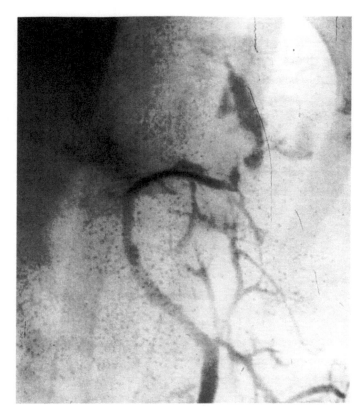

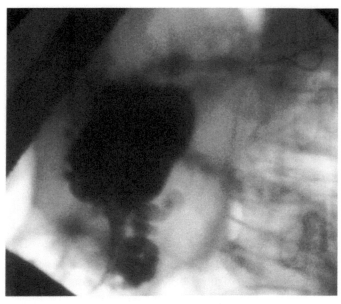

Figure 13.18. A guidewire has been passed beyond the leak into the tail of the pancreas.

Figure 13.16. Pancreatogram showing duct disruption with contrast leaking into the peripancreatic tissues and no filling upstream of this point, indicating discontinuity of the rest of the pancreas. A stent placed downstream of the disruption may suffice as long as the distal part is not draining outside this area.

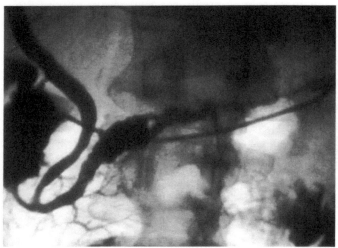

Figure 13.19. This pancreatogram shows a drainage tube that has been inserted over a guidewire down the pancreatic duct across a point of disruption to drain the entire duct system. This tube is then rerouted through the nose using the same technique as is done with nasobiliary drainage (see Fig. 8.4).

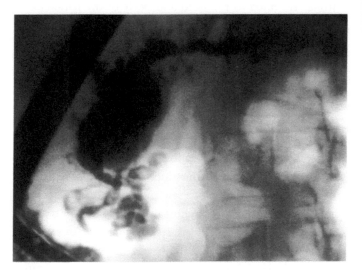

Figure 13.17. This pancreatogram demonstrates the point of duct disruption with leakage of contrast into the peripancreatic tissues. Such a patient would be suitable for stenting or drainage tube insertion past the point of disruption.

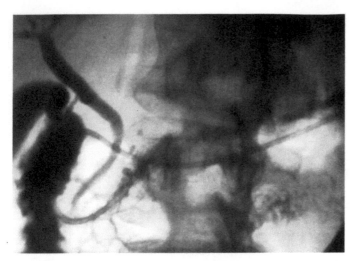

Figure 13.20. This tubogram two weeks later shows sealing of the duct disruption with no leakage of contrast outside the pancreas. At this point the nasopancreatic tube can be removed without further endoscopy.

or drainage tube inserted over a guidewire without prior sphincterotomy. Where follow-up procedures are likely, or in chronic disease where more established pancreatic duct drainage is required, a pancreatic sphincterotomy should be performed.

Pancreatic sphincterotomy

If a cut is performed through the intact papilla into the pancreatic duct it may suffice for initial stent placement, but then tends to close up again and possibly even stenose at a later date. It is also difficult to assess how far to cut safely, as the direction of the cut is towards the 1 o'clock position through the thickness of the ampulla of Vater and on to the adjacent duodenal wall.

To perform this safely, a small biliary sphincterotomy is first performed, after which the roof of the pancreatic duct within the sphincter is opened up just enough to provide drainage or to facilitate stenting.

Small pancreatic stents block within a few months, and there is no way of knowing clinically whether they are patent and the duct is still draining. It is therefore advantageous to use pancreatic drainage tubes which can be conveniently rerouted via the nose, as drainage can then be monitored and follow-up tube pancreatograms can be performed easily to assess whether the leak has healed. Once the situation has settled, the nasopancreatic tube can be removed without the need for further ERCP. Although nasopancreatic drainage confers all these advantages it may

limit the patient to remaining in hospital, whereas pancreatic duct stenting allows the patient to go home, if their clinical condition allows. A pancreatic stent would probably be needed for 1–2 months to allow leaks to settle. If pancreatic leaks or fistulas continue after that period of time it is highly likely that the patient will need a surgical approach, as long-term endoscopic stenting is not applicable in this situation.

In many patients a period of nil-by-mouth and total parenteral nutrition (TPN) is also necessary to encourage leaks to settle and the pancreatic duct disruption to heal. Pancreatic endotherapy is often used when such conservative measures, on their own, have failed to settle the situation.

Pancreatic duct stones

Main pancreatic duct stones are a very common finding in chronic pancreatitis, and in the majority of patients are secondary to the disease process. In some patients the stones may well cause mechanical obstruction and then clinical benefit may follow their removal. There is extensive literature on the technique and results of endoscopic removal of pancreatic duct stones [10–13]. Factors favouring pancreatic stones removal include:

- three stones or less
- stones under 10 mm in diameter
- stones confined to the head and body of the pancreas
- no proximal stricture
- not impacted.

Technical success is therefore better in patients with a few calculi in a dilated duct adjacent to the papilla. Such patients are not that common, but may well have relapsing bouts of pain. Patients with well-established chronic disease with regular pain with widespread calcification tend to be unsuitable for endoscopic removal of stones either due to the number of stones in the duct or to the presence of multiple areas of stricturing. It is not uncommon to find peripapillary fibrosis producing a very proximal stricture which makes endoscopic removal of stones impossible, even though they are within the head of the pancreas.

The majority of series report removal of pancreatic stones by means of direct instrumentation following pancreatic sphincterotomy. However, there are several impressive series of large numbers of patients who have undergone extracorporeal shock-wave lithotripsy to facilitate the spontaneous passage or the direct endoscopic removal of pancreatic duct stones [14,15]. Modern lithotripters with fluoroscopic targetting can satisfactorily fragment stones within the pancreatic duct, allowing fragments and debris to pass through a relatively small pancreatic sphincterotomy. This is particularly valuable in patients where intact stones could not be removed because of size or position. Such techniques may well also be suitable for stones behind pancreatic duct strictures. While waiting for pancreatic duct fragments to pass, a pancreatic stent is sometimes of benefit to ensure good drainage. Very careful clinical follow-up and review of such cases is necessary as the risk of precipitating acute attacks if stones or stone fragments impact is high.

The radiological and endoscopic aspects of pancreatic duct stone removal are illustrated in Figures 13.21–13.27.

The period of follow-up in many of the series is usually limited, but most report symptomatic improvement in 50% to 80% of patients over a period of 15 to 24 months of follow-up. In the majority of patients, as part of the disease process, there will be a tendency toward further stone formation, duct obstruction and a return of symptoms. Some patients will continue with severe symptoms, despite a patent pancreatic duct, which would imply parenchymal disease.

Pancreatic duct strictures

When demonstrating a pancreatic stricture – either single or multiple – in the pancreatic duct in a patient with pain, it is tempting to assume that the patient's symptoms will improve if that stricture was simply stented. Many of these patients probably have incidental strictures which are not the cause of pain but are part of the disease process. It has been known for many years that patients with painless chronic pancreatitis and steatorrhoea have an equal instance of strictures as those with pain [16]. Nevertheless, there are some patients where recurrent bouts of distal pancreatitis are associated with a tight main duct stricture and dilatation upstream. In these patients it originally seemed reasonable to improve the course of the disease by placing an endoscopic stent across the obstruction.

Early reports in the literature, though numerous [10,12,17,18], often dealt with combined numbers of techniques and rarely with isolated groups of patients with

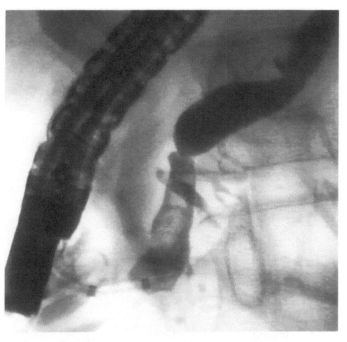

Figure 13.21. The pancreatogram demonstrates several calculi within a dilated duct in the head of the pancreas.

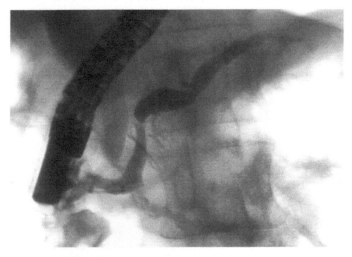

Figure 13.22. Following a pancreatic sphincterotomy, the stones have been removed and the duct is empty of calculi and draining freely.

strictures alone, dealing rather with patients with a combination of strictures and stones. Some authors have reported a dramatic immediate relief of pain in 94% of patients after stenting a duct stricture, with just under half the patients continuing to be helped with stent changes over a 3-year period of follow-up [19].

Recent experience has tended to show that the benefit of stenting for pancreatic duct strictures is limited and may, in

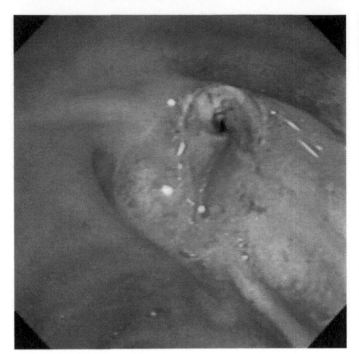

Figure 13.23. The endoscopic view of a pancreatic sphincterotomy which has been made in the 1 o'clock position.

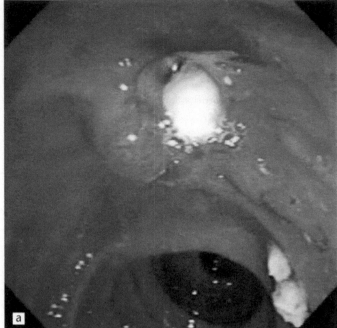

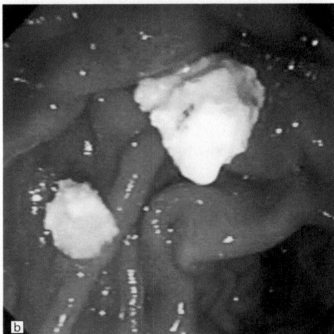

Figure 13.24. Pancreatic calculi in the lumen of the duodenum following endoscopic removal.

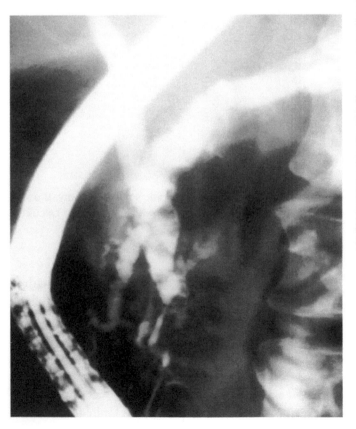

Figure 13.25. Pancreatogram showing pancreatic calculi in the head of the pancreas in a slightly dilated duct system. There is a very proximal stricture of the pancreatic duct adjacent to the papilla, which although short would preclude successful endoscopic management.

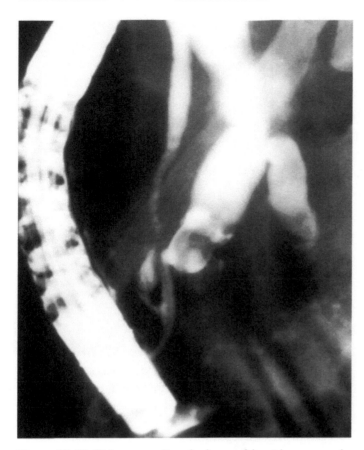

Figure 13.26. This pancreatic calculus could not be removed endoscopically due to a degree of narrowing, but not complete stricturing, of the pancreatic duct adjacent to the papilla. Extracorporeal shock wave lithotripsy (ESWL) was used in this patient to shatter the stone up and allow spontaneous passage following prior pancreatic sphincterotomy.

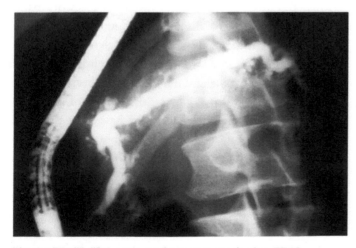

Figure 13.27. The same patient, one week after ESWL, showing a completely patent pancreatic duct system.

some patients, actually cause further damage. Endoscopists have assumed that the results of pancreatic stenting would be similar to experience in the biliary tree, where even small stents can lead to prolonged periods of relief from cholestasis. Unfortunately, small stents inserted in the pancreatic duct occlude very quickly, and up to almost half the patients may have blocked stents within 2 months, with the majority of small stents being completely occluded within 3 months [20]. Unlike stents in the biliary tree, where bacterial biofilm is an important factor in initiating stent clogging, pancreatic duct stents occlude with proteinaceous material. This protein, mainly albumin, may be produced as a result of damage to the duct wall by the stent, as it differs from normal pancreatic protein secretion [21].

There is also an increasing literature on the risks of inducing further main pancreatic duct damage by leaving stents in the duct, even for periods of 3–4 months [12,22–24]. Up to 80% of patients have developed new strictures, often at the site of the upper end of the stent and, worryingly, about half of these strictures appear to then be permanent on follow-up ERCP. Although earlier series reported quite large numbers of endoscopic stents for strictures, there has been an increasing trend, in view of the problems of long-term stenting, to question this advisability. It may well be that the clinical progress after stent insertion in this situation could be used as a prognostic indication as to whether a patient, if they do well following stenting, would therefore respond well to a distal duct drainage procedure.

The decision to attempt endoscopic therapy in patients with a long history of chronic disease should be balanced against the potential problem of endoscopic complications or inducing infection if that patient has subsequently to proceed to surgery.

There have been very few reports concerning the use of self-expanding metal stents in the pancreas. The majority of authors feel that even if you are going to place a stent, it should be a removable polyethylene one. There is a real need for caution, as experience of metal stents in benign biliary strictures raises concerns about inflammatory tissue ingrowth blocking the stent, which then can be extremely difficult to manage. The techniques and appearances of stenting for pancreatic strictures are illustrated in Figures 13.28–13.30.

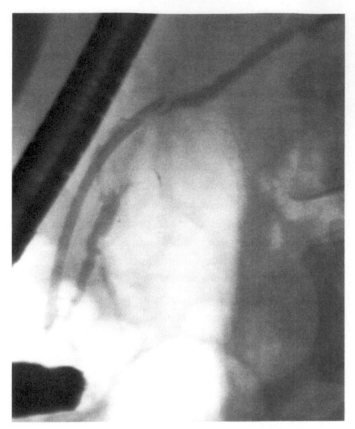

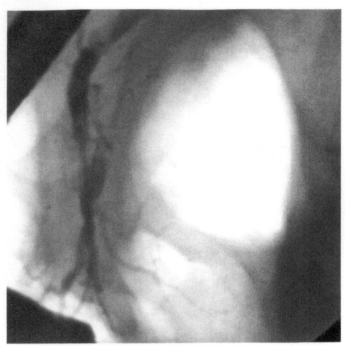

Figure 13.30. Pancreatogram after stent removal showing a second pancreatic duct stricture that has developed at the site of the tip of the stent.

Figure 13.28. This pancreatogram in a patient with a relapsing pancreatitis demonstrates a pancreatic stent that has been placed across a stricture in the head of the pancreas.

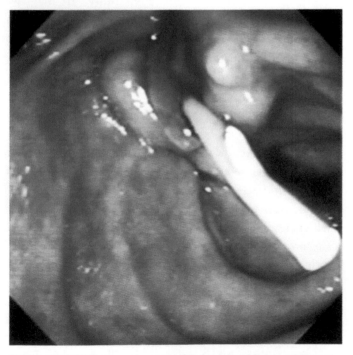

Figure 13.29. The accessory papilla is seen above and lateral to the major papilla and has a very small orifice.

Pancreas divisum

About 4% of the population have the congenital abnormality pancreas divisum, but only a small proportion of those patients get clinical pancreatitis. Despite some initial doubt as to the relevance of this theory of dorsal pancreatic duct obstruction and pancreatitis, it is now widely accepted that this is certainly a factor in the causation of some patients' disease. Early surgical results at accessory papilla sphincteroplasty were disappointing and many patients subsequently underwent further surgical resection. Endoscopic sphincterotomy with or without stenting at the level of the accessory papilla and dorsal duct has been established for many years [25]. Unlike other areas of pancreatic endotherapy, some controlled studies have been performed in this situation and show a clear advantage in the active endoscopic treatment in patients with relapsing bouts of pancreatitis when compared with no endoscopic therapy [26]. Some 75% of patients with acute relapsing pancreatitis showed an improvement, whereas only 26% of those with chronic pain had any benefit over 1.7 years' follow-up [27].

Diagnostic cannulation of the dorsal duct is difficult and is associated with a higher rate of complication, particularly

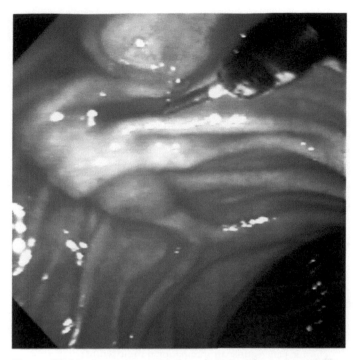

Figure 13.31. An endoscopic view showing the major papilla (below) and the accessory papilla (above). A fine metal tip cannula is being used to cannulate the accessory orifice.

post-procedure pancreatitis. Due to the small size of the papilla and difficult anatomical approach, endoscopic techniques are very complex but successful accessory duct sphincterotomy – usually with a guidewire-assisted sphincterotome and subsequent stenting – are now well established. The anatomy and technique of these procedures are shown in Figures 13.31–13.32.

The same dilemmas exist with this condition as with stenting the main duct in terms of the length of time stents should remain *in situ* and the need for long-term stent changes. Again, a good case can be made for a successful outcome after stenting indicating the probability of a successful outcome after surgery if that patient has a permanent drainage of the dorsal pancreatic duct system.

Sphincter of Oddi dysfunction

It is well known that patients get biliary symptoms and abnormal liver function with this condition, but there is a small group of patients who have proven intermittent attacks of acute pancreatitis or pancreatic-sounding pain.

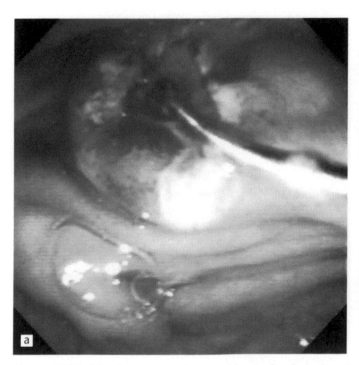
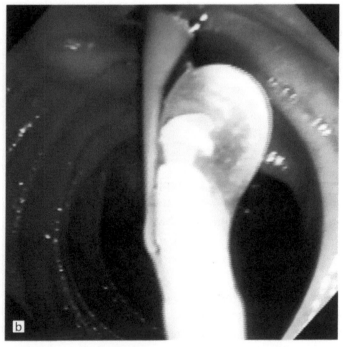

Figure 13.32. (a) After cannulation a guidewire has been inserted into the duct and a small sphincterotomy performed using an over-the-wire sphincterotome. The sphincterotomy must be carefully performed as the diameter of the dorsal pancreatic duct, although dilated, is still small. This view shows the guidewire *in situ* following sphincterotomy. (b) A small pancreatic stent has been inserted into the dorsal duct system over the guidewire through which proteinaceous pancreatic juice can be seen draining. Such stents need to be removed or changed after 3–4 months as they occlude quickly.

While data exist in randomized trials concerning biliary dysmotility, it is not possible to say with any certainty whether a biliary sphincterotomy or, more specifically, a pancreatic sphincterotomy or balloon dilatation, relieves symptoms in patients with abnormal sphincter manometry and pancreatic symptoms. The relationship of these conditions to papillary stenosis is uncertain, and it is even more uncertain that any therapeutic manoeuvres at the level of the papilla are of any benefit. It is well-recognized that attempts at improving drainage at the papilla in these patients are associated with a higher rate of complications, especially with balloon dilatation, which has a 17% incidence of pancreatitis [28]. At present, this area is highly controversial, and much more data are needed before routine endotherapy for 'dyskinesia problems' is warranted.

Biliary obstruction in chronic pancreatitis

Because endoscopic biliary stenting of benign biliary strictures can be performed easily and safely, it clearly has a place in the management of patients with chronic pancreatitis presenting with jaundice. It has little place in the long-term management of such patients unless they are medically unfit for surgery or severe portal hypertension with para-bile duct varices makes biliary bypass impossible [29]. There are some patients who benefit from biliary stent replacement while awaiting more complex surgery, such as pancreatic resection.

SUMMARY

Pancreatic endotherapy is complex and should only be performed in centres with, not only the requisite endoscopic skills, but also the combination of radiological and surgical expertise that is needed to make a multidisciplinary team that is so essential in the successful management of pancreatic disease.

It is extremely important not to treat the radiological abnormalities alone, but to choose the correct clinical indications at an appropriate time in the course of a patient's disease. Decisions about endoscopic therapy need to be made with due consideration of the available surgical alternatives and long-term results.

Pancreatic endotherapy is particularly successful in:
- Pseudocyst drainage.

- Pancreatic duct disruptions with peri-pancreatic collections, pancreatic ascites or fistula, particularly in association with a duct stricture.

Moderately good results are obtained in:
- Removal of pancreatic calculi in the head of the pancreas, particularly when combined with extracorporeal shock-wave lithotripsy.
- Pancreas divisum with acute relapsing pancreatitis.

Poor results are seen in:
- Pancreas divisum with chronic pain.
- Long-term stenting in patients with strictures and/or stones, particularly in patients with chronic pain.
- Papillary stenosis and dysmotility syndromes.

REFERENCES

1. Lowenfels AB, Maisonneuve P, Cavallini G *et al.* Prognosis of chronic pancreatitis: an international multicentre study. International Pancreatic Study Group. *Am J Gastroenterol* 1994; 89: 1467–71.

2. Cremer M, Deviere J, Engelholm L. Endoscopic management of cysts and pseudocysts in chronic pancreatitis: long-term follow-up after 7 years of experience. *Gastrointest Endosc* 1989; 35: 1–9.

3. Sahel J. Endoscopic drainage of pancreatic cysts. *Endoscopy* 1991; 23: 181–184.

4. Smits ME, Rauws EAJ, Guida NJ. The efficacy of endoscopic treatment of pancreatic pseudocysts. *Gastrointest Endosc* 1995; 42: 202–207.

5. Barthet M, Sahel J, Bodiou-Bertel C. Endoscopic transpapillary drainage of pancreatic pseudocysts. *Gastrointest Endosc* 1995; 42: 208–213.

6. Binmoeller KF, Seifert H, Walter A. Transpapillary and transmural drainage of pancreatic pseudocysts. *Gastrointest Endosc* 1995; 42: 219–224.

7. Catalano MF, Geenen JE, Schmalz MJ. Treatment of pancreatic pseudocysts with ductal communication by transpapillary pancreatic duct endoprosthesis. *Gastrointest Endosc* 1995; 42: 214–218.

8. Devière J, Bueso H, Baize M. Complete disruption of the main pancreatic duct: endoscopic management. *Gastrointest Endosc* 1995; 42: 445–451.

9. Kozarek RA, Ball TJ, Patterson DJ. Endoscopic transpapillary therapy for disrupted pancreatic duct and peripancreatic fluid collections. *Gastroenterology* 1991; 100: 1362–1370.

10. Cremer M, Deviere J, Delhaye M. Non-surgical management of severe chronic pancreatitis. *Scand J Gastroenterol* 1990; 25(Suppl. 175): 77–84.

11. Kozarek RA, Traverso LW. Endotherapy for chronic pancreatitis. *Int J Pancreatol* 1996; 19: 93–102.

12. Lehman GA, Sherman S, Hawes RH. Endoscopic management of recurrent and chronic pancreatitis. *Scand J Gastroenterol* 1995; 30(Suppl. 208): 81–89.

13. Sherman S, Lehman GA, Hawes RH. Pancreatic ductal stones: frequency of successful endoscopic removal and improvement in symptoms. *Gastrointest Endosc* 1991; 37: 511–517.

14. Delhaye M, Vandermeeren A, Baize M. Extracorporeal shock-wave lithotripsy of pancreatic calculi. *Gastroenterology* 1992; 102: 610–620.

15. Sauerbruch T, Holl J, Sackmann M. Extracorporeal lithotripsy of pancreatic stones in patients with chronic pancreatitis and pain: a prospective follow up study. *Gut* 1992; 33: 969–972.

16. Girdwood Ah, Bornman PC, Marks IN. Is pancreatic duct obstruction or stricture a major cause of pain in calcific pancreatitis? *Br J Surg* 1980; 67: 425–428.

17. Malfertheiner P, Büchler M. Indications for endoscopic or surgical therapy in chronic pancreatitis. *Endoscopy* 1991; 23: 185–190.

18. Smits ME, Badiga SM, Rauws EAJ. Long-term results of pancreatic stents in chronic pancreatitis. *Gastrointest Endosc* 1995; 42: 461–467.

19. Cremer M, Deviere J, Delhaye M. Stenting in severe chronic pancreatitis: results of medium term follow up in 76 patients. *Endoscopy* 1991; 23: 171–176.

20. Ikenberry SO, Sherman S, Hawes RH. The occlusion rate of pancreatic stents. *Gastrointest Endosc* 1994; 40: 611–613.

21. Smits ME, Groen AK, Mok KS. Analysis of occluded pancreatic stents and juices in patients with chronic pancreatitis. *Gastrointest Endosc* 1997; 45: 53–58.

22. Burdick JS, Geenan JE, Venu RP. Ductal morphological changes due to pancreatic stent therapy – a randomized controlled study. *Am J Gastroenterol* 1992; 87: 155A.

23. Kozarek RA. Pancreatic stents can induce ductal changes consistent with chronic pancreatitis. *Gastrointest Endosc* 1990; 36: 93–95.

24. Sherman S, Hawes RH, Savides TJ. Stent induced ductal and parenchymal changes. *Gastrointest Endosc* 1996; 44: 276–282.

25. Keith RG, Shapero TF, Saibil FG. Dorsal duct sphincterotomy is effective long term treatment of acute pancreatitis associated with pancreas divisum. *Surgery* 1989; 106: 660–667.

26. Lans JI, Geenan JE, Johanson JF. Endoscopic therapy in patients with pancreas divisum and acute pancreatitis: a prospective, randomised, controlled trial. *Gastrointest Endosc* 1992; 38: 430–434.

27. Lehman GA, Sherman S, Nisi R. Pancreas divisum: results of minor papilla sphincterotomy. *Gastrointest Endosc* 1993; 39: 1–8.

28. Kozarek RA. Balloon dilatation of the sphincter of Oddi. *Endoscopy* 1988; 20: 207–210.

29. Barthet M, Bernard JP, Duval JL. Biliary stenting in benign biliary stenosis complicating chronic calcifying pancreatitis. *Endoscopy* 1994: 26: 569–572.

14

Benign obstruction of the colon

R. Leicester
With acknowledgement to M. Lamah

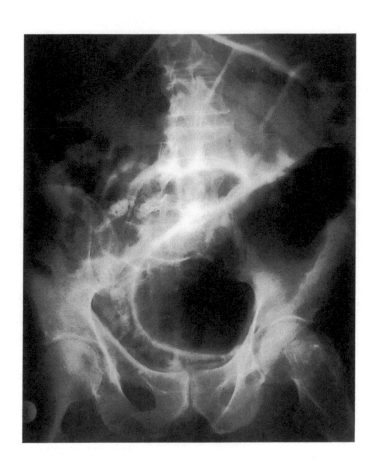

INTRODUCTION

Obstruction of either small or large bowel accounts for a significant proportion of emergency hospital admissions, and is associated with significant morbidity and mortality. Significant advances have been made over the past 50 years, with a decrease in mortality rates from 25%, to less than 10% [1], due largely to the recognition of the need for correction of fluid and electrolyte imbalance and early surgical relief.

Endoscopy offers an alternative therapeutic modality to surgical intervention, particularly in chronic obstruction. All cases should be assessed on the basis of radiological and clinical findings and provided that there is no evidence of ischaemia, sepsis or perforation, the possibility of endoscopic intervention should be considered.

DEFINITIONS AND CLASSIFICATION

Intestinal obstruction is defined as any interference with the normal, proximal to distal passage of intestinal contents, and can be classified according to aetiology, site of obstruction, speed of onset, ischaemic state of the affected bowel, and the completeness of obstruction. Differentiation is clinically important, as management of the various types is substantially different.

Aetiology

Mechanical intestinal obstruction
This may be due to intraluminal, mural, or extrinsic lesions. The spectrum of aetiological factors has changed dramatically over the past few decades: hernias have declined as a cause from about 50% to less than 10%, while adhesions have increased to 70% [2]. Cancer is the third most common cause overall and is the commonest cause of colonic obstruction. Benign causes of large bowel obstruction include volvulus, inflammatory stricture (diverticular or inflammatory bowel disease), congenital disorders in infants, intussusception, pseudo-obstruction, and a variety of rarer conditions such as drug-related strictures following non-steroidal anti-inflammatory drug (NSAID) ingestion [3,4] or long-term use of ergotamine suppositories [5].

Non-mechanical obstruction
This is characterized by inadequate propulsive motility of the bowel, despite an open lumen. This may be transient, as in acute pseudo-obstruction, or permanent as in the syndrome of chronic intestinal pseudo-obstruction. Ileus is properly defined as intestinal obstruction generally, but the term is almost always qualified as adynamic ileus and refers to an atonic physiological state with primary failure of peristalsis.

Diagnosis

When evaluating a patient with suspected bowel obstruction, the degree of obstruction – complete or incomplete, level, pathological nature of the obstructing lesion, whether or not strangulation has occurred and the general condition of the patient need to be assessed.

A careful history and physical examination are fundamental to reaching a diagnosis. Laboratory tests, radiological imaging and endoscopy are essential to confirm or refute the clinical diagnosis.

Clinical presentation

The symptoms and signs of obstruction are the result either of a physical alteration of the bowel in mechanical obstruction, or of a neuromuscular phenomenon which results in defective intestinal propulsion ('pseudo-obstruction'). In advanced cases the patient may be obtunded with signs of shock, dehydration or circulatory collapse.

- *Pain* is the hallmark of mechanical intestinal obstruction and is generally described as intermittent with paroxysms of severe pain at 4- to 5-minute intervals in proximal obstruction (less frequently in distal obstruction) alternating with periods of relief lasting several minutes. Pain that progresses in severity, localizes or becomes constant is an important symptom of progression to strangulation or perforation that requires urgent surgical treatment.
- *Vomiting* follows the onset of pain after an interval that varies with the level of obstruction; initially, the vomiting is reflexive due to intestinal wall distension. Subsequent episodes of vomiting tend to correlate with the level of obstruction, being early, bilious and voluminous with proximal obstruction, and late and faeculent in distal ileal obstruction. In colonic obstruction vomiting may not occur at all if the ileocaecal valve prevents reflux.

- *Constipation* occurs after the bowel distal to the obstructed segment empties and is a universal feature in complete obstruction of the colon. Patients with partial bowel obstruction often continue to report bowel movements and flatus, which may occur as explosive diarrhoea following episodic crampy abdominal pain. Careful physical examination establishes the state of hydration, estimates the degree of physiological compromise and the influence of intercurrent illness, the presence of complications, and sometimes the possible cause. Inspection may reveal an incarcerated inguinal hernia or scars of a previous laparotomy, indicating adhesions or an incisional hernia.
- *Distension* of the abdomen is more pronounced with distal small bowel or colon obstruction, but may be totally absent with a closed loop or proximal small bowel obstruction.
- *Tenderness* may be revealed by palpation in simple obstruction. Marked tenderness, peritoneal signs or a palpable mass suggest a closed loop obstruction, strangulation, or gangrene.
- *Auscultation* is also helpful; early on in simple obstruction, high-pitched tinkling sounds and peristaltic rushes are produced by increased motility and contractile amplitude of the proximal bowel and distinguish the obstructed bowel from the quiet, aperistaltic bowel of adynamic paralytic ileus. Progressive distension however inhibits smooth muscle contraction and the abdomen becomes relatively quiet. Strangulation and peritonitis are marked by a silent abdomen.
- *Rectal and pelvic examinations* are mandatory; the former may reveal blood, or a mass.

DIAGNOSTIC STUDIES

Laboratory findings

Laboratory evaluation is useful in detecting the severity of physiological derangement. A leucocytosis greater than 18×10^9 cells/litre is suggestive, but not confirmatory, of strangulation [6]; similarly, the presence of a metabolic acidosis is an ominous sign, but its sensitivity as an indicator of strangulation is only about 75%.

Radiographical studies

These are an important adjunct to clinical assessment, not only in confirming or refuting the diagnosis but also in determining the site of obstruction, whether it is partial or complete, and whether it involves small and/or large bowel.

Plain radiography

Plain radiographs must be taken before giving any contrast agents, which by introducing air may confuse the diagnosis. Supine and erect views of the abdomen must include the diaphragm and pelvis, and an erect chest film rules out free intraperitoneal air due to perforation. Normally, the small intestine contains only small amounts of swallowed air and is 2–3 cm in diameter; plain radiographs show air in the stomach and colon, but not usually in the small bowel. With obstruction, air is swallowed, gas separates from intraluminal fluid, producing air–fluid levels in the small intestine (Fig. 14.1); their appearance in dilated loops of small bowel allows a diagnosis of bowel obstruction in 70% of cases. Small bowel is differentiated from large bowel by its central location, and by identification of valvulae conniventes that completely cross the bowel. Colonic haustral markings on the other hand occupy only a portion of the transverse diameter of the bowel, and the colon shadow is on the periphery of the abdominal film or in the pelvis. Radiographs in partial or early complete small bowel obstruction may have associated colonic gas, but without colonic distension. 'Beak-like' narrowing of a gas- and fluid-filled loop implies a volvulus of either small or large bowel. The presence of a fixed loop with progressive loss of mucosal detail on serial films suggests ischaemia with impending perforation. Radiographic evidence of passage of gas into the colon, especially when observed on serial films, can be helpful in distinguishing partial from complete bowel obstruction. It is important to note that the presence of intestinal gas in initial radiographs of the abdomen does not exclude complete or strangulated small bowel obstruction, and the patient may continue to have bowel movements or pass flatus until the distal bowel is depleted of its contents. In mechanical small bowel obstruction, plain films show multiple air–fluid levels with minimal colonic gas, which contrasts with paralytic ileus, in which there is copious gas throughout the large and small bowel (Fig. 14.2). The presence of a closed loop can sometimes be surmised from discordance between the clinical features and the radiographic picture, the history

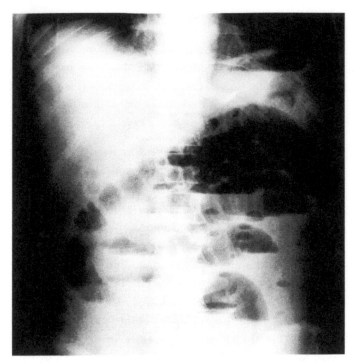

Figure 14.1. Multiple air–fluid levels in mechanical small-bowel obstruction.

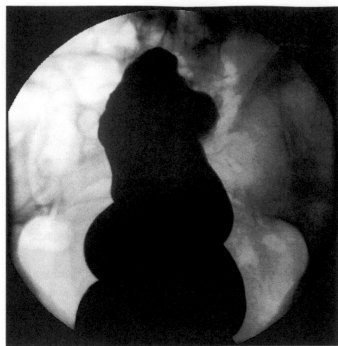

Figure 14.3. Use of barium for partial obstruction.

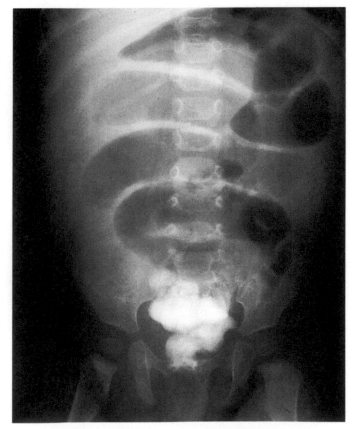

Figure 14.2. Paralytic ileus in a child: copious gas without fluid levels.

strongly suggesting bowel obstruction but the plain radiographs being unimpressive. Preoperative localization of obstruction may prevent unnecessary lysis of otherwise stable adhesions, a procedure that carries the risk of entering bowel or creating new obstructive adhesions.

Contrast radiography

Indications for contrast radiography in suspected acute small bowel obstruction remain controversial [7]. In stable patients in whom the diagnosis is uncertain, or in those who are considered high surgical risks, a contrast study is useful to confirm the diagnosis and determine the site and severity of the obstruction. In the postoperative patient, for example, it will help in distinguishing obstruction from paralytic ileus. The most definitive studies are obtained by small bowel 'enema', infusing barium through a tube placed past the ligament of Treitz under fluoroscopic guidance (Fig. 14.3). Small bowel mucosal abnormalities, intra-luminal masses and points of obstruction may be identified in a highly accurate way. Passage of barium through an area of partial obstruction within 24 hours in a stable patient whose proximal bowel does not appear compromised suggests that a careful trial of intestinal decompression is safe. In contrast, evidence for a high-grade obstruction with thickened, dilated proximal bowel, mucosal disruption, or findings of a closed loop should prompt urgent surgical treatment. Contrast radiography is more commonly employed in large bowel obstruction, where a barium enema also has therapeutic potential (e.g. intussusception or volvulus). Other imaging modalities include ultrasound [8], computed tomography [9] and magnetic resonance imaging. These may be helpful in identifying abdominal wall hernias, fluid-filled loops of bowel, and intraluminal or extraluminal masses.

Other diagnostic procedures

Endoscopy

This can reveal obstructing lesions at both proximal and distal ends of the alimentary tract, and biopsy or brush cytology may be performed. Laparoscopy can rapidly differentiate simple from strangulated obstruction, and when adhesions are not too dense, laparoscopic lysis may be feasible; this avoids the need for open operation and minimizes the propensity for further adhesions. There is no single investigation which can preoperatively detect strangulation, but recent work has shown that radionuclide scanning with technetium diphosphonate shows increased uptake of isotope by ischaemic bowel [10], and there is significant delay of intraperitoneally instilled xenon-133 in strangulated obstruction in experimental animals [11]. The clinical application of these findings awaits further evaluation.

MANAGEMENT

The fundamental principles involved in the management of the acutely obstructed patient are:
- resuscitation by correction of haemodynamic and electrolyte imbalance;
- decompression of the gastrointestinal tract by whatever means possible; and
- timely surgical intervention.

In small bowel obstruction, the timing of operation depends on three factors: (i) duration of obstruction; (ii) the opportunity to improve vital organ function; and (iii) consideration of the risk of strangulation. The mortality from obstruction with gangrenous bowel varies from 4% to 30%, whereas in simple mechanical obstruction relieved within 24 hours, the mortality rate is about 1%.

The compelling reason for operation is that strangulation cannot be excluded with certainty. The surgeon must avoid being lulled into a false sense of security by the improvement in symptoms and signs that invariably occurs after resuscitation. Because no test reliably detects strangulation preoperatively, surgery should be performed as soon as is reasonable. Absence of fever, tachycardia, localized tenderness and leucocytosis indicates that non-operative management is still safe. The presence of any one of these findings, however, mandates surgery [12].

In the case of large bowel obstruction, the approach to management is predicated on the high likelihood that malignancy is the underlying cause, for which surgical intervention is almost always ultimately necessary. However, the more recent introduction of endoscopic manipulation, cutting, ablating, laser recanalization, dilatation and stenting of obstructing strictures has added treatment options for a condition that has traditionally always required emergency surgical intervention [13].

Fluid and electrolyte replacement

In general, fluid and electrolyte deficits should be rapidly restored in all patients; however, when strangulation is suspected, surgical intervention should not be delayed. Intravenous therapy should usually begin with isotonic sodium chloride solution supplemented by potassium after urine flow is restored. Serum electrolytes and arterial blood gas determinations are guides to electrolyte therapy. The amount and rate of intravenous infusion should be guided by clinical signs of hydration and monitoring of central venous pressure, which should be maintained at between 5 and 10 cm of saline. Changes in blood composition take much longer to correct than do volume losses; profound hypokalaemia for example may require up to 24 hours to reverse. With strangulation, a significant amount of blood may be lost into the bowel and peritoneal cavity, and this should be replaced by packed cell transfusion as needed.

Intubation

The initial and simplest measure should be nasogastric suction with the aid of a nasogastric tube. This reduces further intestinal distension by the aspiration of swallowed air, relieves vomiting, and minimizes the risk of aspiration during the induction of anaesthesia. Long intestinal tubes of the double-lumen Miller–Abbott type may also be placed in the small intestine under endoscopic guidance preoperatively to treat small bowel obstruction particularly if nasogastric suction has failed.

Truong *et al.* [14] reported successful placement of a Dennis tube in 97% of 174 patients with paralytic ileus or different kinds of partial small bowel obstruction with no mortality and minimal morbidity. Resolution of symptoms was achieved in over half the cases, although the greatest success rate was in cases of paralytic ileus, where spontaneous resolution might have been expected. In 77 patients with mechanical small bowel obstruction, Snyder *et al.* [15] achieved resolution of obstruction in almost one-third of cases, using an endoscopically and fluoroscopically placed Leonard long intestinal tube, with no complications. The best results were achieved in cases of adhesive obstruction (37%), compared with only 12% resolution in malignant causes and no success in inflammatory obstruction.

Timing and nature of surgical intervention

The most critical decision in managing obstruction is distinguishing between simple and strangulated obstruction. Emergency surgery is required for closed-loop obstruction or suspected strangulation, although there is no single clinical sign or diagnostic test that accurately diagnoses strangulation in 100% of cases [16], and rarely does a patient exhibit all the classic signs of strangulation (fever, localized peritonism, tachycardia, leucocytosis). However, in the absence of all these signs, dead bowel is found in less than 10% of cases.

Patients with complete small bowel obstruction or those suspected of having an intussusception, volvulus, gallstone ileus or obstructing hernia are at an increased risk of strangulation and should receive surgical treatment – either immediate or delayed – almost regardless of their clinical status. In contrast, stable patients with recurrent incomplete adhesive obstruction, early postoperative or multiple recurrent obstruction, Crohn's disease, radiation enteritis and carcinomatosis are less likely to progress to strangulation and may therefore be considered for a trial of non-operative therapy. Close observation and frequent physical and radiological examinations are essential to detect signs of progression. Complete obstruction due to adhesions is much less likely to respond to non-operative therapy, but a cautious trial of conservative therapy may still be worth-

while, as obstruction in one-third of patients thereby resolves. Persistence with non-operative management for longer than 24–48 hours in a patient who shows no improvement is not only unlikely to be successful but also results in increased morbidity. Conservative treatment is also contraindicated in irreducible hernia and small bowel obstruction in a patient without abdominal scars or hernia as the obstruction then is often due to volvulus, internal herniation, or congenital adhesion and is unlikely to resolve spontaneously.

Non-surgical manoeuvres to decompress the colon prior to or instead of surgery, or as definitive treatment of benign strictures have been developed over the past decade [17], and include balloon dilatation of obstructing strictures, stent insertion across the stricture, or laser photocoagulation of an obstructing lesion, especially in the rectum.

Surgical and conservative treatments of bowel obstruction are summarized in Table 14.1.

SPECIFIC ENTITIES

Volvulus (Fig. 14.4)

In this condition, the bowel becomes twisted around its mesenteric axis, resulting in partial or complete obstruction. The sigmoid colon is the most commonly affected part of the colon (60%), followed by the right colon and more rarely the transverse colon and splenic flexure. There is also wide geographical variation, the condition being very common in parts of Africa, Asia and Eastern Europe, but accounting for between 2% and 5% of large-bowel obstruction in Western Europe and North America, where

Table 14.1. Summary of treatment options

Surgical treatment	Conservative treatment
Complete small-bowel obstruction	Incomplete obstruction
	Adhesions
Intussusception	Postoperative or multiple recurrent obstruction
Volvulus	
Gallstone ileus	Crohn's disease
Obstructing hernia	Radiation enteritis
	Carcinomatosis

it is seen most commonly in elderly, institutionalized patients. Plain radiographs are usually diagnostic of a sigmoid volvulus, the dilated sigmoid colon taking the form of the 'ace of spades' or 'bent inner tube' arising from the left lower quadrant (Fig. 14.5). Barium enema may demonstrate complete retrograde obstruction at the level of torsion, but in experienced hands colonoscopy may be used as a diagnostic as well as therapeutic tool, as first described in 1976 [18].

The major cause of mortality in sigmoid volvulus is delayed decompression resulting in bowel ischaemia and, in the absence of peritonitis, decompression of the volvulus should be attempted at the earliest opportunity. Emergency laparotomy is indicated if decompression by conservative means fails, ischaemia is suspected clinically, or if ischaemic change is apparent following endoscopic assessment of the colonic mucosa. When emergency laparotomy is not indicated, initial non-operative reduction of sigmoid volvulus should be attempted either colonoscopically or with the aid of a rigid sigmoidoscope and flatus tube. Brothers *et al.* [19] reported that sigmoidoscopy was not diagnostic in 24% of cases of sigmoid volvulus, whereas colonoscopy was 100% accurate, having the advantage of better visualization of the point of rotation and assessment of the viability of the bowel wall. The point of torsion is usually seen as an oedematous narrow area through which it is difficult to negotiate the endoscope. Gentle onward movement and rotation produces a gush of flatus and fluid, following which the instrument enters an extremely dilated segment of proximal bowel. As well as reducing the volvulus, this also rules out the presence of an intrinsic lesion causing the obstruction. The disadvantages of colonoscopy include the risk of perforation, and it is not easy to leave a tube of adequate calibre in place over the following few days. No matter how good the initial decompression of the volvulus, the subsequent recurrence rate is over 50% [19], and tends to occur early in approximately one-half of the patients. Elective resection of the sigmoid colon should therefore be considered early on after successful decompression. Volvulus of the caecum and right colon accounts for about 25% of all cases of volvulus; laparotomy is usually required, as with few exceptions [20], colonoscopic decompression is generally unsuccessful, Friedman *et al.* [21] reporting no success in attempted colonoscopic decompression of 27 cases of caecal volvulus, compared with an 81% success rate for sigmoid volvulus.

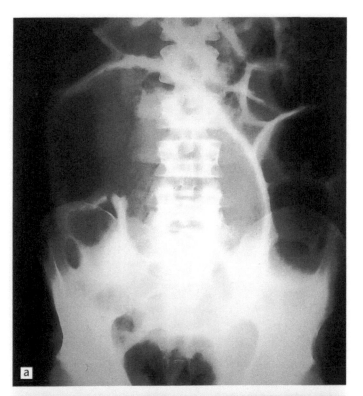
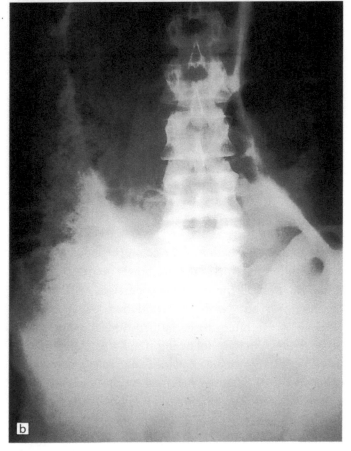

Figure 14.4. (a) Caecal volvulus. (b) Sigmoid volvulus.

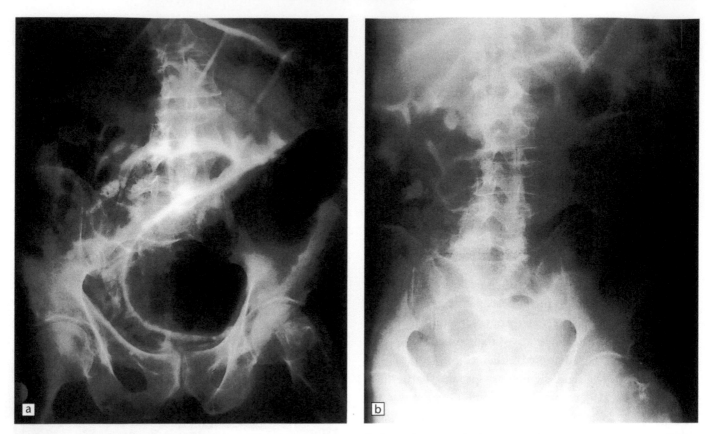

Figure 14.5. Plain abdominal X-ray of sigmoid volvulus before and after colonoscopic decompression.

When the colon is non-viable, resection is mandatory, though where it is found to be viable after reduction the optimal treatment remains controversial. That a definitive procedure should be performed is now generally accepted, as the recurrence rate of the volvulus is otherwise high.

Pseudo-obstruction

Acute pseudo-obstruction of the colon (Ogilvie's syndrome) is a condition in which the large bowel becomes markedly distended with all the symptoms and signs of large bowel obstruction, but with no evidence of mechanical obstruction.. It often arises in bed-ridden patients with other serious illnesses, following trauma or major surgery, particularly orthopaedic. Provided that emergency surgery is not indicated because of perforation or infarction, either a water-soluble contrast enema or colonoscopy should be performed to confirm the diagnosis since the treatment of pseudo-obstruction is rarely surgical. Colonoscopy has the added advantage that it can also be used therapeutically [22]; it is likely to replace radiological examination as the principal diagnostic investigation and should be performed with the aim of decompressing the colon. Very little air insufflation should be used when advancing the instrument, in order to prevent perforation; once the caecum has been reached the instrument is withdrawn while aspirating all air and liquid faeces. Once decompression has been achieved, recurrence is unlikely, but a long tube within the lumen of the colon may be left, after it has been threaded over a guidewire passed down the operating lumen of the colonoscope [23]. The overall success of colonoscopic decompression is high, Geller *et al.* [24] reporting successful decompression in over 90% of cases, after one endoscopy. However, 18% of patients in this series required multiple colonoscopies to achieve success. An alternative approach, provided that there are no medical contra-indications, is the use of neostigmine, which can produce resolution in up to 75% of cases [25]. Surgery is indicated if rupture is thought imminent, and dilatation of the caecum accompanied by peritoneal signs should encourage the surgeon to perform an emergency laparotomy. Either a caecostomy or appropriate colostomy is required, or in some cases subtotal colectomy and ileorectal anastomosis.

Diverticular disease

Diverticular disease as a cause of acute large bowel obstruction is uncommon and is usually secondary to acute diverticulitis or acute-on-chronic inflammation of a diverticular segment. It is difficult to differentiate it from malignant disease either before or at the time of operation, but water-soluble barium enema or endoscopy with biopsy or brush cytology should be performed to try and achieve a diagnosis before any planned surgery. Decompression of the obstructed colon remains the first priority and, while a proximal diverting colostomy (often performed laparoscopically) with minimal morbidity is frequently advocated, endoscopic decompression has now become an option. Colonoscopic decompression entails passing an

expandable metallic (or other) stent over a guidewire, which is manoeuvred through the stricture, preferably under fluoroscopic control. An unprepared water-soluble contrast enema is performed and a guidewire is then manipulated across the stricture. This may be achieved simply using an angiographic catheter under fluoroscopic control or, in patients with more proximal lesions, an endoscope is used to guide the wire across the lesion. The catheter is then exchanged for a self-expandable metallic stent, which is thus deployed across the stricture, and the guidewire withdrawn (Fig. 14.6).

This avoids the need for emergency surgery, and allows decompression of the bowel and preoperative bowel preparation. Elective surgery can then be planned soon after stent insertion, or may be avoided altogether with

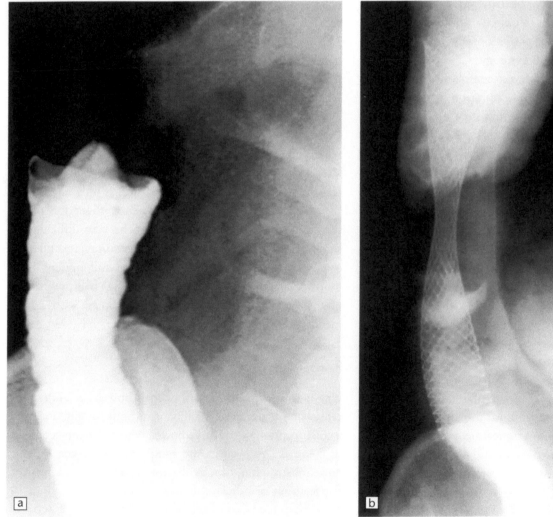
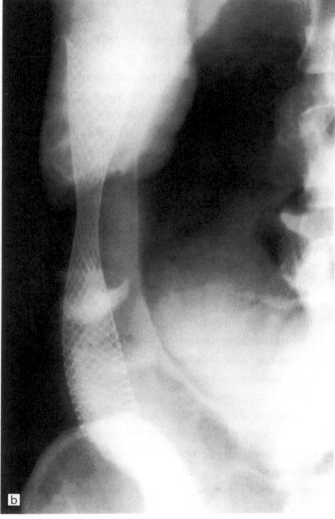

Figure 14.6. (a) Gastrograffin enema showing complete obstruction of the sigmoid colon. (b) Expandable metal stent relieving the obstruction.

benign lesions. Potential stent-related complications include perforation, bleeding, or erosion of the colonic mucosa and stent migration.

This technique is still in its infancy and has been used mainly in the treatment of obstructing colonic cancer, but encouraging results have emerged from several studies [26–28], in one of which a diverticular obstructing stricture was successfully managed this way [30].

Crohn's disease

Stricturing occurs in between 5% and 17% of cases with colonic Crohn's disease and, while usually benign, carcinoma can arise in longstanding strictures [30]. If the stricture is not causing significant obstructive symptoms, management is usually non-interventional, but in cases with worsening symptoms of obstruction, either surgical or endoscopic intervention is required. All Crohn's colonic strictures should be assessed endoscopically for malignancy, using either biopsy or brush cytology.

Recurrent stricturing commonly complicates anastomoses in patients who have undergone resection of their disease. Trnka et al. [31] found a 69% symptomatic stricturing rate in 40 patients undergoing resection for Crohn's ileocolitis followed up over 20 years. Previously, these strictures were dealt with by resection and permanent ileostomy or reanastomosis. Strictureplasty has also been reported for strictures involving ileocolic and ileorectal anastomoses.

Colonoscopic dilatation of anastomotic strictures is now a reasonable alternative, avoiding the need for surgery in most cases. Blomberg et al. [32] reported results in 27 Crohn's patients, using balloon dilatation. The strictures ranged from 0.5 to 3 cm in length, with diameters of 5 to 8 mm. The lumens were expanded to a diameter of at least 12 mm and after an average follow-up of 15 months, 67% of the patients were symptom-free. Complications occurred in three patients – two cases of haemorrhage requiring transfusion and one case of bowel perforation. Although more than one dilatation session was usually required, all of the patients preferred this form of treatment to repeat surgery. Breysem et al. [33] reported successful endoscopic balloon dilatation in 16 of 17 anastomotic strictures, without complication. Half of these patients remained asymptomatic after an average follow-up of 25 months. Dilatation was most successful in those patients with fibrotic, short (<8 cm) strictures, where there was no active disease. More recently, the use of endoscopic steroid injection combined with balloon dilatation has been suggested as a method to reduce the incidence of restenosis [34,35].

Ischaemic stricture

This may arise as a result of disease of the intestinal vessels aggravated by hypotension, occlusion of the inferior mesenteric artery by thrombosis, embolus, or iatrogenic injury, or following an attack of ischaemic colitis. In the latter case, the stricture is situated classically at the splenic flexure, but may also occur in the sigmoid or in the right colon. The conventional treatment is resection of the stricture, some authors also suggesting that the possibility of arterial reconstruction be considered. Coaxial colonoscopic dilatation is an alternative to surgery: using hydrostatic balloon dilatation, Kozarek reported immediate symptomatic relief in up to 90% of cases [37]. It is essential however that histological diagnosis is ascertained before this technique is employed, using biopsy and brush cytology.

Endometriosis

Endometriosis may cause stricture of the ileum, caecum or rectum, and the symptoms tend to be cyclical, but there is a tendency to progressive narrowing of the lumen. For this reason, colonoscopic balloon dilatation is only effective in the short term as most strictures recur. Resection of the rectum and sigmoid colon may also be very difficult and should be combined with total hysterectomy and bilateral oophorectomy where these organs are still present [38]. Hormonal manipulation with danazol may halt progression of the obstructive process, but is associated with a high incidence of side effects.

Intussusception

Unlike intussusception of the small bowel, an underlying cause such as polyp or malignant tumour usually underlies intussusception of the large bowel, which may be ileocaecal or colocolic. As well as the symptoms and signs of large bowel obstruction, bloody diarrhoea may also be a feature. Laparotomy is indicated if the intussusception cannot be reduced, as resection of the presumed malignant lesion will be necessary. Intussusception due to polyps however may be reduced and the polyp snared at colonoscopy.

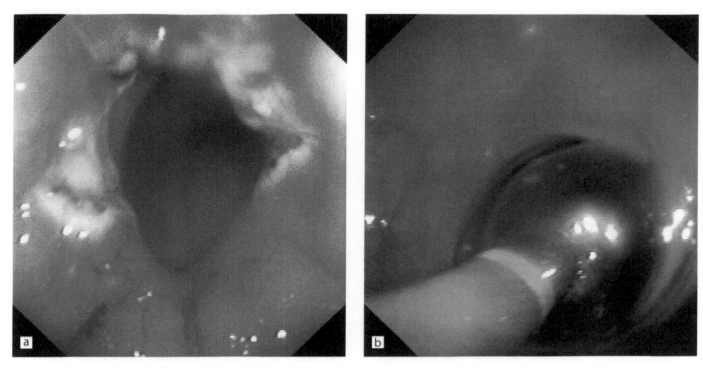

Figure 14.7. Laser incision ('Mercedes' technique) and balloon dilatation of anastomotic stricture.

Postoperative strictures

Anastomotic strictures may occur after colonic anastomoses (more commonly colorectal or coloanal), as a result of ischaemia, adhesions, or recurrent disease, and may present with subacute obstruction. Rectal stenosis may also occur following diathermy treatment of polyps and other benign tumours. Rarely, mucosal webs can cause obstructive symptoms, following closure of a loop stoma. These webs can be divided using either laser or diathermy instruments [38]. Benign strictures can usually be dilated endoscopically or managed with an expandable stent. Venkatesh *et al.* [39] reported results of endoscopic dilatation in 25 patients with benign colorectal anastomotic strictures using a TTS balloon. Most of the strictures were secondary to anastomosis using a circular stapling device and no complications were encountered. Repeated dilatation is often necessary, Dinneen and Motson reporting improvement in only 50% of cases of anastomotic stricture using a similar technique. In this series, a perforation occurred following repeat procedure [40]. Perforation probably occurs due to splitting of the fibrotic bowel at the site of the stricture. This complication can be minimized by using the 'Mercedes' technique. Here three incisions are made in the stricture, using a contact laser fibre (Diomed) prior to dilatation with a Rigiflex® (Boston Scientific) balloon inserted alongside the colonoscope, allowing dilatation to up to 4 cm for rectal strictures. The advantage of this technique lies in the healing of the laser incisions by re-epithelialization, rather than the scarring and subsequent restenosis following simple dilatation (Fig. 14.7). The use of a standard Sengstaken–Blakemore tube has also been advocated [41], but perforation of the balloon can occur when dilating a stapled anastomosis. It is essential that the histological nature of the stricture be ascertained, to exclude local recurrence, before treatment is started.

REFERENCES

1. Davis SE, Sperling L. Obstruction of the small intestine. *Arch Surg* 1969; 9: 424–426

2. McEntee G, Pender D, Mulvin D *et al.* Current spectrum of intestinal obstruction. *Br J Surg* 1987; 74: 976–980.

3. Gargot D, Chaussade S, d'Alteroche L *et al.* Nonsteroidal anti-inflammatory drug-induced colonic strictures: two cases and literature review. *Am J Gastroenterol* 1995; 90(11): 2035–2038.

4. Halter F, Weber B, Huber T *et al.* Diaphragm disease of the ascending colon. Association with sustained-release diclofenac. *J Clin Gastroenterol* 1993; 16: 74–80.

5. Machnig T, May A, Steininger H *et al.* Ergotamine-induced rectal stenosis in a patient with long-term migraine. *Leber, Magen, Darm* 1993; 23: 166–168.

6. Bizer LS, Liebling RW, Delany HM *et al.* Small bowel obstruction: the role of nonoperative treatment in simple intestinal obstruction and predictive criteria for strangulation obstruction. *Surgery* 1981; 89: 407–413.

7. Shrake P, Rex D, Lappas J, Maglinte D. Radiographic evaluation of suspected small bowel obstruction. *Am J Gastroenterol* 1991; 86: 175–178.

8. Ko YT, Lim JH, Lee DH *et al.* Small bowel obstruction: sonographic evaluation. *Radiology* 1993; 188: 649–653.

9. Gazelle GS, Goldberg MA, Wittenberg J *et al.* Efficacy of CT in distinguishing small bowel obstruction from other causes of small bowel dilatation. *Am J Roentgenol* 1994; 162: 43–47.

10. Frantzides CT, Condon RE, Tsiftsis D *et al.* Radionuclide visualization of acute occlusive and nonocclusive intestinal ischaemia. *Ann Surg* 1986; 203: 295–300.

11. Bulkley GB, Gharagozloo F, Alderson PO *et al.* Use of intraperitoneal xenon133 for imaging of intestinal strangulation in small bowel obstruction. *Am J Surg* 1981; 141: 128–135.

12. Stewardson RH, Bombeck CT, Nyhus LM. Critical operative management of small bowel obstruction. *Ann Surg* 1978; 187: 189–193.

13. Oz MC, Forde KA. Endoscopic alternatives in the management of colonic strictures. *Surgery* 1990; 108: 513–519.

14. Truong S, Willis S, Riesener KP *et al.* Value of intraluminal intestinal decompression by endoscopic placement of a Dennis tube in therapy of ileus. Retrospective clinical study of 174 patients. *Langenbecks Arch Chir* 1997; 382: 216–221.

15. Snyder CL, Ferrell KL, Goodale RL, Leonard AS. Nonoperative management of small-bowel obstruction with endoscopic long intestinal tube placement. *Am Surg* 1990; 56: 587–592.

16. Sarr MG, Bulkley GB, Zuidema GD. Preoperative recognition of intestinal strangulation obstruction. Prospective evaluation of diagnostic capability. *Am J Surg* 1983; 145: 176–182.

17. Fruhmorgen P. Endoscopic treatment of non-neoplastic stenoses and benign tumours in the lower gastrointestinal tract. *Endoscopy* 1986; 18: 66–68.

18. Ghazi A, Shinya H, Wolff W. Treatment of volvulus of the colon by colonoscopy. *Ann Surg* 1976; 182: 263–265.

19. Brothers TE, Strodel WE, Eckhauser FE. Endoscopy in colonic volvulus. *Ann Surg* 1987; 206: 1–4.

20. Janardhanan R, Bowman D, Brodmerkel GJ Jr *et al.* Cecal volvulus: decompression and detorsion with a colonoscopically placed drainage tube. *Am J Gastroenterol* 1987; 82: 912–914.

21. Friedman JD, Odland MD, Bubrick MP. Experience with colonic volvulus. *Dis Colon Rectum* 1989; 32: 409–416.

22. Munro A, Youngston GC. Colonoscopy in the diagnosis and treatment of colonic pseudo obstruction. *J R Coll Surg Edinb* 1983; 28: 391–393.

23. Ell C. Colon decompression using an anatomically adapted, large-caliber decompression probe. *Endoscopy* 1996; 28: 456–458.

24. Geller A, Petersen BT, Gostout CJ. Endoscopic decompression for acute colonic pseudo-obstruction. *Gastrointest Endosc* 1996; 44: 144–150.

25. Turegano-Fuentes F, Munoz-Jimenez F, Del Valle-Hernandez E *et al.* Early resolution of Ogilvie's syndrome with intravenous neostigmine: a simple, effective treatment. *Dis Colon Rectum* 1997; 40: 1353–1357.

26. DeFriend DJ, Klimack OE, Humphrey CS, Schraibman IG. Intraluminal stenting in the management of adhesional intestinal obstruction. *J R Soc Med* 1997; 90: 132–135.

27. Saida Y, Sumiyama Y, Nagao J, Takase M. Stent endoprosthesis for obstructing colorectal cancers. *Dis Colon Rectum* 1996; 39: 552–555.

28. Mainar A, Tejero E, Maynar M *et al.* Colorectal obstruction: treatment with metallic stents. *Radiology* 1996; 198: 761–764.

29. Lamah M, Mathur P, McKeown B *et al.* The use of rectosigmoid stent in the management of acute large bowel obstruction. *J R Coll Surg Edinb* 1998; 43: 318–321.

30. Yamazaki Y, Ribeiro MB, Sachar DB *et al.* Malignant strictures in Crohn's disease. *Am J Gastroenterol* 1991; 86: 882–885

31. Trnka YM, Glotzer DJ, Kadon DJ *et al.* The long-term outcome of restorative operation in Crohn's disease. Influence

of location, prognostic factors, and surgical guidelines. *Ann Surg* 1982; 196: 345–355.

32. Blomberg B, Rolny P, Jarnerot G. Endoscopic treatment of anastomotic strictures in Crohn's disease. *Endoscopy* 1991; 23: 195–198.

33. Breysem Y, Janssens JF, Coremans G *et al*. Endoscopic balloon dilatation of colonic and ileocolonic Crohn's strictures: long term results. *Gastrointest Endosc* 1992; 38: 142–147.

34. Ramboer C, Verhamme M, Dhondt E *et al*. Endoscopic treatment of stenosis in recurrent Crohn's disease with balloon dilation combined with local corticosteroid injection. *Gastrointest Endosc* 1995; 42: 252–255.

35. Lee M, Kubik CM, Polhamus CD *et al*. Preliminary experience with endoscopic intralesional steroid injection therapy for refractory upper gastrointestinal strictures. *Gastrointest Endosc* 1995; 41: 598–601.

36. Kozarek RA. Hydrostatic balloon dilatation of gastrointestinal stenosis: a national survey. *Gastrointest Endosc* 1986; 32: 15–19.

37. Parr NJ, Murphy C, Holt S *et al*. Endometriosis and the gut. *Gut* 1988; 29: 1112–1115.

38. Constantinescu MA, Leicester RJ. Colonic mucosal sieve: an unusual endoscopic finding. *Endoscopy* 1997; 29: 52.

39. Venkatesh KS, Ramanujam PS, McGee S. Hydrostatic balloon dilatation of benign colonic anastomotic strictures. *Dis Col Rect* 1992; 35: 789–791.

40. Dinneen MD, Motson RW. Treatment of colonic anastomotic strictures with 'through the scope' balloon dilators. *J R Soc Med* 1991; 84: 264–266.

41. Stigliano V, Fracasso P, Citavlo F *et al*. Endoscopic dilatation of a benign postoperative colonic stenosis with a Sengstaken–Blakemore tube. *Gastrointest Endosc* 1996; 43: 70–72.

15 Cancer surveillance and screening

B.P. Saunders

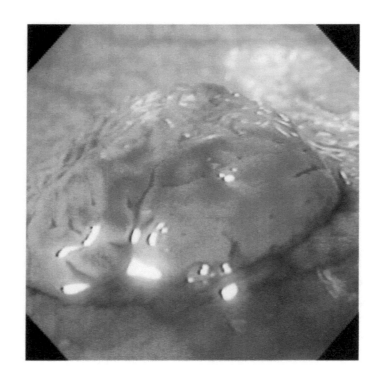

INTRODUCTION

Colorectal cancer (CRC) is the third most commonly diagnosed cancer and the second leading cause of cancer death. In the UK, more than 28 000 new cases are diagnosed, with 19 000 deaths occurring from the disease per year. In America, assuming a life expectancy of 80 years, there is a 6% lifetime risk of developing CRC, and in over 50% of people the condition will prove fatal. Five-year survival rates vary dramatically depending upon the stage of the disease. For localized disease, a 92% 5-year survival rate is expected, for regional disease 62%, and for metastatic disease just 7% [1]. Treatment of CRC is costly and not without considerable morbidity and mortality. CRC prevention or detection at an early stage is, therefore, one of the most important goals of modern health care.

PRINCIPLES OF SCREENING

When discussing screening/surveillance it is important to appreciate the correct use of each term:
- *Screening* refers to a process which identifies individuals who are more likely to have CRC or adenomatous polyps from among those without signs or symptoms of the disease.
- *Surveillance* monitors individuals with previously diagnosed colonic disease, adenomas, CRC or inflammatory bowel disease.

Symptomatic patients (change in bowel habit, rectal bleeding, abdominal pain or anaemia) should be referred promptly for a full colonic examination, either by colonoscopy or sigmoidoscopy plus barium enema.

Most CRCs are thought to be derived from pre-existing adenomas (the adenoma–carcinoma sequence), and it may take 10–20 years of acquired mutations before the benign adenoma develops into a cancer. A window of opportunity therefore exists for CRC prevention by the detection and removal of adenomas. The USA National Polyp study has demonstrated that, with careful colonoscopic surveillance, the incidence of CRC can be significantly reduced. During 8400 person-years of follow-up in 1418 adenoma patients, only five new cases of CRC were detected (all malignant polyps), a reduction in incidence of 76–90%, compared with that predicted from three reference populations [2]. Sporadic CRC is unusual below the age of 50 years, and it has been suggested that screening of 'average-risk' individuals should start at about this age, although there is no current consensus as to the optimal method of population screening.

It is however, widely accepted that colonoscopic follow-up is indicated for certain 'high-risk' groups; that is, those with previous colonic neoplasia, inflammatory bowel disease or a strong family history of cancer.

HIGH-RISK GROUPS

Cancer follow-up

Follow-up is mandatory after colonic resection for cancer, all such patients needing at least one total colonoscopy either before or soon after surgery because of the likelihood of there being synchronous neoplasia. The object of follow-up is primarily to identify and ablate new (or missed) adenomas in those with favourable staging of the original cancer and so, reasonably normal life expectancy. Simply identifying local recurrence is of little use, because the likelihood of successful 'second-look' operations in such patients is generally low [3].

Paradoxically, a single malignancy alone does not confer much increased likelihood of further neoplasms in the patient's remaining lifetime unless there are multiple (three or more) additional adenomas as well as the cancer. Furthermore, their risk – and thus the efficacy of surveillance examinations – is reduced by the fact that the colon has been shortened. Rather than concentrating all resources on the affected patient a more useful exercise – especially in those with multiple neoplasms or in whom the CRC occurred at a young age (under 50 years) – may be to encourage other first-degree relatives to submit for check colonoscopy.

Genetic screening and surveillance

With CRC affecting 1 in 20 of the population it is scarcely surprising that there are a large number of 'worried well' who are fearful of cancer, sometimes demanding the reassurance of colonoscopy. Although overall having a single relative with CRC (index case) increases a related individual's lifetime risk of CRC three-fold, the risk is currently only considered significant if the index case was under 50 years of age or there are two or more first-degree relatives (parents, siblings, children). Having relatives with adenomas, especially if multiple, may be of equal significance (Table 15.1). Current policy for any patient with only a single elderly first-degree relative with CRC is generally to temporize with occult blood testing or a 'one-off' flexible sigmoidoscopy, but it can be difficult to refuse the more accurate modality of colonoscopy when there is anxiety or symptoms (typically dysfunctional and longstanding). Having started such 'surveillance' however, it may be difficult to avoid 3- to 5-yearly follow-up on tenuous grounds, especially if no polyp is found.

The situation will be greatly eased when specific genetic testing becomes available. In the meantime, a careful genetic interview – preferably with a geneticist or trained interviewer – is an essential prerequisite. This is in part due to the potential relevance to colonic sequelae of other somatic abnormalities (skin or bone cysts, etc.) and other non-colonic malignancies (female genital tract, prostate) which can easily be overlooked in a cursory examination, questionnaire or clinic interview. Of prime concern is the existence of families at high risk for colorectal (hereditary non-polyposis colorectal cancer; HNPCC) or other cancers, and exhibiting dominant inheritance characteristics. This diagnosis should be considered whenever there is a single affected relative under 40 years of age or when three or more relatives are affected, especially when in line over several generations. In general, it is considered that in HNPCC families the classic 'adenoma–carcinoma sequence' is followed, but that the rate of conversion from small polyp to cancer may be accelerated. Five-yearly surveillance from the age of 25 to 30 years, reducing the interval to 3-yearly if polyps are found, seems to be a safe practice in most cases. In a few families with younger age onset or multiple cancers it is justifiable to increase follow-up frequency to 1- to 2-yearly.

Polyposis syndromes

Hamartomatous polyposis patients (Peutz–Jeghers syndrome, juvenile) can form surprisingly large polyps relatively fast, and 2-yearly follow-up with removal of any lesion over 2–3 mm is probably appropriate, though malignancy is very uncommon. Metaplastic polyposis is a relatively rare condition where 15–20 metaplastic (hyperplastic) polyps are scattered around the colon proximal to the rectum, sometimes admixed with adenomas. It does (unlike rectal or solitary metaplastic polyps) carry cancer risk, and 3-yearly surveillance is indicated. Adenomatous polyposis (familial adenomatous polyposis; FAP) is usually managed surgically, although the endoscopist may have an important role in diagnosis, in establishing a reasonable date for surgery according to the number and size of polyps, and subsequently in keeping the duodenum and rectum (if any) under review. Rectal malignancy can develop rapidly, and 6-monthly checks are usual. The likelihood of duodenal malignancy is small and 2- to 3-yearly diagnostic

Table 15.1. Summary of risk and screening guidelines for colon cancer in different groups at genetic risk

Life-time risk of death from CRC		Screening strategies
*Average risk	1/50	One-off flexible sigmoidoscopy at 55–60 years
*One first-degree relative > 50 years	1/17	One-off colonoscopy age 55–60 years Annual FOB + flexible sigmoidoscopy 5-yearly from age 50 years Colonoscopy 10-yearly from age 50 years
One first-degree relative < 50 years or Two first-degree relatives any age	1/10	Colonoscopy 5-yearly from age 40, or 10 years before the index case's age
Three first-degree relatives**	1/6	Colonoscopy 5-yearly from age 25 (or 10 years before index case)
Suspected HNPCC**	1/2	Colonoscopy 2-yearly from age 25 years or 5 years before index case

*Currently in the UK, no screening strategy for average-risk individuals or those with a minor family history has been implemented. The author's preferred strategy would be a one-off flexible sigmoidoscopy for average-risk individuals and a one-off colonoscopy for individuals with one first-degree relative.

**These individuals should be referred to a family cancer clinic for genetic assessment.

examinations are probably sufficient, most of the dysplastic areas or polyps being small or flat and too hazardous for conventional endoscopic therapy.

Follow-up after polypectomy

When initial examination has been technically difficult, bowel preparation imperfect, or removal of a large number (five or more) of adenomatous polyps has focused the endoscopist's attention, it is wise to consider an initial follow-up examination at 1 year (and barium enema if total colonoscopy has been impossible). As in the rectum, sessile villous adenomas have a tendency to recur in the longer term, so follow-up is wise at 1- to 2-yearly intervals for the first few years. Tattooing to facilitate early re-check of the site of removal of malignant polyps and larger sessile lesions is discussed in Chapter 16. It has been argued that those having only a single tubular adenoma under 1 cm diameter removed, especially if they are 60–70 years of age, thereafter have lower lifetime colorectal cancer risk than the average population and so may not need follow-up at all [4]. Overall, there is an obligation to offer follow-up after polypectomy, on the basis that up to 50% of patients will be found to have further adenomas long-term, albeit over 90% under 1 cm in size and of uncertain lifetime risk.

With these exceptions, there is general agreement and some positive evidence [5–7] that the interval for first follow-up after polypectomy can be at 3 years. Most endoscopists continue at 3-yearly intervals thereafter, but the first two colonoscopies are those with the highest yield and a case can be made for increasing the interval to 5-yearly once one to two follow-up examinations have been normal [8]. Similarly, there is little likelihood of the 'adenoma–carcinoma sequence' occurring in the remaining lifetime of follow-up patients attaining 75 years of age, who we discharge from follow-up. At any age, however, there is the small possibility of the endoscopist missing a lesion, and a few reported cases where aggressive malignancy appears to have developed fast or apparently 'de novo'. Follow-up patients should therefore be told to make contact, and repeat colonoscopy be considered, if bleeding or any unexpected change of bowel habit occurs.

Inflammatory disease

Small shiny mucosal tags are common after any form of colitis (ulcerative, Crohn's, ischaemic) and have no malignant potential. Polyps of $\geq$ 1 cm diameter should be removed however, both because of their potential for blood or protein loss and because it can be difficult to differentiate a chance adenoma. If a polyp appears difficult or hazardous to remove, a forceps biopsy will show its type.

Only extensive (to the splenic flexure or more) or total colitis appears to give significant long-term risk of malignancy. The risk is established for ulcerative colitis over 8–10 years from onset, even in the absence of recurrent symptoms or activity. Crohn's colitis probably has similar risk. The occurrence of flat dysplasia – difficult and sometimes impossible to visualize in a generally damaged surface – is a worry for the endoscopist, particularly so as more rapid malignant change can occur than in conventional dysplastic polyps. Taking multiple (at least eight to ten) biopsies at intervals around the colon, with extra specimens of any elevated or 'odd-looking' area, is the best that can currently be done – unless the patient is advised and accepts prophylactic colectomy.

Average risk screening

As 20–30% of a Western population will have one or more adenomas by the age of 55–60 years, perhaps with a long (perhaps 5–10 years or longer) probable interval before cancer formation, there is an undoubted opportunity for screening, with intervention by polypectomy when indicated. Mass screening by indirect methods such as occult blood testing has shown some efficacy, but fails to detect up to 40–50% of those with adenomas (and some with CRC). The concept of 'once-only' flexible sigmoidoscopy around the age of 55 years (followed by colonoscopy and polypectomy if there are 'high risk' adenomas 71 cm, 72, villous histology) has been proposed and is the subject of a prospective study in the UK. Flexible sigmoidoscopy has been shown to be acceptable to patients, as it can also be performed competently by nurse endoscopists and so may become a realistic screening approach, including therapy of any smaller lesions present. Some have argued for screening total colonoscopy, on the basis that many patients with proximal cancers have no 'marker' polyps distal to the splenic flexure to be identified on flexible sigmoidoscopy. Very few countries at present have either the endoscopic skills or resources available to contemplate screening colonoscopy. Increasing population awareness of suspicious symptoms, particularly rectal bleeding (especially dark, mixed-in or repeated blood loss), and ensuring the presence of readily available colonoscopy services, is an essential and achievable interim aim until new technology or new teaching methods improve the situation.

PRACTICALITIES OF SCREENING AND SURVEILLANCE METHODS

Faecal occult blood testing

Cancers and large polyps tend to bleed more frequently than normal mucosa, and therefore detection of blood in the stool may provide an early warning of serious pathology. Faecal occult blood (FOB) testing, usually on an annual basis, is simple and cheap and has been proposed as an effective means of population screening. Large, prospective trials have shown a reduction in mortality from CRC, although much of the benefit may be derived from the result of colonoscopy occurring after a positive FOB test [9]. Used alone, FOB has poor sensitivity for neoplasia detection, and many patients with a positive test will undergo unnecessary colonoscopy. In the USA, the standard of practice is to offer annual FOB testing, supplemented by flexible sigmoidoscopy at 5-yearly intervals for average-risk individuals, starting at an age of 50 years [4].

Flexible sigmoidoscopy

Following a phosphate enema to clear the distal bowel, flexible sigmoidoscopy to the sigmoid/descending junction can be performed safely, in unsedated patients, by doctors or trained technicians. Approximately 60% of all colorectal neoplasms are within the reach of the 60-cm flexible sigmoidoscope, making this examination attractive as a possible means of population screening for CRC. A single examination at age 55–60 years to clear the left colon of colonic polyps, with follow-up surveillance colonoscopy, only in those patients with 'high-risk' polyps (villous histology, more than two in number, or >1 cm in size) has been proposed as the most cost-effective means of population screening. A large multicentre trial testing this hypothesis is currently under way [11].

Barium enema

In the author's opinion, barium enema has no place in CRC screening or surveillance programmes, apart from the occasional use to complete technically difficult colonoscopies. Barium enema has a low complication rate, and in experienced hands will detect most colonic cancers. However, it is much less sensitive than colonoscopy in the detection of colonic polyps.

Virtual colonoscopy (CT-colography)

This is a new and evolving technology combining spiral computed tomography (CT) with advanced virtual reality software. CT volume data are reconstructed by a computer to produce a representation of the colon that can be examined from the luminal surface in a fly-through technique which resembles conventional video colonoscopy. Currently, the patient must undergo a full bowel preparation and the colon must be inflated with air before the CT scan. The advantages of virtual colonoscopy are that it is quick, non-invasive and that it images the entire colon and surrounding structures. Currently virtual colonoscopy is less sensitive than conventional colonoscopy for detecting small (<1 cm) polyps [12]. In the future, this technology may become the preferred technique for CRC population screening.

Colonoscopy

The aim of the endoscopist during colonoscopy is to scrutinize as much of the colonic mucosa as possible. Careful observation is particularly important during screening examinations when small polyps may be the only, but nevertheless important, finding. Because of the slight discomfort that may occur during colonoscope insertion and the short duration of action of intravenous analgesia, rapid caecal intubation is desirable, but should be followed by meticulous examination on withdrawal – with time allowed to suction fluid pools and repeatedly examine poorly visualized colonic segments. Irrigation with a simethicone/water mixture may also prove useful to disperse bubbles. Small polyps (<1 cm) seen during the insertion phase are best removed immediately as they may prove difficult to find later in the examination.

Routine premedication with anti-spasmodic (hyoscine *n*-butyl bromide, 10–20 mg; or glucagon, 0.5 mg) helps to reduce colonic contraction and maximize views during insertion and withdrawal. Occasionally, if the insertion has been prolonged, an additional bolus of antispasmodic is required. On withdrawal, optimal views are obtained by gentle insufflation and by maintaining the colonoscope tip in the centre of the lumen. Patient repositioning may also improve views. In general, the caecum and ascending colon are best observed in the left lateral position, the hepatic flexure and transverse colon in the supine position, the splenic flexure and descending colon in the right lateral position, and the sigmoid and rectum with the patient back in the left-lateral position [8]. When an abnormality is detected, additional washing and scope or patient rotation, aid visualization.

RECOGNITION OF PRECANCEROUS LESIONS

Most colonic adenomas are reddish, stalked or sessile polypoid lesions that extend into the bowel lumen (Fig. 15.1). As such they usually prove easy to detect, but recently there has been considerable interest in less clearly defined, flat or depressed colonic adenomas. These so-called 'flat adenomas' were first described in Japanese

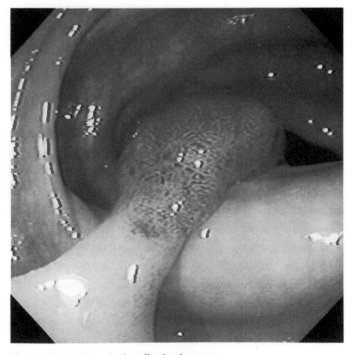

Figure 15.1. A typical stalked adenoma.

patients [13], and recent studies have confirmed their presence in the Western colon [14,15]. Flat adenomas may have a higher incidence of severe dysplasia [8], and although they probably account for (at most) 12% of all colonic neoplasia [14], they may represent an accelerated pathway towards carcinogenesis. Indeed, small, flat (3–10 mm), endoscopically resectable carcinomas have been described [16]. Macroscopically, flat adenomas may appear as reddish, flat or slightly elevated lesions often with a central depression, and may become more visible after suctioning air to decompress the bowel wall [13]. Flat or slightly raised lesions are often better defined by dye-spray techniques (Fig. 15.2). Indigo carmine (0.2–0.8%) is the most commonly used dye and can be injected directly down the biopsy channel or sprayed over the colonic surface using specially designed dye-spray catheters. Attempts have even been made to stain the entire colonic surface using a slow-release capsule containing indigo carmine (100 mg) taken with the bowel preparation [17]. Indigo carmine highlights tissue topography by pooling in epithelial crevices and depressions. It defines the edge of flat or depressed lesions and therefore aids detection and helps guide completeness of resection. Recently, there has been much interest in the use of dye-spray in combination with a magnifying colonoscope (Figs 15.3, 15.4) or high-resolution (410 000 versus 180 000 pixels) video systems, to distinguish hyperplastic (pitted surface pattern) from adenomatous ('sulcal' pattern) polyps (Fig. 15.5). Preliminary results suggest a high level of accuracy for polyp differentiation [18], and these new technologies may become standard for screening examinations to maximize the detection of adenomas and reduce the additional morbidity caused by unnecessary resection of hyperplastic polyps.

Marking and identifying colonic lesions

Tattooing with India ink is the preferred method to facilitate intraoperative [19] or repeat colonoscopic localization of small cancers or suspicious polyps (Fig. 15.6) [20]. Autoclaved India ink, diluted to 1/10 concentration, can be injected, via a stiff variceal injection needle, submucosally, adjacent to the site of the lesion. A single 0.5-ml injection is sufficient for endoscopic recognition, but if surgery is likely then four (0.5–1 ml) injections in each quadrant of the colon ensure easy visualization from

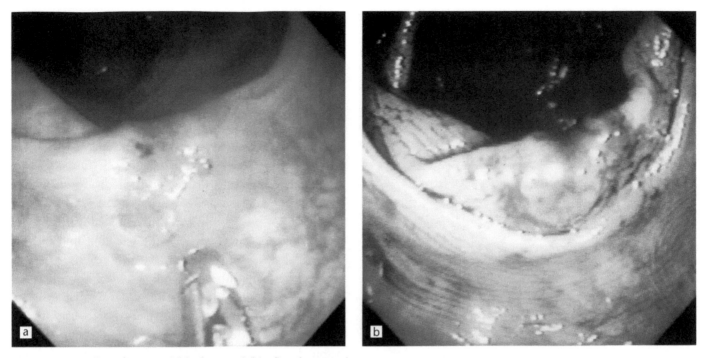

Figure 15.2. A flat adenoma (a) before and (b) after dye-spraying.

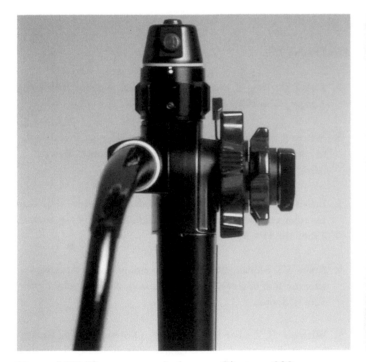

Figure 15.3. The zoom control on an Olympus 100 × magnifying colonoscope.

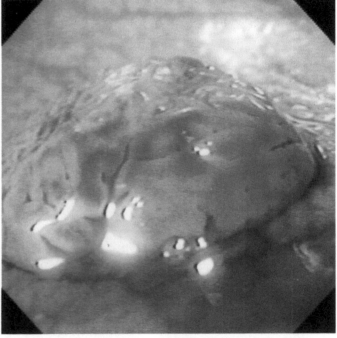

Figure 15.4. Surface appearance of an adenomatous polyp using magnification and dye-spray (note the sulcal pattern).

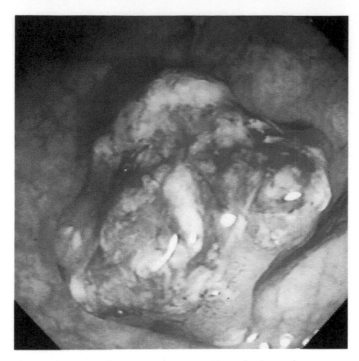

Figure 15.5. A 1.2-cm rectal cancer. Note the irregular, ulcerated surface. This lesion felt fixed on palpation and was not suitable for endoscopic resection. Histology after resection confirmed muscle invasion.

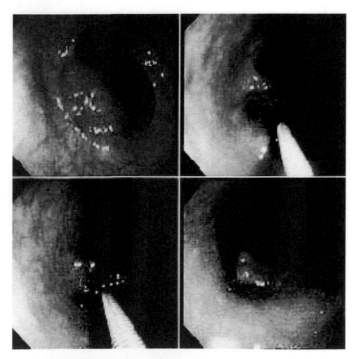

Figure 15.6. A methylene blue/saline mixture has been injected alongside this sessile lesion. It fails to lift (non-lifting sign), confirming malignant invasion. Endoscopic resection is not advisable.

the serosal surface at laparotomy. In order to avoid spilling ink within the colon or peritoneal cavity, we prefer to raise a 1- to 2-ml submucosal saline bleb to define the submucosal space, before ink injection. India ink tattoos appear to be permanent and can be placed without significant side effects [21]. Metal clips attached to the mucosa have also been used to mark colonic lesions, but have the disadvantage that they tend to fall off if left *in situ* for more than a few days [22]. Tattooing is of particular relevance in management of the 5% of polyps found to contain invasive malignancy, most of which prove to be well- or moderately-well differentiated histologically, with at least 2–3 mm between the resection line and the margin of invasion – which are the criteria generally accepted as permitting conservative non-operative management [23]. If the histological diagnosis of malignancy comes as a surprise it is necessary to re-endoscope for tattooing purposes within about 10 days before the ulcerated polypectomy site heals over, sometimes invisibly.

REFERENCES

1. Parker SL, Tong T, Bolden S *et al.* Cancer Statistics, 1996. *CA Cancer J Clin* 1996; 65: 5–27.

2. Winawer SJ, Zauber AG, May Nah Ho MS *et al.* Prevention of colorectal cancer by colonoscopic polypectomy. *N Eng J Med* 1993; 329 : 1977–1981.

3. Ballantyne GH, Modlin IM. Editorial: Postoperative follow-up for colorectal cancer: who are we kidding? *J Clin Gastroenterol* 1988; 10: 359–364.

4. Atkin WS, Morson BC. Long-term risk of colorectal cancer after excision of rectosigmoid adenomas. *N Engl J Med* 1992; 326: 658–662.

5. Winawer SJ, Zanber AG, Stewart E, O'Brien MJ. The natural history of colorectal cancer. *Cancer* 1991; 67: 1143–1149.

6. Bond JH. Polyp guideline: diagnosis, treatment and surveillance for patients with nonfamilial colorectal polyps. *Ann Intern Med* 1993; 119: 836–843.

7. Winawer SJ, St John DJB, Bond JH *et al.* Prevention of colorectal cancer: guidelines based on new data. *WHO Bulletin* 1995; 73: 7–10.

8. Cotton PB, Williams CB. *Practical Gastrointestinal Endoscopy.* Blackwell Scientific, London, 1996.

9. Mandel JS, Bond JH, Church TR *et al.* Reducing mortality for colorectal cancer by screening for fecal occult blood. *N Eng J Med* 1993; 328: 1365–1371.

10. Winawer SJ, Fletcher RH, Miller L *et al.* Colorectal cancer screening: clinical guidelines and rationale. *Gastroenterology* 1997; 112: 594–642.

11. Atkin WS, Cuzak J, Northover JMA, Whynes DK. Prevention of colorectal cancer by once-only flexible sigmoidoscopy. *Lancet* 1993; 341: 736–740.

12. Hara AK, Johnson CD, Reed JE *et al.* Detection of colonic polyps with CT-colography: initial assessment of sensitivity and specificity. *Radiology* 1997; 205: 59–65.

13. Muto T, Kamiya J, Sawada T *et al.* Small 'flat adenoma' of the large bowel with specific reference to its clinico-pathologic features. *Dis Colon Rectum* 1985; 28: 847–851.

14. Jaramillo E, Watanabe M, Sklezak P, Rubio C. Flat neoplastic lesions of the colon and rectum detected by high resolution video endoscopy and chromoscopy. *Gastrointest Endosc* 1995; 42: 114–122.

15. Lanspa SJ, Rouse J, Smyrk T *et al.* Epidemiologic characteristics of the flat adenoma of Muto: a prospective study. *Dis Colon Rectum* 1992, 35: 543–546.

16. Tada S, Iida M, Matsumoyo T *et al.* Small flat cancer of the rectum: clinicopathological and endoscopic features. *Gastrointest Endosc* 1995; 42: 109–113.

17. Mitooka H, Fujimori T, Maeda S *et al.* Minute flat depressed neoplastic lesions of the colon detected by contrast chromoscopy using an indigo carmine capsule. *Gastrointest Endosc* 1995; 41: 453–459.

18. Axelrad AM, Fleischer DE, Geller AJ *et al.* High-resolution chromoendoscopy for the diagnosis of diminutive colorectal polyps: implications for colon cancer screening. *Gastroenterology* 1996; 110: 1253–1258.

19. Hyman N, Waye JD. Endoscopic four quadrant tattoo for the identification of colonic lesions at surgery. *Gastrointest Endosc* 1991; 37: 56–58.

20. Shatz BA, Thavorides V. Colonic tattoo for follow-up of endoscopic sessile polypectomy. *Gastrointest Endosc* 1991; 37: 59–60.

21. Lightdale CJ. India ink colonic tattoo: blots on the record. *Gastrointest Endosc* 1991; 37: 99–100.

22. Lehman GA, Maveety PR, O'Connor KW. Mucosal clipping: utility and safety testing in the colon. *Gastrointest Endosc* 1985; 31: 273–276.

23. Cooper HS, Deppisch LM. Gourley WK *et al.* Endoscopically removed malignant colorectal polyps: clinico-pathological correlations. *Gastroenterology* 1995; 108: 1657–1665.

16 Colon cancer prevention

C.B. Williams

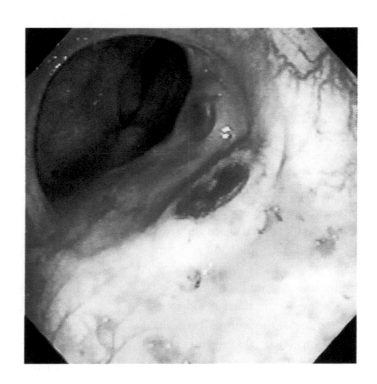

INTRODUCTION

As discussed in Chapter 15, the prevention of colorectal cancer (CRC) is based on the premise of a polyp–cancer sequence, and the assumption that the removal of polyps will prevent cancer. This assumption also underlies the basis of screening all groups at risk of developing CRC. Here, we concentrate on what should be done when precancerous lesions are seen at endoscopy.

ENDOSCOPIC RESECTION OR SURGERY?

When a lesion is seen at colonoscopy a decision must be made regarding the feasibility of endoscopic resection. Almost all stalked polyps are amenable to snare resection, but the decision can be more difficult for sessile lesions which may or may not be malignant. Endoscopic ultrasound with a 20-MHz miniprobe passed through the biopsy channel can define the layers of the colonic wall and assess invasion [1]; however, this modality is not widely available and often the endoscopist must rely upon the look and feel of the lesion in assessing endoscopic resectability. Any lesion that is ulcerated, irregular or feels hard and fixed to the underlying muscle layer during palpation with the biopsy forceps is probably not suitable for endoscopic resection. Another useful indicator of invasion is to inject saline submucosally (see below) into normal, adjacent mucosa and observe whether or not the lesion lifts on the saline cushion. Sessile lesions that fail to lift after submucosal saline injection (non-lifting sign) [2] are likely to be malignant and endoscopic resection should not be attempted.

There are no strict limits regarding the size of polyp that can be endoscopically resected, and much will depend upon the position and relative ease of endoscopic access. As a general rule of thumb however, few polyps greater than one-third the circumference of the colonic lumen or that pass over two haustral folds are manageable endoscopically [3]. If endoscopic resection is feasible but the polyp is large or positioned awkwardly, referral for a second endoscopy performed by an expert may be the most appropriate course of action. It should also be borne in mind that sessile polyps in the mid and distal rectum are accessible to the surgeon and transanal dissection under direct vision may be more appropriate.

SAFETY ISSUES BEFORE POLYPECTOMY

Bowel preparation

Adequate bowel preparation is necessary before polypectomy, partly to ensure visualization but also in order to remove potentially explosive hydrogen and methane gas [4]. If a polyp is seen in a poorly prepared bowel a repeat examination after further cleansing is often the safest course. If polypectomy is attempted, care should be taken to exchange the colonic gas several times before electrocoagulation. Build-up of potentially explosive gases may be a particular problem following mannitol preparation due to fermentation of the sugar by colonic bacteria into hydrogen. Use of carbon dioxide (which does not support combustion) rather than air as the insufflating gas removes the risk of explosion during diathermy, and its use is mandatory following mannitol preparation [5].

Anticoagulants

Aspirin reduces platelet stickiness and results in an increased risk of post-polypectomy bleeding. The drug is therefore best stopped for 7–10 days before, and 10 days after polypectomy. Patients taking warfarin for 'low-risk' indications (atrial fibrillation, venous thrombosis) are usually safe to stop the drug 4 days before polypectomy, allowing enough time for the INR to normalize, and then to restart it soon after the procedure. Those patients taking warfarin for 'high-risk' reasons (prosthetic heart valves, recent vascular graft) require hospitalization before polypectomy for formal conversion to heparin, which can then be stopped, 4 hours before the examination, and restarted soon afterwards [6].

Antibiotic prophylaxis

Although the incidence of transient bacteraemia during routine colonoscopy is approximately 4%, and may be higher following polypectomy, it appears to be without clinical significance in normal individuals [7]. Antibiotic prophylaxis is indicated for patients at high risk of endocarditis (prosthetic heart valves, previous endocarditis, recent vascular grafts) and for those with severe immunosuppression where symptomatic bacteraemia is more likely.

Checking the equipment

Before carrying out snare polypectomy it is important to check that the snare handle moves freely and that it opens sufficiently to take a 2- to 3-cm polyp head. A mark using an indelible pen should be placed on the snare handle corresponding to the point of complete snare closure into the catheter, thus preventing the endoscopy assistant from closing the snare too far and cheese-wiring through the polyp stalk. In addition, the snare loop should close at least 15 mm into the catheter so that the snare can still tighten completely, even allowing for some crumpling of the plastic catheter during diathermy. The patient return plate should be secured to the thigh and the circuit and power settings checked. Almost all polypectomies can be achieved with low power settings (15–20 W) and coagulating current is preferred to encourage adequate dessication of blood vessels within the polyp stalk [8].

PRACTICAL ASPECTS

Colonoscopic snare resection of stalked polyps was first described in the early 1970s by Deyhle *et al.* [9] in Europe and by Wolff and Shinya [10] in America, and 'hot biopsy' for the destruction of diminutive polyps by Williams in 1973 [11]. These basic techniques have changed very little over the years and polypectomy has become a routine and invaluable part of diagnostic colonoscopy. Recently, several new developments have improved detection of colonic neoplasia and facilitated the endoscopic resection of larger, sessile polyps and even early cancers.

Small polyps

Small polyps under 5 mm in diameter comprise over 90% of polyps encountered in the colon, and usually prove histologically to be adenomatous [12]. Without magnification or high-resolution, the endoscopist usually cannot predict on visual grounds which small polyp will be an adenoma, as opposed to a non-neoplastic hyperplastic polyp which might be ignored [12]. Therefore, resection of all polyps is the only way of ensuring a 'clean colon', the exception being the often multiple, tiny, rectal hyperplastic polyps, where one or two cold biopsies are sufficient to confirm histology.

When removing small polyps at colonoscopy there are a variety of options, including hot biopsy, mini-snare, cold snare, bipolar forceps and the argon beamer. The latter two methods destroy all polyp tissue and do not provide histology, which limits their use (see below).

Hot biopsy removal

Provided that good technique is rigorously applied, hot biopsy – in the author's opinion – remains the first-line method for the removal of diminutive (2–4 mm) polyps. The technique of hot biopsy involves grasping the polyp with the insulated hot biopsy forceps, tenting up the underlying mucosa, and then electrocoagulating the pseudo polyp-stalk to cause visible whitening; the so-called 'Mount Fuji effect' (Fig. 16.1) [8]. Heating is maximal in the pseudo-stalk because this is the narrowest point between the flow of current from the forceps to the patient return plate (monopolar); moreover, the polyp grasped in the jaws of the forceps is protected from heating. Once adequate diathermy has been applied – usually 1–2 seconds of low-power (15 W) coagulating current – the biopsy can be pulled off and retrieved for histology. The remaining polyp will slough off as the mucosa ulcerates at the site of hot biopsy (Fig. 16.2). Small polyps are easy to target with the

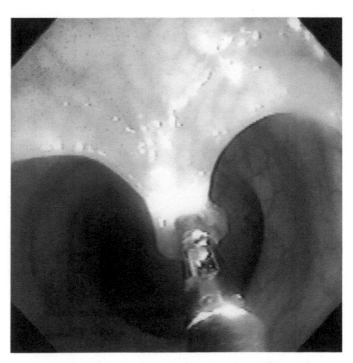

Figure 16.1. Hot biopsy technique. Note the visible whitening (destruction) of the tissue beneath the polyp – the 'Mount Fuji effect'.

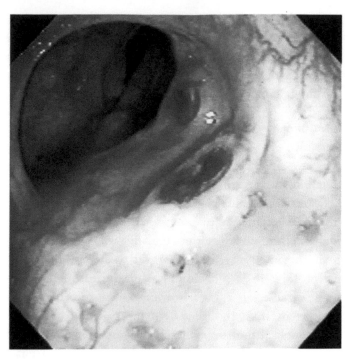

Figure 16.2. Appearance of the polyp approximately 15 min after hot biopsy. Note the ulceration and extent of tissue injury.

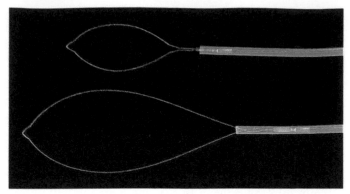

Figure 16.3. A mini snare (2 cm diameter) alongside a conventional (5 cm) snare.

hot biopsy forceps, making it a quick and easily applied technique. Hot biopsy is not suitable for polyps over 5 mm in size as the degree of heating required fully to remove these larger lesions may risk full-thickness burns in the proximal colon, or deep ulceration predisposing to delayed haemorrhage. Conversely, undercoagulation of larger lesions may leave residual polyp tissue [13]. Some authors have suggested that hot biopsy results in a higher incidence of delayed haemorrhage [14], particularly when applied in the right colon and when the patient has recently taken aspirin. A higher than expected incidence of bleeding following hot biopsy was not however seen in a large series of 1730 polypectomies [15].

Snare polypectomy
Alternative approaches include use of mini snares and cold snare mechanical strangulation. Conventional snares are 5–6 cm in length and can prove difficult to manipulate when tackling small polyps, particularly at tight bends when full extension and opening of the snare tends to lose position. Mini snares 2–3 cm in length (Fig. 16.3) are easier to control and can be placed accurately around the polyp base [16]. The strangulated polyp is then lifted away from the colonic wall and diathermy used to cut through the polyp base. Even with mini snares, snaring very small

polyps may prove difficult and time-consuming, and therefore hot biopsy is often preferred.

An alternative for diminutive polyps is the cold snare technique. Here, the snare is closed tightly around the base of the polyp to cheese-wire through the underlying mucosa [17]. The cold snare technique is unlikely to be complicated by delayed, secondary haemorrhage; however, due to the lack of cautery there is an inevitable, slightly increased risk of immediate haemorrhage which may slow the examination as the endoscopist waits to observe for bleeding after each polypectomy.

Polyp retrieval
Retrieval of small polyps after cold or hot snaring may prove troublesome and inevitably some polyps may be lost – another potent argument in favour of hot biopsy where histology is practically ensured. Commercially available suction traps (Endodynamics Inc., Westbury, New York) are most useful for small polyp retrieval following snare resection. Each polyp is suctioned back through the colonoscope and caught in one of four numbered compartments. An alternative is the use of single-chamber 'sputum traps'; however, if overfilled these allow polyp fragments to wash out through the exit tubing and need to be changed if multiple polyps at different sites are encountered.

Large stalked polyps

Large stalked polyps require conventional 5–6 cm oval or hexagonal snares for resection. Manipulating the snare over the polyp head may prove difficult, particularly if the polyp lies at one of the flexures. Changes in patient position may improve the view, and endoscope rotation will bring the

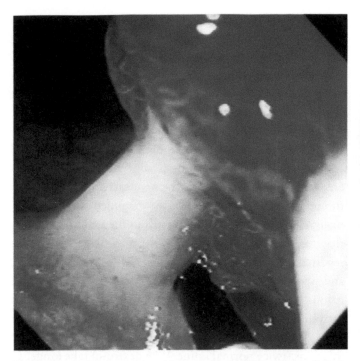

Figure 16.4. A long, variceal injection needle is used to inject 1 : 10 000 adrenaline into a large stalked polyp before to snare resection.

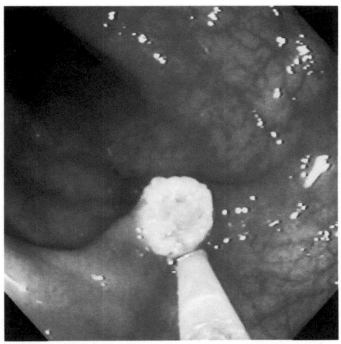

Figure 16.5. A nylon endo-loop is closed over the polyp stalk after snare resection.

polyp into the correct, 5 o'clock axis (opposite the biopsy channel) for polypectomy. If the polyp stalk is broad, then it is likely to contain large central blood vessels and there is a correspondingly increased risk of bleeding. Injection with adrenaline (1 : 10 000) into the polyp stalk before diathermy (Fig. 16.4), or the use of a commercially available nylon endo-loop (Olympus Optical Corporation, Tokyo) (Fig. 16.5), may help to prevent bleeding.

Lassoo snare polypectomy

Once the polyp head has been lassooed, the snare should be closed around the mid part of the stalk; too close to the head risks incomplete resection, particularly if the polyp contains a focus of malignancy, while too close to the base risks serosal damage during diathermy. Low-power (15–20 W) coagulating current is used with gradual closing of the snare. It is important to cut through the polyp stalk slowly, giving adequate time for the central, blood vessel-containing part of the stalk to coagulate, thus avoiding immediate haemorrhage. Once the polyp head has been severed it can be retrieved using the snare, baskets, specialized tripod grasping forceps, or simply by sucking the polyp to the tip of the colonoscope and maintaining suction during withdrawal. We prefer to retrieve large polyps

with the snare, not only because it provides a better grip when traversing the anal canal, but also so that the polyp can be held away from the colonoscope tip on withdrawal, thereby allowing a complete examination and avoiding the need to repass the colonoscope.

Large sessile polyps

Possibly the greatest challenge to the endoscopist is the safe and complete removal of large, sessile colonic polyps. In the relatively thin-walled, right colon, the endoscopic approach requires considerable skill and should not be attempted by the inexperienced. Sessile lesions up to 1 cm can be safely resected in one piece, and up to 2 cm if submucosal injection is employed (see below); however, larger polyps should be removed piecemeal. Fragments from a piecemeal polypectomy can be retrieved via a suction trap and larger, basal pieces can be withdrawn after regrasping with the snare. If there are multiple large fragments, commercially available retrieval nets (Roth, United States Endoscopy Group Inc., Ohio, USA) can be employed (Fig. 16.6). A wire 'snare loop' attached to the net is repeatedly opened and closed over the polyp fragments, forcing them into the netting basket. This is then withdrawn with the colonoscope.

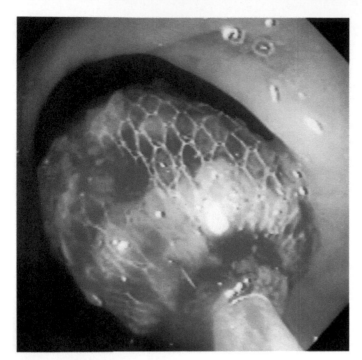

Figure 16.6. The Roth retrieval net is used to gather up multiple fragments following piecemeal polypectomy.

Saline injection techniques and submucosal polypectomy

Recently, submucosal saline injection before polypectomy has made excision of large sessile polyps technically easier, and probably both safer and more frequently complete [18]. The colonic submucosa is the only layer in the colonic wall to contain loose areolar tissue. This property means that when fluid is injected in the correct plane, the muscle layer is separated from the mucosa by a 2- to 3-mm protective fluid cushion. The mucosa can then be 'stripped' from the muscle by current from a polypectomy snare, the fluid cushion preventing deep thermal burning and damage to the serosal surface. The terms 'strip biopsy' and submucosal injection polypectomy have been coined to describe this technique.

Submucosal injection polypectomy was first described in 1971 by Dehyle *et al.* [9], but has been developed in recent years by Japanese endoscopists, particularly for resection of flat adenomas and early carcinomas [19–21]. The technique is useful for sessile lesions of all sizes. A long, sclerotherapy needle is used for the injection, and it is important that it has a stiff outer sheath that can traverse the full length of the colonoscope without crumpling. Once in position the needle is extended from its sheath and

passed tangentially into the colonic wall. The first injection should be proximal to the lesion in order to lift it towards the colonoscope without obscuring the view, as can happen if the distal part is elevated first. If injection fails to produce an immediate bleb, then the needle may have passed right through the bowel wall. Injection of sterile saline into the peritoneal cavity does not appear to be of any significance, but the needle should be immediately withdrawn and injection repeated more superficially. Multiple injections are often required and it may be necessary to inject directly through the lesion. This is best avoided in obviously malignant lesions. There is no limit to the amount of saline that can be used and volumes of up to 56 ml have been reported [22]. Saline tends to dissipate within a few minutes, and therefore repeat injections – particularly for large lesions – may be necessary. Adrenaline plus saline has been used in an attempt to prevent haemorrhage, although there is no clear evidence of benefit over saline [23]. Hypertonic solutions (twice normal saline/10% dextrose) take longer to dissipate and may be advantageous, particularly when tackling a large polyp where polypectomy is likely to be prolonged.

After submucosal injection, polyps of up to 2 cm in size can be resected safely in one piece (Fig. 16.7), while larger polyps are best removed piecemeal. Standard, 3 cm diameter, oval or hexagonal polypectomy snares are usually adequate, but have a tendency to slip over the saline mound as the snare is closed. This problem has led to the development of modified snares with tiny barbs, positioned at regular intervals around the snare loop, designed to add grip. A further modification is the inclusion of a small spike at the tip of the snare which is dug into the mucosa proximal to the polyp, allowing wide opening of the snare around the polyp as the snare is advanced. Kanamori *et al.* have suggested using a needle-knife to cut circumferentially into the mucosa around the polyp in order to produce a groove to seat the opened snare prior to resection [22]. The incision also acts as a mark of total excision.

Once the snare has been positioned, resection proceeds as usual, using standard (15 W, coagulating current) diathermy settings. Occasionally increased power settings are appropriate, particularly when resecting sessile lesions in the very thin-walled caecum, where a more rapid cut guards against the possibility of heat penetration to the serosal surface. With submucosal injection polypectomy, larger individual pieces can be resected (1–2 cm) and it is possible to retrieve all segments of the polyp, which can then be pieced together and pinned out on a cork block, confirming total excision and facilitating subsequent histological assessment.

Non-contact, thermal destruction
For several years lasers (Nd-YAG) have been used for tissue destruction under direct vision at colonoscopy, and have proved useful for debulking stenosing colon cancers [24]

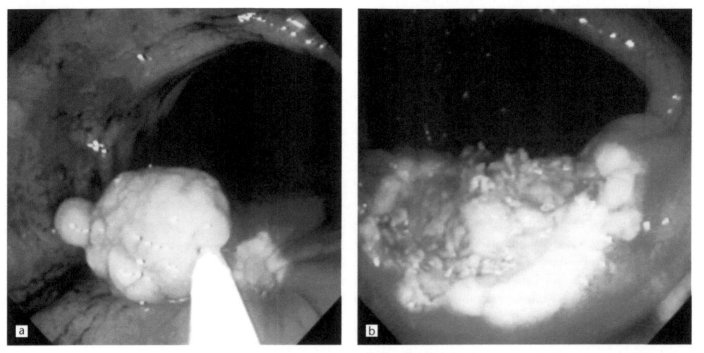

Figure 16.7. Saline injection, snare polypectomy of a 2 cm sessile polyp in one piece. (a) Before resection; (b) polypectomy base after resection.

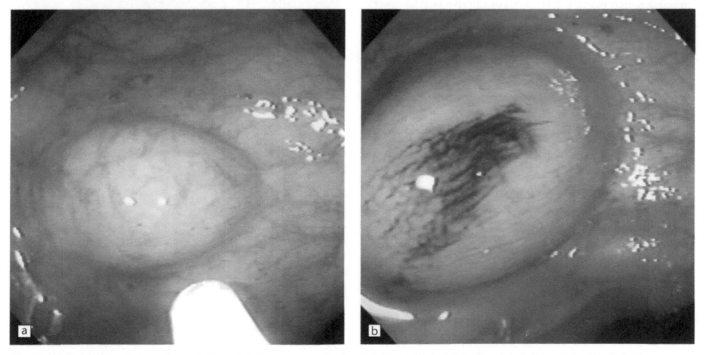

Figure 16.8. Method for placing a tattoo: (a) A submucosal saline bleb is raised; (b) India ink is injected directly into the submucosal space.

and ablating sessile polyps [25]. Lasers however have some inherent disadvantages in that they are expensive and the depth of tissue destruction may be difficult to control.

Recently, a new method of thermal ablation has been developed – the argon beamer – which has the advantages of being cheap, portable, easy to use and provides controlled tissue destruction [26]. Argon plasma coagulation (APC) is a mono-polar, high-frequency technique in which ionized and thus electrically conductive argon (argon plasma) is generated. The system essentially consists of a wire-containing catheter connected to a diathermy unit and an argon gas cylinder. The catheter is passed down the colonoscope and directed to within a few millimetres of the tissue to be coagulated. Just inside the catheter tip is a wire electrode which, when activated, transmits high frequency currrent (65 W) towards the colonic surface. As the electrode is fired, argon gas flowing around the electrode becomes electrically charged, allowing a spark of high-frequency current to flow from the electrode onto adjacent colonic mucosa; this generates heat and causes tissue destruction (Fig. 16.9). The depth of penetration is limited to approximately 3 mm and remains uniform, even when applied over a wide area. This is because, as soon as the colonic surface loses its electrical conductivity as a result of desiccation, the plasma stream automatically redirects itself to the nearest area of normal mucosa which is still electrically conductive (see Chapters 4 and 17).

Intraluminal argon gas tends to build up rapidly with repeat applications causing distension and therefore frequent withdrawal of the catheter to allow suction of gas is mandatory. Complete ablation of sessile polyps is made considerably easier with APC. Often, during snare resection of sessile lesions, small areas of tissue remain at the periphery of the lesion. These are easily targeted and destroyed with APC (Fig. 16.10) [27]. APC should not be used to ablate the entire lesion as it does not provide the opportunity for histology. Occasionally however histology is unimportant and the ability for rapid targeting and multiple applications makes APC the destructive method of choice, such as when fulgurating the many tiny rectal polyps in patients with familial adenomatous polyposis and an ileorectal anastomosis. In the author's experience 40–50 polyps can be targeted and destroyed in about 10 min. APC has also been used to fulgurate colonic tumours. The limited tissue penetration makes it less effective than laser in recanalizing malignant strictures; however, it can be usefully applied to the surface of bleeding lesions and can be used to treat tumour ingrowth through metal stents [28].

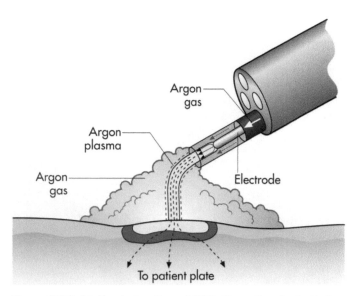

Figure 16.9. Method of action of APC. Once the electrode is activated, argon plasma sparks towards the colonic wall, directing current from the electrode to diathermy the mucosal surface.

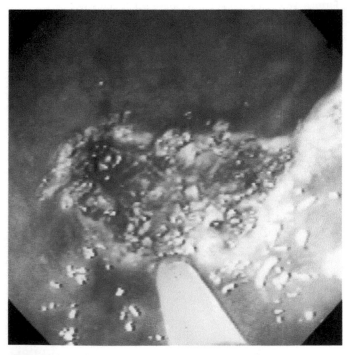

Figure 16.10. Following piecemeal resection of a sessile polyp, the argon beamer is used to diathermy the polypectomy site, preventing bleeding and ensuring that all remaining polyp fragments are destroyed.

COMPLICATIONS

Early bleeding

Bleeding is the most common major complication and may be immediate or delayed for up to 14 days after polypectomy. Minor, immediate oozing from the polypectomy site is relatively common and usually stops spontaneously within a few minutes. If it continues, irrigation of the polypectomy site with water or a dilute adrenaline/saline (5 ml of 1 : 10 000 adrenaline with 50 ml saline) mixture is often sufficient to encourage haemostasis. Continued bleeding can be stopped by adrenaline (1 : 10 000) injection at the polypectomy site, in much the same way as for the treatment of a bleeding peptic ulcer, or by repeat cautery. In our experience, the heater probe and argon beamer are both quick and effective methods for cauterizing the polypectomy base; hot biopsy forceps can also be used, but tend to produce deeper coagulation (rather than the surface charring of the heater probe or beamer) which, although effective in the acute situation, may increase the subsequent risk of secondary haemorrhage. Dramatic spurting from a severed arteriole mainly occurs after inadequate coagulation of a thick-stalked polyp. If it occurs, rapidly re-snaring the stalk and applying mechanical tamponade for several minutes is often sufficient to stop the bleeding. Adrenaline injection or application of a metal clip or a constricting nylon 'Endoloop' (see above) may also prove effective.

Late bleeding

Delayed or secondary haemorrhage occurs as a result of sloughing of destroyed tissue at the polypectomy site and exposure of an underlying vessel. The patient presents with the frequent, and often urgent, passage of clots and altered blood per rectum. Most secondary haemorrhages stop spontaneously, but hospitalization for observation (and occasionally transfusion) is an essential precaution. Should haemorrhage continue, localization of the bleeding site can be achieved by repeat endoscopy, red cell scanning or angiography. Endoscopic therapy or selective infusion of vasopressin [29] at angiography are often sufficient to stop bleeding, although very occasionally laparotomy and segmental resection is necessary.

Pain

Post-polypectomy syndrome is due to a full-thickness burn at the polypectomy site causing serosal irritation and localized peritonitis. The patient complains of pain and tenderness over the polypectomy site and may have a mild fever associated with a leukocytosis. Symptoms usually resolve with conservative treatment (close observation, bed rest and parenteral antibiotics); however, persistent or worsening symptoms may necessitate laparotomy, so surgeon and endoscopist should consult closely.

Perforation

Perforation is more likely when resecting large sessile polyps, particularly in the relatively thin-walled right colon. It may be immediately apparent with direct visualization of the peritoneal cavity, but presentation with abdominal pain, peritonism and free gas on a plain abdominal film may be delayed for up to 2 weeks. If the patient's condition remains stable and the bowel preparation was good, the likelihood of heavy faecal contamination of the peritoneal cavity is small and conservative treatment can be instituted with close observation, nil-by-mouth, intravenous fluids and parenteral antibiotics [30]. Most large perforations however will require immediate surgery to oversew the defect and prevent faecal peritonitis.

Complication rates

It is difficult to assess the true complication rate for colonoscopic polypectomy as most reported series come from specialist units whose results are invariably skewed by complicated patients referred from others. Waye *et al.* [15] in a personal account of 777 patients with 1730 polyps of all sizes, reported minor immediate bleeding in 1.4% of polypectomies and delayed haemorrhage in 2% at 1–12 days. Post-polypectomy syndrome occurred in 1% of cases, with delayed perforations (1 and 9 days) in only 0.3%. The overall therapeutic complication rate was therefore 3.4%, but only 2% of patients required hospitalization. A German study [31] of 30 000 colonoscopies reported that the perforation rate for therapeutic colonoscopy was 0.83% and that in their authors' experience 25% of bleeding complications could be managed conservatively, whereas over

25% of perforations or full-thickness burns after polypectomy were submitted to surgery. A recent comprehensive review of the complications of colonoscopy [32] comments that recent series show a lowering of the complication rate for both diagnostic and therapeutic (0.4%) colonoscopy.

REFERENCES

1. Saitoh Y, Obara T, Einami K *et al.* Efficacy of high-frequency ultrasound probes for the preoperative staging of invasion depth in flat and depressed colorectal tumours. *Gastrointest Endosc* 1996; 44: 34–39.

2. Uno Y, Munakata A. The non-lifting sign of invasive colon cancer. *Gastrointest Endosc* 1994; 40: 485–489.

3. Waye JD. How big is too big? *Gastrointest Endosc* 1996; 43: 256–257.

4. Bigard MA, Gaucher P, Lassaile C. Fatal colonic explosion during colonoscopic polypectomy. *Gastroenterology* 1979; 77: 1307–1310.

5. Taylor EW, Bentley S, Youngs D *et al.* Bowel preparation and the safety of colonoscopic polypectomy. *Gastroenterology* 1981; 81: 1–4.

6. *Patients undergoing endoscopy taking anticoagulants.* British Society of Gastroenterology Guidelines, September 1996.

7. *Antibiotic prophylaxis in gastrointestinal endoscopy.* British Society of Gastroenterology Guidelines, September 1996.

8. Cotton PB, Williams CB. *Practical Gastrointestinal Endoscopy.* Blackwell Scientific, London, 1996.

9. Deyhle P, Seuberth K, Jenny S, Demling L. Endoscopic polypectomy in the proximal colon. *Endoscopy* 1971; 3: 103–115.

10. Wolff WI, Shinya H. A new approach to colonic polyps. *Ann Surg* 1973; 178: 367–378.

11. Williams CB. Diathermic biopsy: a technique for the endoscopic management of small polyps. *Endoscopy* 1973; 5: 215–218.

12. Church JM, Fazio VW, Jones IT. Small colorectal polyps: are they worth treating? *Dis Col Rectum* 1988; 31: 50–53.

13. Williams CB. Small polyps – the virtues and dangers of hot biopsy. *Gastrointest Endosc* 1991; 37: 394–395.

14. Dyer WS, Quigley EMM, Noel SM *et al.* Case Report. Major colonic haemorrhage following electrocoagulating (hot) biopsy of diminutive colonic polyps: relationship to colonic location and low-dose aspirin therapy. *Gastrointest Endosc* 1991; 37: 361–364.

15. Waye JD, Lewis BS, Yessayan S. Colonoscopy: a prospective report of complications. *J Clin Gastroenterol* 1992; 15: 1–4.

16. McAfee JH, Katon RM. Tiny snares prove safe and effective for removal of diminutive polyps. *Gastrointest Endosc* 1994; 40: 301–303.

17. Tappero G, Gaja E, Degiuli P *et al.* Cold snare excision of small colorectal polyps. *Gastrointest Endosc* 1992; 38: 310–313.

18. Waye JD. Saline injection colonoscopic polypectomy. *Am J Gastroenterol* 1992; 89: 305–306.

19. Karita M Cantero D, Okita K. Endoscopic diagnosis and resection treatment of flat adenoma with severe dysplasia. *Am J Gastroenterol* 1993; 88: 1421–1423.

20. Karita M, Tada M, Okita K *et al.* Endoscopic therapy for early colon cancer: the strip biopsy resection technique. *Gastrointest Endosc* 1991; 37: 128–132.

21. Karita M Tada M, Okita K. The successive strip biopsy, partial resection technique for large early gastric and colonic cancers. *Gastrointest Endosc* 1992; 38: 174–178.

22. Kanamori T, Itoh M, Yokoyama Y, Tsuchida K. Injection-incision-assisted snare resection of large sessile colorectal polyps. *Gastrointest Endosc* 1996; 43: 189–195.

23. Shirai M, Nakamura T, Matsuura A *et al.* Safer colonoscopic polypectomy with local injection of hypertonic saline-epinephrine solution. *Am J Gastroenterol* 1994; 89: 334–338.

24. Arrigoni A, Pennazio M, Spandre M, Rossini FP. Emergency endoscopy: recanalisation of intestinal obstruction caused by colorectal cancer. *Gastrointest Endosc* 1995; 40: 553–556.

25. Mathus-Vliegen EMH, Tytgat GNJ. The potential and limitations of laser photoablation of colorectal adenomas. *Gastrointest Endosc* 1991; 37: 9–17.

26. Farin G, Grund KR. Technology of argon plasma coagulation with particular regard to endoscopic applications. *Endoscopy* 1995; 2: 71–77.

27. Grund KE, Storek D, Farin G. Endoscopic argon plasma coagulation (APC) first clinical experiences in flexible

endoscopy. *Endoscopic Surgery and Allied Technologies* 1994; 2: 42–46.

28. Grund KE, Farin G. New principles and applications of high-frequency surgery, including argon plasma coagulation. In: Cotton PB, Tytgat GNJ, Williams CB, Bowling TE (eds), *Annual of Gastrointestinal Endoscopy*, 10th edn, London: Rapid Science, 1997, 15–24.

29. Gibbs DH, Opelka FG, Beck DE *et al*. Postpolypectomy colonic haemorrhage. *Dis Colon Rectum* 1996; 39: 806–810.

30. Seow-Choen F, Look MC, Ho YH. Non-surgical management of colonoscopic bowel perforation. *Int J Colorect Dis* 1995; 10: 77–78.

31. Jentschura D, Raute M, Winter J *et al*. Complications in endoscopy of the lower gastrointestinal tract. *Surg Endosc* 1994; 8: 672–676.

32. Waye JD, Kahn O, Auerbach ME. Complications of colonoscopy and flexible sigmoidoscopy. *Gastrointest Endosc* 1996; 6: 343–377.

17 Palliation of malignant lower gastrointestinal disease

S.G. Bown

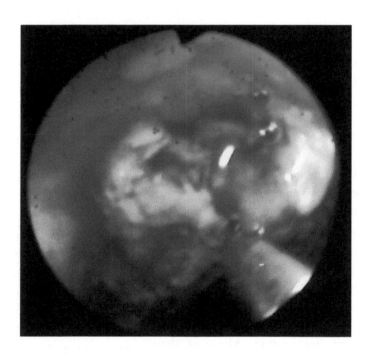

INTRODUCTION

Patients with advanced colorectal cancers – particularly those in the rectum and distal sigmoid colon – can suffer from a variety of local symptoms including bleeding, mucus discharge, tenesmus, constipation (from tumour obstructing the lumen), diarrhoea, urgency, incontinence and pelvic pain. These may be due to tumour in the bowel wall or lumen, or due to local spread in the pelvis.

Surgery is the treatment of choice for most cancers of the colon and rectum, particularly for patients in whom there is any prospect of cure. However, there is a significant number of patients for whom potentially curative surgery is not possible either because of the extent of their disease (local spread or distant metastases) or because of their poor general condition [1]. For these individuals, the therapeutic goals are limited to palliation.

OBJECTIVES OF PALLIATION

Until relatively recently, the main aim of palliative therapy was to prolong life for as long as possible, but it is now recognized that the quality of life is just as important – if not more so – than the quantity.

The aim of palliative therapy is to control symptoms with a minimum of general upset to the patient. This requires the use of methods which carry a low morbidity and mortality. Furthermore, methods should be chosen that provide palliation for as long as possible to minimize the need for subsequent intervention. Many of these patients are old and frail, and the aim is to keep them in comfort at home or in a hospice or other institution for as long as possible, with few visits to hospital. To do this most effectively requires close collaboration between hospital and hospice staff, the patient's general practitioner, community-based carers (particularly nurses), and the patient and his or her family. An especially effective arrangement is to have a nurse coordinator based in the hospital who can coordinate in-patient and out-patient management. If such an individual is closely involved in the patient care and is also easily accessible by telephone or otherwise to the patient, family, carers and community-based doctors and nurses, it can remove a great deal of the anxiety and worry associated with advanced malignant disease and so relieve the pressures on everyone involved.

Total patient care is essential for optimizing the quality of the remaining life for these unfortunate individuals, but the first task is to relieve their physical symptoms as simply and rapidly as possible. The local aims of palliative therapy can be summarized as follows:

- Removing or bypassing as much of the tumour bulk as possible.
- Removing the parts of the tumour that are causing the worst symptoms (usually the exophytic parts of the tumour in the bowel lumen).
- Slowing down the progression of tumour that cannot be removed.

These therapeutic options are not mutually exclusive, and in many cases combinations may provide the best overall management. Removing or bypassing the tumour bulk requires surgery. For patients in good general condition in whom it is reasonable to remove the vast majority of a cancer in the colon or rectum, this is nearly always the best option. The tumour bulk is reduced and it minimizes the risk of later complications such as bleeding and obstruction [2]. Adjuvant radiotherapy or chemotherapy can be given for unresectable parts of the tumour in the pelvis, and chemotherapy for multiple hepatic metastases. A range of options including surgical and non-surgical techniques is now available for isolated hepatic metastases. Even though few of these patients are likely to be cured, many have an excellent quality of life for an extended period. The choice of therapy becomes more difficult when it is not feasible to remove the primary tumour. Then, all surgery can offer is a bypass procedure. This occurs most frequently with rectal and rectosigmoid cancers when there is no room for a distal anastomosis and a defunctioning colostomy is required. This relieves obstruction, but cannot help bleeding, rectal discharge and tenesmus.

ENDOSCOPIC PALLIATION

Almost all the techniques for debulking exophytic tumours in the rectosigmoid region are applied endoscopically. These are the most widely applied methods of palliating these cancers, and most are effective although there are considerable variations in the requirements for equipment and skills and in the associated morbidity and mortality.

Palliation techniques

Nd-YAG laser (Fig. 17.1)

Endoscopic Nd-YAG laser treatment in the lower gastro-intestinal tract was first described by Brunetaud *et al.* in 1985 [3] for the management of inoperable, sessile villous adenomas, but several other groups started using it at about the same time for local palliation of advanced cancers and further reports have been appearing ever since [3–14]. Treatment can usually be done as a day case on patients who are in reasonable general condition with little or no sedation. The concept is straightforward, as discussed previously in Chapter 4. The high-power, infra-red laser beam (typically 50–80 W) is transmitted down a flexible fibre delivery system which can be passed through the operating channel of a standard flexible sigmoidoscope or colonoscope. The laser beam can be dangerous if used carelessly, but as long as the laser is only activated when the fibre has been passed through the endoscope in a patient, the only precaution required is a filter on the eyepiece of the endoscope to protect the doctor's eye from any beam reflected back up the endoscope. Even this may not be necessary with videoscopes, but not all videoscopes are suitable for use with lasers. The effect of the laser beam on tissue is purely thermal and depends on the power used, the length of each shot and the distance of the fibre tip from the tissue. With a typical 1-s shot at 60 W, with the fibre tip 5–10 mm from the target tumour, a small amount of tumour will be vaporized, another 2 mm or so will be coagulated and will slough off over a few days, and below that an inflammatory response will be initiated which may lead to fibrosis. This is the real attraction of laser therapy. The effect is much more predictable and controllable than that of diathermy and most of the other modalities, and it is safe to use it for lesions above the peritoneal reflection. The laser beam is targeted under direct vision, the amount of tissue that has been vaporized can be seen immediately and it is known that, after treatment, another 2–3 mm of necrosed tissue will slough over the subsequent few days. However, one must be sure that there is enough tissue under the treated area for this to happen safely, or there will be a risk of a delayed perforation, which makes it wiser just to treat exophytic lesions.

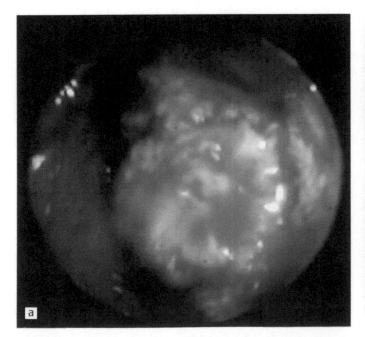 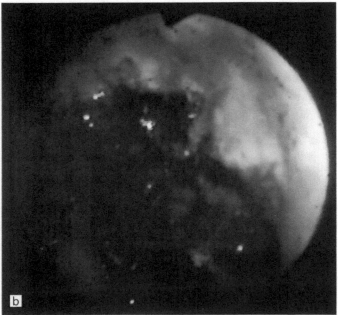

Figure 17.1. Advanced rectosigmoid cancer (a) before and (b) after debulking with the Nd-YAG laser. The coagulated tissue on the surface of the tumour after treatment will slough away over the subsequent days.

Argon laser

The argon laser should not be confused with the argon photocoagulator (APC) discussed below. The argon laser produces a bright blue-green laser beam which can be transmitted via a flexible fibre and used endoscopically. The biological effect is actually quite similar to that of the APC as the penetration of the argon laser beam into tissue is much less than that of the Nd-YAG laser and its use has been described in the lower gastrointestinal tract [3], although most groups just use the Nd-YAG laser.

Argon photocoagulator (APC)

This is a new instrument (sometimes known as the argon beamer) (see Chapter 4 and 16) which is a convenient form of electrofulguration [15]. A slow flow of argon gas is passed through a thin catheter containing a wire which goes down to a tungsten electrode at its distal tip, and this is inserted through an endoscope operating channel. The electrode is activated by a high-frequency surgical diathermy unit and the electrical circuit completed by an earth plate fixed to a neutral site on the patient. When the catheter tip is close enough to the target tissue (up to 10–15 mm), the argon gas is ionized and an electrical discharge flows through it, causing fulguration in the tissue. The method is simple and safe, but the effect is superficial and it takes longer than the laser to debulk tumour tissue [15]. Actual vaporization of tumour tissue is much more difficult than with the laser. It has one advantage over the laser in that the discharge goes from the catheter tip to the nearest tissue, which may be at the side of the catheter rather than in front, so it can effectively fire sideways. The laser can only fire straight ahead, which sometimes makes aiming more difficult.

Photodynamic therapy

Photodynamic therapy (PDT) is a technique for producing localized tissue necrosis with light after prior administration of a photosensitizing drug [16] (see Chapter 4). For endoscopic applications, the most convenient light source is a laser, but unlike Nd-YAG laser therapy, the effect is photochemical and not thermal. There is no increase in tissue temperature during treatment and the biological effect is produced because the laser light activates the photosensitizing drug which leads to production of the cytotoxic intermediate, singlet oxygen. The attraction of PDT is the nature of the tissue damage as connective tissue like collagen is largely unaffected.

Electrocoagulation

The first attempts at endoscopic treatment of rectal cancers to debulk them and reduce bleeding and discharge using diathermy fulguration and curettage via a rigid endoscope date back to the 1930s. However, the extent of tissue destruction is difficult to predict and it is not a technique that can be recommended.

Cryotherapy

Cryotherapy with a liquid nitrogen probe is relatively easy to apply to lesions below the peritoneal reflection, and can be done without general anaesthesia, although targeting is not as accurate as with a laser [17–19]. There is not much postoperative pain and it can be effective for tumour debulking, although necrosed tissue may continue to slough for a couple of weeks after treatment. Like electrocoagulation, the extent of tissue destruction is unpredictable.

Injection therapy (Fig. 17.2)

The local injection of toxic agents is a simple, cheap and often effective way of producing necrosis in bulky tumours. The agent used most frequently is absolute alcohol. This has proved effective for endoscopic use in palliating advanced oesophageal cancers [20]. A sclerotherapy needle is advanced into the tumour under direct vision and, after aspiration has confirmed that the needle is not in a blood vessel, alcohol is injected causing necrosed tissue to slough over

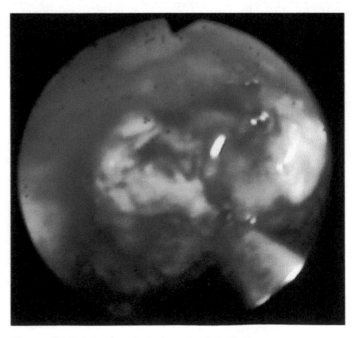

Figure 17.2. Injection technique to debulk tumour.

the following week or so. Treatment can be repeated as necessary to produce progressive debulking of tumour. The interval before retreatment is required is comparable with that seen with laser therapy.

Transanal resection

This is the most recent and effective way of using diathermy to debulk rectal tumours. The diathermy loop designed for transurethral resection of the prostate in the management of benign prostatic hypertrophy is modified for use in the rectum through an operating proctoscope. Slices of tumour can be removed under direct vision. This requires spinal or general anaesthetic, but is particularly valuable for bulky tumours as large volumes of tissue can be removed in a relatively short time [21–23].

The technique is undoubtedly effective, but the complication rate is disturbingly high. This may be because too much tissue is removed during one procedure, so there is a greater risk of cutting a blood vessel that is too large to be coagulated by the diathermy current. The depth of tissue coagulation is also difficult to predict, and this may increase the risk of full-thickness damage to the rectal wall and hence of perforation, although this is not so serious if treatment is applied only below the peritoneal reflection. It would probably be safer to remove a smaller volume of tissue at one procedure, but complete treatment would then require several sessions and consequently several general anaesthetics, which is not an attractive prospect in this patient group.

Snare polypectomy (Fig. 17.3)

Piecemeal removal of bits of tumour with a polypectomy snare at flexible sigmoidoscopy should also be included in this section. This is crude debulking, but for soft, fleshy lesions which have lots of polypoid nodules, it can be of value although there is a risk of starting significant bleeding.

Stents

The insertion of endoprostheses has been one of the routine options for palliation of malignant dysphagia for many years (see Chapter 3). The first to become well established were the silicon rubber tubes. In the early days, these were inserted surgically, but now almost all are placed endoscopically. With a typical internal lumen of 10–12 mm, they permit easy swallowing of liquids and semi-solids, and with care many solids can be eaten if they are cut up small, well-chewed and washed down with plenty of fluids. However, a lumen of this size was not

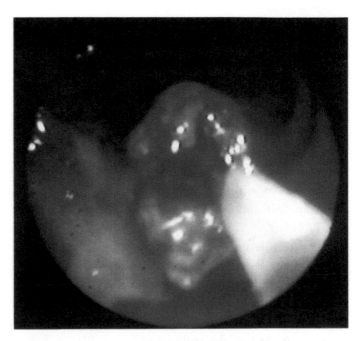

Figure 17.3. Technique of piecemeal snare polypectomy for large lesions.

considered large enough for the passage of solid faeces and so these tubes have not been used for the palliation of obstructing rectal cancers.

In the past few years, most interest has focused on expanding metal stents. These are simpler and safer to insert as they are supplied in a compressed form and require an initial lumen of only about 10 mm, so less dilatation is required. However, when expanded, the lumen can expand to up to 30 mm.

Choice of technique

The choice of technique will be influenced by several factors, as listed in Table 17.1.

Table 17.1. Factors influencing choice of palliative technique

Size and nature of lesion
Location of lesion
Frailty of patient, concomitant medical conditions, fitness for anaesthesia
Preference for in-patient, out-patient treatment
Prognosis or predicted longevity
Availability of modality and expertise
Evidence of efficacy

Size and nature

Optimum palliation of bulky rectal cancers requires initial removal of exophytic bulk as rapidly as possible, for which the best techniques are probably snare polypectomy or transanal resection. However, these are relatively crude techniques, and for smaller volumes (or after removal of the largest lumps), more precise techniques like the Nd-YAG laser are better.

Friable lesions require a method which produces deep haemostasis, for which the best options are electrocoagulation, injection (with adrenaline or a sclerosing agent) and the Nd-YAG laser.

Scirrhous lesions are difficult to inject and often inconvenient shapes for snaring, so high-power Nd-YAG laser or electrocoagulation are best. If there is no suitable endoscopic target and there is a risk of obstruction, then the only option short of surgery is a stent, but stents cannot be used too close to the anal margin.

Location

All the methods described can be used in the rectum, but the constraints are much greater for any lesion that extends above the peritoneal reflection, as the consequences of an accidental perforation are so much worse. Above the peritoneal reflection, the Nd-YAG laser and the APC are the safest, as treatment is delivered under direct vision and the extent of the necrosis produced is most predictable. However, on difficult corners, targeting can be a problem and in this situation stenting is often the best option. Treatment is also difficult for lesions encroaching on the anus as a general anaesthetic is often required, so it is important to remove as much tumour as possible in one treatment.

Frailty and concomitant conditions

The aim must be to minimize the stress caused by each treatment, so the most attractive options are those that can be delivered with a flexible sigmoidoscope with little or no sedation and which have a low risk of complications. These would include injection therapy, APC, the Nd-YAG laser and, for bulky lesions, piecemeal snare resection. As expanding metal stent technology improves, this will probably become the treatment of choice for tight strictures, but careful patient selection is essential.

Preference for out-patient treatment

The same considerations apply as for frail patients with other serious pathology, but in the present state of knowledge, it would be unwise to insert stents as an out-patient procedure. It is important to be sure that stents do not slip and that they have expanded well enough to permit a comfortable bowel evacuation before discharge from hospital. Piecemeal snare resection is unwise as an out-patient procedure on friable tumours because of the risk of bleeding.

Predicted longevity

The better the overall prognosis, the longer one should try and make the intervals between palliative treatments. In an ideal world, stent insertion is a one-off procedure, but in practice, follow-up procedures are likely to be necessary for tumour overgrowth, stent slippage or faecal blockage. Probably the best long-term plan is to use one of the endoscopic, debulking procedures and follow this with a palliative course of external radiotherapy as this has been shown to reduce the need for repeat intervention without causing any significant morbidity.

EVIDENCE

Thermal ablation

The largest number of papers on endoscopic palliation of advanced rectosigmoid cancers report results using the Nd-YAG laser [3–14]. This is not surprising as the technique is basically simple, safe and effective – even if the capital cost of the equipment is somewhat more than that required for most of the other options. For small, non-circumferential lesions that have not spread beyond the bowel wall, laser therapy may even occasionally be curative, but the general conclusion is that 80–90% of patients with advanced cancers can be palliated initially and that local symptoms can be controlled for the remainder of the patient's life in 75% of the total by repeating laser treatment when symptoms recur. McGowan *et al.* confirmed that relief of rectal symptoms did indeed improve the quality of life [7]. The overall morbidity and mortality rates are remarkably low, typically under 5% and under 2%, respectively. One drawback is that it is usually necessary to repeat treatments. Some groups recommend regular treatments at 1- to 2-month intervals and others advise waiting until symptoms recur. The data do suggest that it may be wiser to treat regularly as, if one waits for symptoms to recur, the tumour bulk may make treatment technically difficult, or even impossible [8]. The speed of vaporization can be increased by raising the laser power, but for extra-large, bulky rectal cancers some other form of crude debulking first may reduce the number of laser treatments required. One suggested modification was to use a sapphire tip on the end of the laser fibre and use it in contact with the tissue, but this was shown to be expensive and ineffective and was soon abandoned [9].

Three studies have been reported comparing Nd-YAG laser treatment with palliative surgery for managing advanced rectal cancers. None was randomized, but they provide useful comparisons. Tacke et al. [10] analysed the results of treating 196 patients with rectal cancer; these included 37 patients treated with endoscopic laser therapy and 42 with palliative surgery, the rest having potentially curative surgery. The laser group averaged four treatments each, with good results in 95% and a mean survival of 8 months with no complications. Palliative surgery gave good results in 98% of cases, but complications occurred in 7% and there was one death. These authors concluded that if curative surgery was not an option, then laser therapy may be preferable to palliative surgery as the time in hospital was less and there were fewer complications. Loizou et al. [11] undertook a similar analysis, comparing 47 patients treated with palliative surgery and 35 treated with the Nd-YAG laser. Patients in the laser group were older, and more had locally advanced cancers less than 7 cm from the anus, so would have required a colostomy if treated surgically. Thirty-four surgical cases had a resection and the other 13 just had a defunctioning colostomy. Long-term symptomatic palliation was achieved in 85% of the surgical cases and 74% of the laser ones (67% for relief of obstruction and 80% for relief of rectal bleeding, discharge and tenesmus). Procedure-related mortality (9% versus 0%), morbidity (44% versus 8%) and lifetime, procedure-related hospitalization time (40 versus 10 days) were all considerably higher in the surgical group. For those with locally advanced disease, there was no difference in the survival time. For those with hepatic metastases, survival was longer in the surgical group, but this probably reflected selection of patients with a better prognosis for surgery. Like Tacke et al., these authors concluded that laser palliation may be preferable to palliative surgery for at least some of these patients, particularly those with advanced local disease. Mellow et al. compared laser and surgery with regard to complications and costs and concluded that for palliation, the laser results were better on both counts [12].

Argon beamer

A recent report from Regula et al. in Poland [24] described the use of APC after piecemeal polypectomy of colorectal adenomas in patients unsuitable for surgery. Complete tumour ablation was documented in 30 of 36 cases, including four of five with proven malignant change. Between one and 11 endoscopic sessions were required, but there were no complications.

Photodynamic therapy (PDT)

This technique makes it safe to treat deeper into the bowel wall, as even with full-thickness necrosis, preservation of collagen preserves the mechanical integrity. This can even be true in tumour areas as there is often more collagen in tumour tissue than in the adjacent normal areas, although of course tumours may perforate spontaneously. However, in the present context, there are major drawbacks to using PDT. It is suitable for treating only small volumes of diseased tissue, and administration of a photosensitizing drug leaves patients generally sensitive to bright lights for a period that may vary from a few days up to 2–3 months, depending on which photosensitizer is used (see Chapter 4).

Several reports have described the use of PDT with the photosensitizer Photofrin for palliating malignant dysphagia. The results are comparable with those achieved using the Nd-YAG laser, but with more complications because of the generalized skin photosensitivity which reduce the quality of life for these patients with such a limited life expectancy [16]. Preliminary reports have appeared using PDT for palliation of rectal cancer [25]. The technique can be used in this way, but this application is unlikely to become established as other options are simpler and more effective. One possible way in which PDT might find a useful role in palliating advanced rectal tumours is after debulking with the Nd-YAG laser or some other technique. As it is safe to treat deeper with PDT than with any of the thermal techniques, PDT might prolong the period of palliation produced by the other methods, but this has yet to be reported. PDT is much more appropriate – and indeed may be the treatment of choice – for early tumours of the upper and lower gastrointestinal tract in patients who are unsuitable for surgery.

Electrocoagulation, cryotherapy and injection therapy

Electrocoagulation

In 1983, Madden and Kandalaft reported their results of electrofulguration in 77 patients [26]. They achieved good relief of symptoms in many, but there were significant complications (29%), one-third of which were bleeds severe enough to require transfusion. Other problems included rectovaginal and rectovesical fistulae, perforation into the abdominal cavity and rectal strictures. These were most likely attributable to the nature of the electrocoagulation equipment available which made it difficult to predict or control the extent of the tissue destruction produced. This technique has been superseded by laser methods.

Cryotherapy

In a recent series of cryotherapy, Meijer et al. [17] reported complete relief of local symptoms in nine of 20 patients with local recurrence after an anterior resection for rectal cancer after an average of two or three treatments, although three of these individuals later required a colostomy for complete obstruction. However, there is significant morbidity. In an earlier series [18], there were complications in 11 of 68 patients (18%) which included haemorrhage in seven and fistulae in three (two rectovaginal and one rectovesical). Heberer et al. [19] reported long-term palliation of rectal discharge and tenesmus in 65% of patients and avoidance of a colostomy in 78%. Perforation and mortality was only 5%, but 34% of patients had other complications.

Injection therapy

Alcohol injection is most suitable for soft, bulky, exophytic tumours. As yet, alcohol injection has not been reported for palliation of rectal tumours, but one would anticipate similar results to those reported in the oesophagus. For large exophytic tumours, alcohol injection can lead to recanalization of the lumen comparable with that achieved with laser therapy at a fraction of the cost, although the success rate is not so high. The problem is that it is difficult to control exactly where the alcohol goes once it is in the tumour as, having left the end of the needle, it passes along the line of least physical resistance. This is fine in soft, vascular tumours, but in hard, scirrhous lesions the alcohol simply returns along the needle track and achieves very little. This difficulty of control also makes it more likely that some necrosis will be produced in immediately adjacent normal tissue, which can cause pain and increase the risk of perforation or fistulation.

Another reported option is injection of polidocanol. This is a sclerosing rather than a necrosing agent, and so it is not clear why its injection leads to debulking, though this effect has been described. In five patients with inoperable rectal cancers causing bowel obstruction and treated with intratumoral injection of polidocanol, the obstruction was relieved in all cases, with no major complications [27].

Transanal resection and stenting

Berry et al. [21] reported the use of transanal resection in 137 treatments in 81 patients with inoperable small and large rectal cancers and adenomas. In the 31 advanced cancers, bleeding was abolished or improved in 66% of cases, diarrhoea controlled in 77%, and tenesmus and incontinence improved in 50%. However, in the whole series, there was a postoperative complication rate of 15% and a 30-day mortality rate of 11%. Another group [23] treated 40 patients with endoscopic transanal resection (including seven with advanced cancers, of whom five were well palliated) with no deaths within 30 days, although six were complicated by bleeding and one by septicaemia. These authors reported complete ablation of 22 of 23 benign adenomas. Another option would be to treat the main bulk of exophytic tumour with transanal excision, but not to shave the tumour back too close to the rectal wall and instead finish the procedure with endoscopic laser treatment, which is safer and more precise.

Insertion of an endoprosthesis for colon tumours is a relatively recent development. The clinical data on how many of these stents really do expand to the size claimed by the manufacturers (with or without additional dilatation) are very limited and will depend on the rigidity of the stricture being treated and on the design of each type of metal stent. However, the prospect of a lumen considerably larger than that achievable with the silicon rubber stents has encouraged an increasing number of groups to use them for palliating obstructing rectal cancers. The results are encouraging. In an early study on 12 patients with inoperable rectal or rectosigmoid carcinomas, expanding metal stent insertion was possible in 11 after initial Nd-YAG laser recanalization. In three cases the stent migrated, but could be replaced after removal of the first stent. The interval between laser treatments was increased from an average of 5 to an average of 10 weeks [28]. In a more recent larger series, obstruction was relieved in 23 out of 24 patients, although complications were seen in 10 including bleeding, abdominal pain, faecal impaction and tumour ingrowth.

COMBINATION OF ENDOSCOPIC TREATMENT WITH RADIOTHERAPY

Most of the endoscopic techniques described in this chapter are designed to reduce the intraluminal bulk of advanced rectal cancers as simply and rapidly as possible, and with the minimum of general upset to the patient. However, none of them can really tackle tumour in the wall of the rectum or beyond – which radiotherapy and chemotherapy can. Chemotherapy can be effective for patients with relatively limited disease in the pelvis or elsewhere, such as in the liver, but is rarely appropriate for patients requiring relief of symptoms from large, inoperable rectal cancers, even as part of multimodal therapy.

Radiotherapy (external or intraluminal) can give excellent results as primary treatment for small rectal cancers. It can relieve pain due to pelvic infiltration of advanced cancers, but is not effective for debulking large tumours [29]. External beam radiotherapy to large rectal cancers may even cause obstruction, and necessitate a temporary or permanent defunctioning colostomy. However, if the main bulk of intraluminal tumour has been removed by another technique, then it is logical that radiotherapy might slow down local regrowth, although to be of value for patients with advanced cancers, the dose of radiation must be low enough for the side effects to be minimal.

Sargeant et al. [30] reported a pilot study using external radiotherapy to enhance laser palliation of advanced rectal and rectosigmoid cancers. Thirteen patients received external beam radiotherapy (30–55 Gy in 10–20 fractions) after successful laser recanalization. The additional treatment was tolerated well in all except one patient, and the median time interval between laser endoscopies was increased from 4 weeks before radiotherapy to 20 weeks afterwards. One drawback of this approach is that multiple fractions of radiotherapy were used. No data are available to see if the same results can be achieved with less fractions.

With the development of new after-loading instruments for delivering high local doses of irradiation in short periods of time, the role of brachytherapy (intraluminal radiotherapy) is increasing rapidly. As the radiation from ^{192}Ir penetrates a few centimetres into tissue, it is possible to give intense local treatment (10 Gy in less than 30 min) without affecting tissues more than a couple of centimetres or so away. Brachytherapy as primary treatment for oesophageal cancer was first reported in 1985 and a single treatment has been shown to be highly effective in prolonging laser palliation of these cancers after laser treatment. However, the only results so far reported in the rectum have been a bit disappointing. Conio et al. [31] treated nine patients with the Nd-YAG laser followed by 20-Gy brachytherapy in two fractions, a week apart. The need for further laser treatment was reduced, but four of the nine patients complained of acute perineal pain and tenesmus. Further studies may be appropriate using a lower dose of brachytherapy.

CONCLUSIONS

All the endoscopic techniques described here can palliate symptoms of advanced rectal cancers due to exophytic tumour in the bowel lumen, but there is considerable variation in their costs and efficacy. The most important aspects for each technique are compared in Table 17.2. In some cases there is not yet enough evidence to judge how effective or safe a new approach is. This is particularly true for expanding metal stents, where very little information is yet available on their short- or long-term safety and efficacy in the rectosigmoid region. Transanal resection puts the greatest strain on the patient as general anaesthesia is required and the complication rate is highest, but it is the fastest way to debulk a large tumour. Injection therapy is undoubtedly the cheapest option, but is relatively crude. It is likely to work best for soft, fleshy tumours and least well for hard, craggy lesions. Photodynamic therapy is unlikely to find a role in the palliation of advanced rectal cancers because of the problems of prolonged photosensitivity, unless it is able to prolong the effect of one of the other techniques. Photodynamic therapy is much better suited to complete ablation of small tumours in patients who are unsuitable for surgery.

In the current state of the art, for most of these patients, the Nd-YAG laser is probably still the treatment of choice. The argon beamer can perform the same job just as safely, but more slowly. Laser purchase costs are certainly high, but for a department seeing many of these patients, the running costs are very reasonable. Whichever endoscopic debulking technique is used for rectal cancers, the duration of effect

Table 17.2. Summary of the 'pros' and 'cons' of techniques, and which lesions are most suitable for each method

Technique	Advantages	Disadvantages	Suitable cases	Unsuitable cases
Nd-YAG laser	safe, easy to control, extent of necrosis predictable	expensive	large and small lesions above and below peritoneal reflection	extrinsic lesions, lesions around tight corners, very bulky lesions
Argon laser	safe	expensive, slow, equipment often needs technical support	small lesions, especially above peritoneal reflection	bulky lesions, extrinsic lesions
Argon beamer	cheap, safe, can aim sideways	slow	small lesions, especially above peritoneal reflection	bulky lesions, extrinsic lesions
PDT	safe	prolonged skin photosensitivity, slow response	small lesions, above or below peritoneal reflection	bulky lesions or lesions close to obstruction, extrinsic lesions
Electrocoagulation	cheap	difficult to control extent of necrosis	bulky lesions	lesions above peritoneal reflection, extrinsic lesions
Cryotherapy	cheap	difficult to control extent of necrosis, prolonged discharge	bulky lesions	lesions above peritoneal reflection, extrinsic lesions
Injection	cheap, simple, readily available	difficult to control which areas are necrosed	soft, bulky lesions	hard tumours or lesions above peritoneal reflection, extrinsic lesions
Transanal resection	rapid removal of large volumes of tumour	requires general anaesthetic, high incidence of complications	bulky, distal lesions	lesions above peritoneal reflection, extrinsic lesions
Snare piecemeal	rapid removal of large volumes of tumour	risk of bleeding	bulky, soft, polypoid tumours	hard, sessile lesions, extrinsic lesions
Stenting	one stage procedure	expensive	stenosing lesions above the mid-rectum, extrinsic compression	lesions extending below the upper rectum, lesions causing significant bleeding or tenesmus

can probably be prolonged by the addition of a palliative course of external beam radiotherapy.

The symptoms of advanced, inoperable rectosigmoid cancer can be very distressing, but with currently available endoscopic techniques, good palliation can be achieved in most patients for the remainder of their life.

REFERENCES

1 Goligher J. *Surgery of the Anus, Rectum and Colon*. 5th edn. Bailliere Tindall, 1994, 731–733.

2. Moran MR, Rothenberger DA, Lahr CJ *et al*. Palliation for rectal cancer: resection? Anastomosis? *Arch Surg* 1987; 122: 640–643.

3. Brunetaud JM, Mosquet L, Houcke M *et al*. Villous adenoma of the rectum. Results of endoscopic treatment with argon and Nd YAG lasers. *Gastroenterology* 1985; 89: 832–837.

4. Mathus-Vliegen EM, Tytgat GN. Nd-YAG laser photocoagulation in gastroenterology: its role in palliation of colorectal cancer. *Lasers Med Sci* 1986; 1: 75–80.

5. Bown SG, Barr H, Matthewson K *et al*. Endoscopic treatment of inoperable colorectal cancers with the Nd-YAG laser. *Br J Surg* 1986; 73: 949–952.

6. Brunetaud JM, Manoury V, Durcotte P *et al*. Palliative treatment of rectosigmoid carcinoma by laser endoscopic photoablation. *Gastroenterology* 1987; 92: 633–638.

7. McGowan I, Barr H, Krasner N. Palliative laser therapy for inoperable rectal cancer. Does it work? A prospective study of quality of life. *Cancer* 1989; 63: 967–969.

8. Van Custem E, Boonen A, Geboes G *et al.* Risk factors which determine long term outcome of neodymium YAG laser palliation of colorectal carcinoma. *Int J Colorectal Dis* 1989; 4: 9–11.

9. Rutgeerts P, Vantrappen G, D'Heygere F, Geboes K. Endoscopic contact ND: YAG laser therapy for colorectal cancer: a randomized comparison with non-contact therapy. *Laser in Medical Science* 1987; 2: 69–72.

10. Tacke W, Paech S, Kruis W *et al.* Comparison between endoscopic laser and different surgical treatment for palliation of advanced rectal cancer. *Dis Colon Rectum* 1993; 36(4): 377–82.

11. Loizou LA, Boulos PB, Komborozos V, Bown SG. Palliation for incurable rectal and rectosigmoid cancer: surgery or laser? *Gut* 1989; 30: A1478.

12. Mellow MH. Endoscopic laser therapy as an alternative to palliative surgery for adenocarcinoma of the rectum – comparison of costs and complications. *Gastrointest Endosc* 1989; 35: 283–287.

13. Loizou LA, Grigg D, Boulos PB, Bown SG. Endoscopic ND:YAG laser treatment of rectosigmoid cancer. *Gut* 1990; 31: 812–816.

14. Farouk R, Ratnaval CD, Monson JR, Lee PW. Staged delivery of ND:YAG laser therapy for palliation of advanced rectal carcinoma. *Dis Colon Rectum* 1997; 40(2): 156–60.

15. Grund KE, Storek D, Farin G. Endoscopic argon plasma coagulation (APC) – first clinical experiences in flexible sigmoidoscopy. *End Surg* 1994; 2: 1–6.

16. Bown SG, Millson CE. Photodynamic therapy in gastroenterology. *Gut* 1997; 41(7): 5–7.

17. Meijer S, de Rooij PD, Derksen EJ *et al.* Cryosurgery for locally recurrent rectal cancer. *Eur J Surg Oncol* 1992; 18(3): 255.

18. Mlasowsky B, Duben W, Jung D. Cryosurgery for palliation of rectal tumours. *J Esp Clin Cancer Res* 1985; 4: 81–83.

19. Heberer G, Denecke H, Demmel N, Wirsching R. Local procedures in the management of rectal cancer. *World J Surg* 1987; 11: 499–503.

20. Nwokolo CU, Payne-James JJ, Silk DB *et al.* Palliation of malignant dysphagia by ethanol induced tumour necrosis. *Gut* 1994; 35(3): 299–303.

21. Berry AR, Souter RG, Campbell WB *et al.* Endoscopic transanal resection of rectal tumours – a preliminary report of its use. *Br J Surg* 1990; 77: 134–137.

22. Dickinson AJ, Savage AP, Mortensen NJ, Kettlewell MG. Long-term survival after endoscopic transanal resection of rectal tumours. *Br J Surg* 1993; 80(11): 1401–4.

23. Wetherall AP, Williams NM, Kelly MJ. Endoscopic transanal resection in the management of patients with sessile rectal adenomas, anastomotic stricture and rectal cancer. *Br J Surg* 1993; 80(6): 788–93.

24. Regula J, Wronska E, Nasierowska A *et al.* Endoscopic argon plasma coagulation (APC) after piecemeal polypectomy of colorectal adenomas. Two-years follow-up study. *Gastrointest Endosc* 1997; 45(4) (abstract).

25. Kashtan H, Haddad R. Yossiphov Y *et al.* Photodynamic therapy of colorectal cancer using a new light source: from *in vitro* studies to a patient treatment. *Dis Colon Rectum* 1996: 39(4): 379–383.

26. Madden JL, Kandalaft SI. Electrocoagulation as a primary curative method in the treatment of carcinoma of the rectum. *Gynecol Obstet* 1983; 157: 164–79.

27. Marini E, Frigo F, Cavarzere L *et al.* Palliative treatment of carcinoma of the rectum by endoscopic injection of polidocanol. *Endoscopy* 1990; 22(4): 171–173.

28. Rey JF, Romanczyk T, Greff M. Metal stents for palliation of rectal carcinoma: a preliminary report on 12 patients. *Endoscopy* 1995; 27(7): 501–504.

29. Allum WH, Mack P, Priestman TJ, Fielding JWL. Radiotherapy for pain relief in locally recurrent colorectal cancer. *Ann R Coll Surg Eng* 1978; 69: 220–221.

30. Sargeant IR, Tobias JS, Blackman G *et al.* Radiation enhancement of laser palliation for advanced rectal and rectosigmoid cancer: a pilot study. *Gut* 1993; 34: 958–962.

31. Conio M, Picasso M, Orsatti M *et al.* Combined treatment with laser therapy (ND-YAG) and endocavitary radiation in the palliation of rectal cancer. *Hepatogastroenterology* 1996; 43(12): 1518–1522.

18 Management of lower gastrointestinal bleeding

S.G.J. Williams

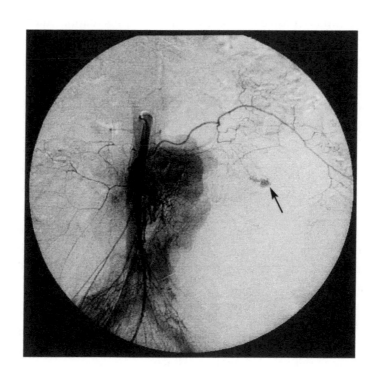

INTRODUCTION

Lower gastrointestinal bleeding includes any source of bleeding distal to the ligament of Treitz [1]. However, upper gastrointestinal bleeding may mimic a lower gastrointestinal bleed, presenting with similar symptoms and signs in up to 10% of patients [2].

The key aspect of managing lower gastrointestinal bleeding is establishing the source of blood loss to allow appropriately directed therapy. Within the spectrum of presentation of these patients it is important to distinguish two groups – the more unusual presentation with an acute onset and the more common problem of occult gastrointestinal bleeding presenting with anaemia or being detected on the basis of positive faecal occult blood testing.

ACUTE LOWER GASTROINTESTINAL BLEEDING

Presentation

All patients presenting with acute colonic bleeding should be appropriately resuscitated with fluid replacement. An acute presentation with haemodynamic instability and a requirement for blood and colloid infusion may require urgent investigation and intervention. Reassuringly, 80–90% of these patients will stop bleeding spontaneously [3–5], though it is not possible to predict which will stop bleeding and which will require urgent intervention.

The plan of investigation will depend on the severity of bleeding at presentation. Laboratory investigation before resuscitation may be of some value in the initial assessment. Patients with an acute bleed may have a normal haemoglobin concentration, haematocrit and mean corpuscular volume, while those with an acute-on-chronic bleed are likely to have a fall or reduction in these parameters. Some 95% of patients with upper gastrointestinal haemorrhage are likely to have a serum urea : creatinine (mmol/l) ratio above 100 : 1 [6].

Exclusion of upper gastrointestinal bleeding

Patients with haemodynamic instability, hypotension or requiring substantial blood transfusions should have an upper gastrointestinal endoscopy to exclude the upper gastrointestinal tract as a possible bleeding source as soon as their condition is stable [2]. While the aspiration of gastric contents via a nasogastric tube has been advocated as a means of establishing an upper gastrointestinal bleeding source, there are concerns that blood from the duodenum may not reflux into the stomach and that bleeding from a gastric ulcer may arrest resulting in an absence of blood from the aspirate. Direct visualization of the ulcer in the case of the second scenario will allow the endoscopist to make an assessment of the ulcer for stigmata of recent haemorrhage and to apply appropriately directed therapy.

Following confirmation that the patient is not bleeding from the upper gastrointestinal tract, the choices for further investigation depend on the severity of bleeding at presentation and the local expertise available.

Investigation of lower gastrointestinal bleeding

Barium studies

Barium enemas have previously been advocated as an appropriate first-line investigation, but it is now accepted that there is no role for them as they do not allow confirmation of the bleeding source, do not detect such abnormalities as arteriovenous malformations, and prevent other interventions such as colonoscopy and angiography in the immediate period after they have been performed. They may still have a role in the assessment of occult gastrointestinal bleeding.

Surgery

Surgical intervention with partial or subtotal colectomy was also a common approach. While surgery may still, on occasions, be necessary for the patient who continues to bleed, it has major limitations including an associated mortality rate of up to 50% and rebleeding rates as high as 33% [7,8].

Colonoscopy

Colonoscopy is the initial investigation of choice. It was, for a long time, considered of little use during the acute bleeding phase due to the technical difficulties performing the test and visualizing the colonic mucosa in the face of a blood-filled lumen. However, it has been demonstrated that following oral purge, a colonic lesion can be identified in over 70% of patients [2,9,10]. In contrast, a selected cohort of patients in two of these studies underwent angiography, which identified the bleeding source in less than 15% of cases [2,10]. Preparation of the colon is best performed using a sulphate-based purgative with polyethylene glycol, as this results in minimal salt and water absorption [11]. If necessary, the purgative can be administered via a nasogastric tube.

The major advantage of endoscopic investigation is that it allows visualization of the colonic mucosa for active sources of bleeding, and allows appropriately directed therapeutic intervention [2] (see below). The presence of adherent clot or active bleeding from a lesion confirms it as the source of haemorrhage. It is reasonable to assume that a lesion detected without stigmata of recent haemorrhage, but in the absence of other potential sources of bleeding, is the source of blood loss. Should colonoscopy fail to locate the source of bleeding the choice for further investigation lies between visceral angiography and ^{99m}Tc-red blood cell (RBC) scans.

Selective visceral angiography (Fig. 18.1)

In general, selective visceral angiography is unlikely to be diagnostic unless blood loss is faster than 0.5 ml/min [12], i.e. 1 litre of blood transfusion to maintain haemoglobin or a 2 g/dl drop in haemoglobin concentration over 24 hours. Studies comparing the pick-up rate of colonoscopy and angiography suggest that the former technique is more sensitive (see above). However, positive angiography has been reported in up to 87% of studies [13]. Clearly, there is some dependence on local expertise. Should colonoscopy

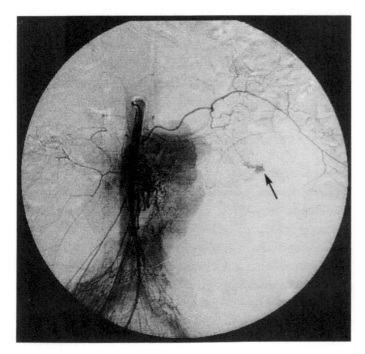

Figure 18.1. Superior mesenteric angiogram demonstrating a bleeding point (arrow) in the transverse colon.

fail to demonstrate a source of bleeding or prove technically impossible an angiogram is the 'next step' investigation in a patient who is bleeding sufficiently briskly.

Angiographic technique involves selective superior mesenteric artery cannulation as the majority of lower gastrointestinal bleeding originates from the right hemicolon. If this is negative, the study should be extended to include the inferior mesenteric artery and, if necessary, the coeliac axis. If a bleeding source is identified there is also the potential for therapeutic intervention (see below).

Identification of the actual bleeding site with angiography may improve the outcome of surgical intervention, when this is required, as it allows the surgeon to perform a limited resection [14]. Localization of the lesion can be helped by injecting methylene blue through the angiography catheter.

The diagnostic yield of angiography (bleeding may be intermittent) has been improved by the infusion of heparin, other thrombolytics or vasodilators [15]. While it may be considered that these manoeuvres are placing the patient at additional risk, the reported series suggest limited complications which are easily outweighed by identifying the bleeding source in the patient with ongoing bleeding and haemodynamic instability.

Radionuclide scanning

Two types of nuclear scanning have been used in the assessment of gastrointestinal bleeding. The first involves the use of technetium-99m sulphur colloid (^{99m}Tc-SC). This radioisotope is rapidly cleared by the reticuloendothelial system, and has the theoretical advantage that it allows identification of a bleeding site with improved contrast against the relatively low background activity. However, the patient must be actively bleeding at the time of injection due to the rapid clearance of the radiotracer from the circulation. There is also the problem posed by uptake by the liver and spleen which obscures bleeding from gastrointestinal sources close to these organs [16].

The second nuclear scan used to localize bleeding is the ^{99m}Tc-RBC scan (Fig. 18.2). This has the advantages that it does not require such brisk bleeding as angiography to achieve a diagnosis (0.1 ml/min), and that it will detect a lesion that is bleeding intermittently. This is because, following injection of the labelled red blood cells, scanning can be repeated over 24–36 hours [17]. However, interpretation of the scans may be hampered by a persisting high level of background activity due to the continuing

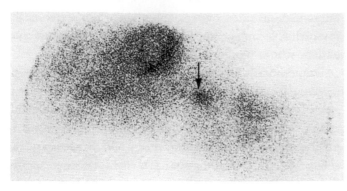

Figure 18.2. Technetium scan demonstrating uptake of isotope in a Meckel's diverticulum.

presence of labelled red cells within the circulation, and delayed scans may also be difficult to interpret as extravasated red cells may move anterogradely and retrogradely in the window between bleeding and scanning, creating some confusion about the exact site of blood loss.

Initial data on radionuclide scanning suggested that the techniques were more sensitive in detecting bleeding than angiography. However, more recent data suggest that ^{99m}Tc-RBC is a poor technique for localizing bleeding [17]. Recent retrospective series have indicated a sensitivity as low as 20% when the site of bleeding had been localized by angiography, endoscopy or surgery [18].

It seems, therefore that nuclear scanning is likely to be the least beneficial of the three investigations in the acute phase of bleeding. If, however, the other investigations have been unhelpful, in my opinion, it is worth doing. Equally, if the local expertise does not allow colonoscopy or arteriography in the acute phase, then it would be a reasonable line of investigation.

Adjunctive investigations
Failure to identify a bleeding source using the modalities described above may result in the need to move to surgical intervention. If, however, the clinical status of the patient allows it may be appropriate to perform a Meckel's scan, small bowel barium series or enteroscopy. These investigative tools are described in further detail below.

OCCULT LOWER GASTROINTESTINAL BLEEDING

Presentation

Occult lower gastrointestinal bleeding usually presents with

the signs and symptoms of anaemia, the incidental detection of iron deficiency or the detection of occult blood within the stool.

Investigation

Upper gastrointestinal endoscopy with distal duodenal biopsies remain important in the work-up of these patients. In patients with gastrointestinal symptoms the investigations are appropriately targeted towards the pathological processes that explain both the blood loss and the symptoms. In a patient presenting with occult gastrointestinal bleeding, the detection of a potential source in the upper gastrointestinal tract does not, on the whole, preclude the need for evaluation of the colon. Further investigation will then depend on a clinical decision regarding the severity, persistence and recurrence of the anaemia and the age and co-morbid problems of the patient.

Preparation
Bowel preparation for elective colonoscopy or barium enema may be performed using one of a number of available preparations. An older preparation, sodium picosulphate (Picolax, Nordic) produces results as acceptable as one of the polyethylene glycol preparations (Klean-Prep, Norgine) [19]. Concerns about the volume of preparation necessary for bowel cleansing with the polyethylene glycol-based preparations have been addressed by other recent studies comparing these with sodium phosphate (Phospho-soda, Fleet). These suggest that sodium phosphate is at least as effective in cleansing the bowel, with better patient tolerance [20]. Sodium phosphate is, however, associated with transient hyperphosphataemia.

Contrast radiology
Barium enema should visualize 80% of colorectal carcinomas and 80% of polyps greater than 1 cm in diameter [13]. Its advantages include its safety and availability. Its disadvantages include inadequate visualization of the rectum due to the presence of the catheter and thickness of the barium column, difficulties in interpreting images in the sigmoid colon where bowel loops may overly one another, where the presence of other pathology such as diverticulosis may obscure the presence of other lesions and where the detection of polyps results in the need for therapeutic colonoscopy.

The standard barium follow-through has a yield in the order of 5% when used in the investigation of obscure gastrointestinal bleeding [21], with positive results being limited to obvious pathology such as regional enteritis.

Enteroclysis or the small bowel enema improves the diagnostic yield to 10% [22]. It is, however, more unpleasant for the patient as it involves the radiological placement of a tube in the duodenum and the introduction of air, barium and water. This results in a double-contrast study with a concomitant improvement in the number of positive investigations.

Angiography

As previously indicated, an angiogram is most likely to be positive in the context of active bleeding. In a patient with occult bleeding the diagnostic pick-up is likely to fall to 25% [23].

Nuclear scanning

The use of a ^{99m}Tc-RBC scan has also been advocated, but again it is most sensitive when active bleeding is present. However, the long half-life of the labelled red cells increases the possibility of obtaining a positive scan, albeit that localization of the bleeding point may be difficult.

The Meckel's scan (Fig. 18.2) uses ^{99m}Tc pertechnetate, which binds to parietal cells; this may also be an appropriate investigation in the 'work-up' of obscure gastrointestinal bleeding, but should only be considered once further evaluation of the small bowel has been completed. It has a reported sensitivity of 75–100% with false-positive scans in 15% of cases and false-negatives in 25% [24].

Surgery

Surgical exploration alone has been advocated for obscure gastrointestinal bleeding. The yield from this approach is, however, unacceptably low (about 10%) and it should be combined with intraoperative endoscopy.

The creation of multiple enterostomies at laparotomy has also been used in the patient with recurrent overt gastrointestinal bleeding. This may help to localize bleeding to a particular segment of bowel, allowing a limited resection [25].

Other techniques include the use of intraoperative angiography (although this is demanding, particularly in terms of equipment), Doppler ultrasonography for the localization of angiodysplasia and intraoperative scintigraphy [26].

The role of endoscopy

Colonoscopy

Colonoscopy is the investigation of choice in patients with a suspected colonic source of occult bleeding [27]. It is extremely sensitive for detecting small mucosal lesions [13], and it allows therapeutic intervention. Its sensitivity for the detection of colorectal tumours and polyps larger than 1 cm is in the region of 95%. Its failure to detect some lesions is caused by problems with acute angulation, polyps concealed behind folds and poor preparation. Completion of the procedure is dependent on operator skill, with rates varying between 80% and 99%. It also carries a 1 in 1000 perforation rate.

If colonoscopy is negative and the patient has also had a normal upper gastrointestinal endoscopy, then further investigation should – if clinically appropriate – be directed at the small bowel.

Enteroscopy

Enteroscopy is the endoscopic evaluation of the distal duodenum, jejunum and ileum. It is currently performed using one of three techniques: push, sonde or intraoperative enteroscopy.

Push enteroscopy

Specifically designed enteroscopes are now available, although most initial experience with this technique involved the use of the adult or paediatric colonoscope.

Table 18.1. Characteristics of instruments available for small-bowel enteroscopy

Instrument	Paediatric colonoscope	Adult colonoscope	Olympus SIF 230	Pentax VSB-P2900
Diameter	11 mm	14 mm	11.2 mm	11 mm
Length	135 cm	165 cm	200 cm	240 cm
Depth of insertion*	60 cm	90 cm	120 cm	120 cm

*Beyond the ligament of Treitz.

These latter instruments allow examination beyond the ligament of Treitz, but do not allow intubation as far as the enteroscope, particularly when these are used in conjunction with the overtube to limit looping in the stomach and duodenal bulb (Table 18.1). The use of push enteroscopy in patients with obscure gastrointestinal bleeding has resulted in diagnostic yields as high as 38% [28], with angiodysplasias accounting for the majority of diagnoses. Enteroscopy allows therapeutic intervention through the working channel of the endoscope. This includes cauterization of bleeding sites using the methods described below and snare resection of bleeding polyps. Therapeutic intervention is, however, hampered by a lack of instruments specifically designed for use with the enteroscope. Complications of push enteroscopy have usually been reported in association with the overtube. These include oesophageal tears [29], although recent modification of the overtubes to incorporate a 10-cm GoreTex tip seems to have overcome some of the problems.

Sonde enteroscopy

This involves the use of a long flexible instrument (2560 mm long, with a tip diameter of 5 mm) with a balloon at its tip which is passed through the distal small bowel using peristalsis. Originally, the instrument was passed with the patient in the right lateral decubitus position and followed with fluoroscopy. More recently, the push entero- scope has been used to hasten the placement of the sonde enteroscope in the jejunum by pulling the sonde enteroscope by grasping (using biopsy forceps) a suture attached to the tip of the instrument. Passage of the instrument takes 6–8 h, while the endoscopic examination, which is performed as the instrument is withdrawn, takes 45–60 min. Its limitations include the lack of tip manoeuvrability which can only be achieved with abdominal palpation coupled with inflation and deflation of the tip balloon. This may limit mucosal visualization to 50–70% [30]. The absence of a working channel prevents biopsy and therapeutic intervention. In addition, the instrument only reaches the ileum in 75% of examinations and the terminal ileum in 10% [30]. The sonde enteroscope may provide a positive diagnosis in 33% of patients [31]. A combination of push and sonde enteroscopy may increase the yield to 42%, with over half of these lesions being distal to the area covered by the push enteroscope [28]. Vascular lesions account for the majority of positive examinations. Small bowel tumours, the

next most common diagnostic category, have been detected in patients with negative small bowel radiology.

Intraoperative enteroscopy (Fig. 18.3)

If sonde enteroscopy is unavailable, examination of the remainder of the small bowel can be achieved using intra- operative enteroscopy. A colonoscope, passed perorally, is usually used for this procedure. The endoscope is passed into the proximal jejunum before the laparotomy due to potential technical difficulties negotiating the ligament of Treitz once the laparotomy has been performed. Following laparotomy, a non-crushing clamp is placed across the ileocaecal valve to prevent distension of the colon. The surgeon holds the tip of the endoscope and also a portion of small bowel which is then examined and pleated onto the endoscope (Fig. 18.3a). Trauma to the mucosa, following pleating, has been reported in up to 50% of examinations and may mimic angiodysplasia [32]. This precludes examination of the bowel during extubation. Identified lesions are marked with a serosal suture by the surgeon and resected at the end of the procedure. Perforations have been reported in up to 5% of cases [32]. The other potential complication is a prolonged ileus. Modifications of the intraoperative enteroscopy technique include enterotomy in the mid small bowel to allow anterograde and retrograde examination of the small bowel (Fig. 18.3b), and retrograde examination of the small bowel using the technique described following a caecostomy and passage of the endoscope through the ileocaecal valve (Fig. 18.3c). Both techniques require the use of a sterilized endoscope or an endoscope covered by a sterile plastic sheath. Intraoperative enteroscopy is widely available as it does not require the use of special endoscopes and is reported to yield positive results in 83–100% of cases [26]. Although haemostasis may be applied using laser or heater probe these may not provide long-term cessation of bleeding [32]. Consequently, surgical resection is considered to be the definitive treatment.

MANAGEMENT AND TECHNIQUES

The most common detected sources of bleeding are diverticulosis, vascular ectasias/angiomata, colonic polyps and tumours. The diagnoses for 80 patients included in a recent series of patients with presumed lower gastrointestinal bleeding are shown in Table 18.2. Some examples are shown in Figures 18.4–18.6. The various therapeutic techniques

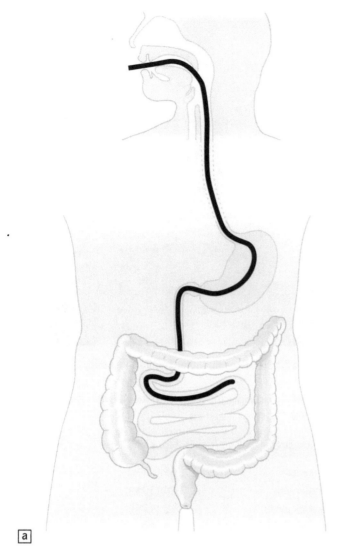

Figure 18.3. Intraoperative enteroscopy technique. (a) The bowel is 'pleated' onto the enteroscope; (b) enterotomy allows anterograde and retrograde examination; (c) caecostomy allows retrograde examination of the small intestine.

that can be applied to sources of acute blood loss in the lower gastrointestinal tract are detailed in Table 18.3.

Injection/contact devices

Adrenaline injection

The simplest and most readily available technique is the use of a sclerotherapy needle and 1 : 10 000 adrenaline.

The needle is inserted to its full depth and approximately 3 ml of the adrenaline is injected adjacent to or into the bleeding source as the needle is withdrawn. Up to five aliquots are injected. This results in the injection of adrenaline deep into the tissues, with the intention of producing a vasoconstrictor effect to the vessels supplying the bleeding site, and also producing a bleb of fluid submucosally. The hope is that this will produce initial

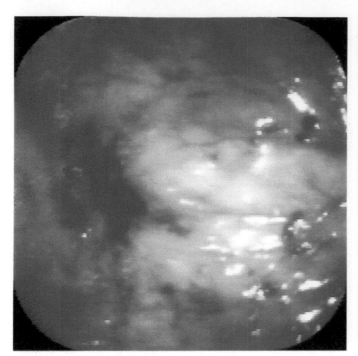

Figure 18.4. Colonic angiodysplasia.

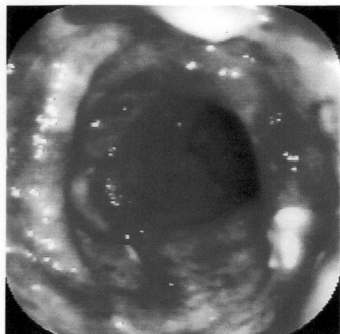

Figure 18.6. Moderately active ulcerative colitis.

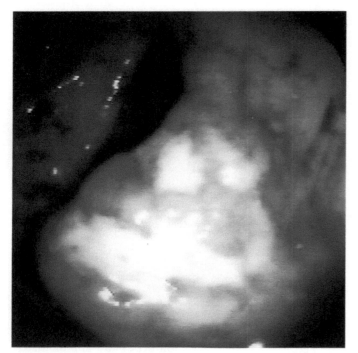

Figure 18.5. Ulceration on the fold adjacent to the ileo-caecal valve.

Table 18.2. Final diagnosis in 80 patients with severe rectal bleeding

Lesion site	No. of patients
Colonic:	59 (74%)
Angiomata	24 (30%)
Diverticulosis	13 (17%)
Active bleeding	6 (8%)
Adherent clot	7 (9%)
Polyps or cancer	9 (11%)
Focal colitis or ulcers	7 (9%)
Rectal lesions	3 (4%)
Bleeding polyp stalk	2 (2%)
Upper gastrointestinal	9 (11%)
Small bowel*	7 (9%)
No site found	5 (6%)

*Presumed small bowel bleeding following normal endoscopy and colonoscopy, with fresh blood and/or clots coming from the ileocaecal valve. Reproduced with permission from [2].

haemostasis simply by exerting some pressure locally. This technique can be used to stop bleeding from a diverticulum, a vessel within an ulcer (much as it is applied in the upper gastrointestinal tract), or bleeding from the base of a polyp post-polypectomy (Fig. 18.7). In general, the use of alternative injectates such as the sclerosants that might be employed in the upper gastrointestinal tract should not be considered in the colon as the wall is

Table 18.3. Therapeutic modalities available for treating lower gastrointestinal bleed

Technique	Therapeutic modality
Endoscopic	Adrenaline injection
	Heater probe
	BICAP probe
	Hot biopsy forceps
	Laser
	Argon plasma coagulation
	Polypectomy
Angiographic	Vasopressin infusion
	Embolization
Surgery	

much thinner and there is a risk of deep ulceration and perforation.

The alternative to inducing haemostasis by adrenaline injection is the use of various heat-producing devices. These are probably best applied to arteriovenous malformations/angiodysplasia with the desired end-point being whitening of the mucosa or superficial coagulation necrosis. Contact probes can be moved over the surface of a lesion with light pressure while the heat is applied. A similar technique is used for laser ablation. Many patients rebleed and they may require the application of several treatments.

Heater probe

The heater probe is a Teflon-coated, non-stick thermal device which delivers heat (250°C) in 0.2 s, under computer control, that effectively seals blood vessels. It has the advantage that the control unit incorporates a strong water jet that allows the area being treated to be washed, and this improves visualization. A setting of 10–15 J is usually sufficient. The probe is applied with gentle pressure because of the concerns of full-thickness necrosis.

BICAP probe

The BICAP probe acts in much the same way as the heater probe. The heat generated must be applied with care, with a setting of 2 or 3 on a 50-W BICAP generator usually being sufficient. This probe also has an integral washing jet.

Hot biopsy forceps

If neither the heater probe nor BICAP probe is available, heat can be applied using the monopolar technique with hot biopsy forceps or a snare which has the last few millimetres protruding from the protective sheath (Fig. 18.8). Hot biopsy forceps can either be applied directly to the surface of the lesion or in the case of angiodysplasia can be used to grasp the lesion or surrounding mucosa. If the lesion is large and there are concerns about bleeding, a ring of treatment should be applied around it, followed by one or more applications to the centre (Fig. 18.9). In the case of small lesions, current is applied to grasped mucosa with the mucosa tented away from the wall of the colon so that the thermal injury is applied as superficially as possible. Following minimal visible coagulation the forceps are opened to release the mucosa.

Laser

Both argon and Nd-YAG lasers have been applied to angiodysplasia with some success. The Nd-YAG laser is usually set at 60–80 W at a 1-cm treatment distance, and with a pulse duration of 0.3–0.5 s and low flow CO_2 in the colon. Long-term follow-up of 107 patients with angiodysplasia treated with Nd-YAG laser revealed haemostasis

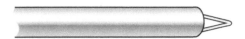

Figure 18.8. Snare with the tip just protruding to be used for cauterizing bleeding points.

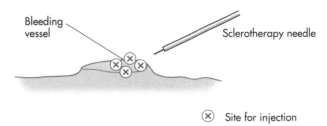

Figure 18.7. Sites for adrenaline injection to control post-polypectomy bleeding.

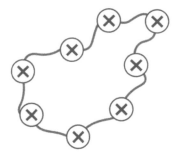

Figure 18.9. Treatment points for large angiodysplasia, before treating the centre of the lesion.

in 78% of patients and a recurrent bleeding rate of 34% [33]. However, there are reports of caecal perforations, suggesting caution using this technique in the right hemi-colon.

Argon plasma coagulation (APC)

This technique uses monopolar electrocoagulation, applying high-frequency electrical current to tissue by means of ionized argon gas, and allowing contact-free coagulation (see Chapter 4 and 17). The constant flow of argon gas ensures that blood is blown away, which permits a better view of the treatment area. The plasma beam that is generated automatically directs itself (independent of the argon flow direction) to the area of tissue with the lowest electrical resistance. This prevents excessive treatment to a particular area as the resistance will rise as the tissue desiccates. APC can be applied to angiodysplasia, residual tissue post-polypectomy and to exophytic tumours. It causes less tissue damage than the techniques described above, with a coagulation depth of approximately 2–3 mm reducing the risk of perforation [34].

To date, there have been no direct comparisons of these therapeutic modalities [35]. The chosen therapeutic approach is, therefore, dependent on availability and local expertise.

Polypectomy

The approach to colonic polypectomy depends on the size and configuration of the polyp (see Chapter 16). Small polyps are usually removed using hot biopsy forceps. The head of the polyp is grasped and tented away from the mucosa. Current is applied until there is a 1- to 2-mm zone of white thermal injury around the polyp base. The specimen is then retrieved and should be suitable for interpretation by the histopathologist.

An alternative approach is to snare the polyp and 'cheese-wire' it, without electrical current. This approach is safe due to the small nutrient blood vessels, which leads to minimal bleeding after the polypectomy.

The chance of bleeding after polypectomy is increased in pedunculated polyps with a large stalk. These should either have their stalks injected before polypectomy with 1 : 10 000 adrenaline, using a sclerotherapy needle, or alternatively have an endo-loop (Olympus Optical Co., Hamburg, Germany) placed around the base of the stalk, below the proposed point of resection [36].

Pedunculated polyps are removed by snare resection, the snare being ideally placed about the mid-portion of the stalk (Fig. 18.10). If the polyp is so large that the snare cannot be placed satisfactorily, it can be removed piecemeal until the residuum is small enough to allow snare placement.

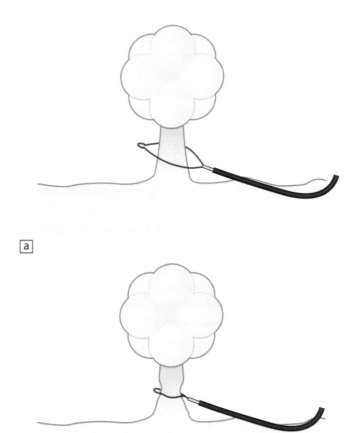

Figure 18.10. Polypectomy of a pedunculated polyp: (a) Snare placed over the polyp; (b) snare closed with sheath advanced to the mid-portion of the stalk.

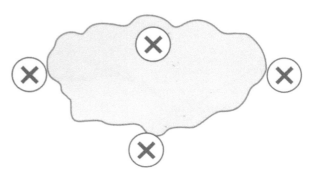

Figure 18.11. Injection sites before the resection of a sessile polyp.

Sessile polyps can also be removed using snare resection. The polyp is elevated from the submucosa by the injection of 2–10 ml of saline, via a sclerotherapy needle, in several aliquots to try to increase the distance of the polyp from the serosa (Fig. 18.11).

Post-polypectomy bleeding

Immediate bleeding after polypectomy occurs in approximately 1% of cases [37] and can be controlled by the endoscopist. The most immediate method is placement of the snare around the pedicle and holding it under pressure for about 5 min until the bleeding stops. If bleeding recurs, a further 5 min of strangulation should result in haemostasis. Alternatives include the injection of 1 : 10 000 adrenaline, cautery using a snare tip or hot biopsy forceps, or the placement of an endo-loop.

Delayed bleeding occurs post-polypectomy in about 2% of cases [36], usually about 1 week after the procedure. However, this complication may occur between 6 h and 14 days after polypectomy. The continued passage of bloody stools indicates continued bleeding and demands immediate colonoscopy [38]. Once the site of bleeding has been identified, bleeding can generally be controlled using adrenaline injection, cautery using the devices described above, or laser. If the bleeding has apparently slowed it suggests that bleeding has ceased, and so colonoscopy should not be attempted. These patients will usually not rebleed.

Angiographic therapy

Selective catheterization of a vessel confirmed as the source of bleeding allows the application of specific therapy aimed at arresting haemorrhage. The available options include the infusion of a vasoconstrictor such as vasopressin, or selective embolization.

Vasopressin is infused at 0.2–0.4 U/min, the response being seen within 20–30 min. A continuous infusion will arrest haemorrhage in approximately 70% of cases [16], but rebleeding rates when the infusion has stopped have been as high as 50%. Attempts at reducing rebleeding have included a gradual tapering of the vasopressin over 12 hours. The catheter can be left *in situ* during this period and the infusion restarted should it be necessary. Other complications include the systemic vasoconstrictor effects of vasopressin which include peripheral vascular ischaemia, myocardial ischaemia and colonic infarction.

Colonic infarction has been reported more commonly (approximately 15%) with embolization due to the relatively sparse vascularity and poorer collateral pathways [16]. The process is, therefore, more technically demanding in that subselective catheterization is necessary. There is, however, no evidence of how distal the embolization should be to stop the bleeding and yet maintain tissue viability. The choice of agent for embolization is unclear, with some authors advocating a temporary agent such as gelatin sponge (Gelfoam), while others have used a permanently occlusive agent such as polyvinyl alcohol particles. Other agents such as collagen suspensions may cause distal thrombosis, while Gelfoam powder and absolute alcohol should be avoided as they may cause mucosal injury and necrosis. 'Blind' or prophylactic embolization in a patient with normal angiography is not recommended.

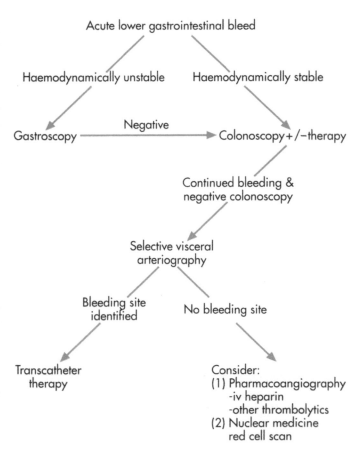

If bleeding continues and bleeding source identified, but intervention has failed then proceed to surgery, or bleeding source unknown, consider surgery with intraoperative enteroscopy

Figure 18.12. Algorithm for the management of acute lower gastrointestinal bleeding.

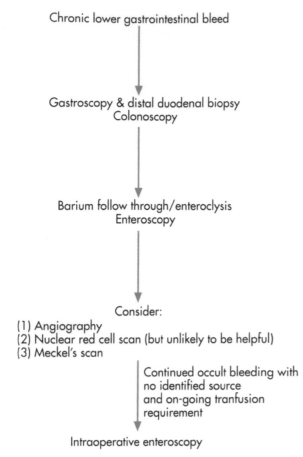

Chronic lower gastrointestinal bleed

↓

Gastroscopy & distal duodenal biopsy
Colonoscopy

↓

Barium follow through/enteroclysis
Enteroscopy

↓

Consider:
(1) Angiography
(2) Nuclear red cell scan (but unlikely to be helpful)
(3) Meckel's scan

Continued occult bleeding with
no identified source
and on-going tranfusion
requirement

↓

Intraoperative enteroscopy

Figure 18.13. Algorithm for the management of chronic lower gastrointestinal bleeding.

Surgical intervention

Emergency colectomy has previously been advocated in patients who continue to bleed but in whom a bleeding site cannot be identified. If this procedure is undertaken it carries a high complication rate, a mortality of 30–50% [13,39], and the possibility remains that the bleeding was from a more proximal source. Given these reservations and the fact that the majority of patients with lower gastrointestinal haemorrhage will stop spontaneously, surgery should be reserved for those with persisting haemodynamic disturbance and continued transfusion requirements.

Surgical intervention is also appropriate following the identification of a bleeding site and the failure to arrest bleeding with endoscopic and/or radiological intervention. Operative mortality rates may fall to 20–30% if the bleeding point has been localized angiographically [40], and become less than 10% if a segmental resection is possible.

Medical therapy

The use of hormonal (oestrogen–progesterone) treatment to treat diffuse angiodysplasia has some advocates. The available data are, however, unclear and suggest that hormonal therapy is most effective in patients with renal failure and Osler–Weber–Rendu syndrome. In contrast, its use in an unselected cohort of 64 patients with small bowel angiodysplasia resulted in no improvement in transfusion requirements and no cessation of bleeding [41].

CONCLUSIONS

Algorithms for the management of overt and occult lower gastrointestinal bleeding are shown in Figures 18.12 and 18.13. The application of available techniques is dependent on local expertise and facilities, but should allow haemostasis to be achieved in the majority of patients. Surgery should only be required for a minority.

In those with continued occult gastrointestinal haemorrhage it may not be possible to define a source of blood loss. These patients can sometimes be managed by continued iron supplementation, but it may be necessary to resort to surgical intervention and intraoperative enteroscopy.

REFERENCES

1. Greenburg AG, Saik RP, Bell RH *et al.* Changing patterns of gastrointestinal bleeding. *Arch Surg* 1985; 120: 341–344.

2. Jensen DM, Machicado GA. Diagnosis and treatment of severe hematochezia. The role of urgent colonoscopy after purge. *Gastroenterology* 1988; 95: 1569–1574.

3. Schrock TR. Colonoscopic diagnosis and treatment of lower gastrointestinal bleeding. *Surg Clin North Am* 1989; 69: 1309–1325.

4. Reinus JF, Brandt LJ. Upper and lower gastrointestinal bleeding in the elderly. *Gastroenterol Clin North Am* 1990; 19: 293–318.

5. Waye JD. Diagnosis and treatment of lower gastrointestinal bleeding. In: Tytgat GNJ, van Blankenstein M (eds), *Current Topics in Gastroenterology and Hepatology.* Thieme Medical Publishers, New York, 1990.

6. Snook JA, Holdstock GE, Bamforth J. Value of a simple biochemical ratio in distinguishing upper and lower sites of gastrointestinal haemorrhage. *Lancet* 1986; i: 1064–1065.

7. Wright HK. Massive colonic haemorrhage. *Surg Clin North Am* 1980; 60: 1297–1304.

8. McGuire HH Jr, Haynes BW Jr. Massive haemorrhage from diverticulosis of the colon: guidelines for therapy based on bleeding patterns observed in fifty cases. *Ann Surg* 1972; 175: 847–855.

9. Wang CY, Won CW, Shieh MJ. Aggressive colonoscopic approaches to lower intestinal bleeding. *Gastroenterol Jpn* 1991; 26(Suppl. 3): 125–128.

10. Church JM. Analysis of the colonoscopic findings in patients with rectal bleeding according to the pattern of their presenting symptoms. *Dis Colon Rectum* 1991; 34: 391–395.

11. Davis GR, Santa Ana CA, Morawski SG *et al*. Development of a lavage solution associated with minimal water and electrolyte absorption and secretion. *Gastroenterology* 1980; 78: 991–995.

12. Colacchio TA, Forde KA, Patsos TJ *et al*. Impact of modern diagnostic methods on the management of active rectal bleeding. Ten year experience. *Am J Surg* 1982; 143: 607–610.

13. Moncure AC, Tomkins RG, Athanasoulis CA *et al*. Occult gastrointestinal bleeding: newer techniques and diagnosis and therapy. *Adv Surg* 1989; 22: 141–177.

14. Uden P, Jiborn H, Jonsson K. Influence of selective mesenteric arteriography on the outcome of emergency surgery for massive lower gastrointestinal haemorrhage: a 15 year experience. *Dis Colon Rectum* 1986; 29: 561–566.

15. Koval G, Benner KG, Rosch J *et al*. Aggressive angiographic diagnosis in acute lower gastrointestinal haemorrhage. *Dig Dis Sci* 1987; 32: 248–253.

16. Shapiro MJ. The role of the radiologist in the management of gastrointestinal bleeding. *Gastroenterol Clin North Am* 1994; 23: 123–181.

17. Smith RK, Arterburn G. Detection and localization of gastrointestinal bleeding using 99mTc-pyrophosphate *in vivo* labeled red blood cells. *Clin Nucl Med* 1980; 5: 55–60.

18. Voeller GR, Bunch G, Britt LG. Use of technetium-labelled red blood cell scintigraphy in the detection and management of gastrointestinal haemorrhage. *Surgery* 1991; 110: 799–804.

19. Heymann TD, Chopra K, Nunn E *et al*. Bowel preparation at home: prospective study of adverse effects in elderly people. *Br Med J* 1996; 313: 727–728.

20. Cohen SM, Wexner SD, Binderow SR *et al*. Prospective, randomized, endoscopic-blinded trial comparing precolonoscopy bowel cleansing methods. *Dis Colon Rectum* 1994; 37: 689–696.

21. Rabe FE, Becker GJ, Besozzi MJ *et al*. Efficacy study of the small bowel examination. *Radiology* 1981; 140: 47–50.

22. Rex DK, Lappas JC, Maglinte DD *et al*. Enteroclysis in the evaluation of suspected small intestinal bleeding. *Gastroenterology* 1989; 97: 58–60.

23. Browder W, Cerise EJ, Litwin MS. Impact of emergency angiography in massive lower gastrointestinal bleeding. *Ann Surg* 1986; 204: 530–536.

24. Brown CK, Olskhaker JS. Meckel's diverticulum. *Am J Emerg Med* 1988; 6: 157–164.

25. Irgau I, Reilly PM, Abdel-Misih RZ. Paired temporary loop ileostomies in the localization of small bowel haemorrhage of obscure origin. *Am Surg* 1995; 61: 1099–1101.

26. Lewis BS. Small intestinal bleeding. *Gastroenterol Clin North Am* 1994; 23: 67–91.

27. Irvine EJ, O'Connor J, Frost RA *et al*. Prospective comparison of double contrast barium enema plus flexible sigmoidoscopy v colonoscopy in rectal bleeding: barium enema v colonoscopy in rectal bleeding. *Gut* 1988; 29: 1188–1193.

28. Berner JS, Mauer K, Lewis BS. Push and sonde enteroscopy for the diagnosis of obscure gastrointestinal bleeding. *Am J Gastroenterol* 1994; 89: 2139–2142.

29. Yang R, Laine L. Mucosal stripping: a complication of push enteroscopy. *Gastrointest Endosc* 1995; 41: 156–158.

30. Lewis BS, Waye JD. Total small bowel enteroscopy. *Gastrointest Endosc* 1987; 33: 435–438.

31. Lewis B, Waye J. Chronic gastrointestinal bleeding of obscure origin: role of small bowel enteroscopy. *Gastroenterology* 1988; 94: 1117–1120.

32. Lewis BS, Wenger JS, Waye JD. Small bowel enteroscopy and intraoperative enteroscopy for obscure gastrointestinal bleeding. *Am J Gastroenterol* 1991; 86: 171–174.

33. Mathus-Vliegen EMH. Laser treatment of intestinal vascular abnormalities. *Int J Colorec Dis* 1989; 4: 20–25.

34. Grund KE. Argon plasma coagulation (APC): Ballyhoo or breakthrough? *Endoscopy* 1997; 29: 196–198.

35. Sharma R, Gorbien MJ. Angiodysplasia and lower gastrointestinal tract bleeding in elderly patients. *Arch Intern Med* 1995; 155: 807–812.

36. Rey J-F, Marek TA. Endo-loop in the prevention of the post-polypectomy bleeding: preliminary results. *Gastrointest Endosc* 1997; 46: 387–389.

37. Waye JD, Lewis BS, Yessayan S. Colonoscopy, a prospective report of complications. *J Clin Gastroenterol* 1992; 15: 347–351.

38. Nivatvongs S. Complications in colonoscopic polypectomy: lessons to learn from an experience with 1576 polyps. *Am Surg* 1988; 54: 61–63.

39. Wagner HE, Stain SC, Gilg M *et al.* Systematic assessment of massive bleeding of the lower part of the gastrointestinal tract. *Surg Gynecol Obstet* 1992; 175: 445–449.

40. Sabiston DCJ. *Textbook of Surgery: The Biological Basis of Modern Surgical Practice.* 14th Edition. New York: W.B. Saunders, New York, 1991.

41. Lewis BS, Salomon P, Rivera-MacMurray S *et al.* Does hormonal therapy have any benefit for bleeding angiodysplasia? *J Clin Gastroenterol* 1992; 15: 99–103.

Index

aspiration pneumonia after endoscopy 21
aspirin and polypectomy 242
Atkinson tube *32*
Atlanta classification of acute pancreatitis 182

bacteraemia after endoscopy 21
balloon catheters for stone removal 133–4
balloon dilatation 16–17, 18–19
   see also under sphincter of Oddi
   for achalasia 14–15, 20
   for biliary obstruction 160
   of colonic strictures 226, 227
   in ERCP 149
   over-the wire 18, *28*
   through-the-scope 18–19, *28*
balloon tamponade for bleeding varices 86, 88, 90
band ligation for bleeding varices 84–5, *87*, 88, 90, 91, 92
barium studies
   for benign colonic obstruction 220–1
   for colorectal cancer 235
   for lower gastrointestinal bleeding 266–7
   of lower gastrointestinal bleeding 264
   of malignant oesophageal obstruction 26–7
   for dysphagia 11–12
   vs endoscopy 12
Barrett's oesophagus
   endoscopic appearance 13
   incidence 54, 57
   screening 56–9, 64
basket for stone removal 132–3
   impaction 138, 139–40
benign colonic obstruction 219
benzodiazepines before endoscopy 3–4
benzporphyrin derivative 47
beta-blockade for variceal re-bleeding prevention 90–1
BICAP for GI bleeding 77, 271
bile duct
   cancer markers 167
   stones 121–42
      acute pancreatitis 182, 184, 185, 190–3
      clearance for bile duct stones 126
      complications 138–40
      controversial issues 140–1
      CT 169
      diagnosis 122–5
      difficult problems with 127–8
      evidence-based management 125–7
      management in children 137
      mimicking biliary stricture *144*

practical aspects 128–35
prevalence with age *122*
recurrent 140
retrieval 132–5
special cases 135–7
symptoms 122
ultrasound 168
bile reflux in acute pancreatitis 183
biliary atresia 145
biliary obstruction and leaks 143–64
   assessment 146
   choice of treatment 161–2
   in chronic pancreatitis 214
   classification 145–6
   diagnosis 145–6
   investigation 146–8
   management and evidence 148–9
   practical aspects 158–61
   presentation 144–5
   prevention of complications 162
   special cases 150–7
biliary stricture
   malignant 165–80
      causes 166
      controversial issues 176–7
      cytology and histology 172–4
      diagnosis 167–70
      management, endoscopic vs percutaneous 170
      presentation 166
   traumatic 150, *151*
Billroth anastomosis, previous, and bile duct stones 128, 135–6
Billroth gastrectomy *62*
   causing gastric malignancy 62–3
biopsy for biliary obstruction 148
Bismuth classification of hilar strictures *167*
bleeding *see* haemorrhage
blood, faecal occult 234, 235
blood tests
   acute pancreatitis 183–4
   bile duct stones 123
   biliary obstruction 146
   biliary tree malignant strictures 167
   chronic pancreatitis 199
   dysphagia 11
   GI bleeding 70
   malignant oesophageal obstruction 27
blood transfusion
   for bleeding oesophageal varices 82
   for GI bleeding 70

upper GI malignancy 45
vs injection therapy 15
dilators 14–15, 16–17
see also specific types
size limitation 19
diode lasers for upper GI malignancy 44–5
dissolution therapy for bile duct stones 127–8
diverticula and bile duct stones 128
diverticular disease 224–5
Dormia basket for stone removal 132, *133*
duodenum
diverticula 156
malignancy risk 233–4
pseudocysts 190
stenosis and ERCP 171
ulcer
see also peptic ulcer
bile duct obstruction and 157
causing GI bleeding 69, 77
dye-spray technique for colonic adenomas 236, *237*
dyes for scanning for biliary obstruction 147
dysphagia 96–7
causes 8
clinical syndromes 9–10
investigations 26–7
malignant
diagnosis 10, 26–7
investigations 26–7
relief 28
symptoms 26
symptoms 8–9
upper GI malignancy 42
diagnosis 42–3

Echinococcus granulosis causing biliary obstruction 157
echoendoscopy *30*
Eder–Puestow dilator *18*
elderly patients, preparation for endoscopy 2, 3
electohydraulic fragmentation for bile duct stones 127
electrocoagulation
debulking of colorectal tumours 254, 258, 260
GI bleeding 76
electrofulguration for debulking of colorectal tumours 254, 258
electrolyte replacement in benign colonic obstruction 221
electrosurgical units for sphincterotomy 129–30
Endocoil stent *32*
endo-loops 245, 272
endometriosis causing colorectal stricture 226
endoprostheses

see also stents/stenting
for bile duct stones 128
insertion, complications 5
for malignant oesophageal obstruction 33–4
for malignant upper GI malignancy 50
endoscope, mother and baby 127
endoscopic drainage of pseudocysts 189–90, 201
endoscopic needle, wide-bore *203*
endoscopic retrograde cholangiography for bile duct stones 125
endoscopic retrograde cholangiopancreatography (ERCP)
acute pancreatitis 182, 188–9
bile duct stones 123, 126, 140
biliary obstruction 148–9, 158–9, 162
chronic pancreatitis 200
for diagnosis, complications in 5
technique in biliary tree malignant strictures 171–6
vs percutaneous route for biliary tree malignant strictures 170
endoscopic sphincterotomy
acute pancreatitis 189
bile duct stones 125–6
endoscopic therapy for malignant oesophageal obstruction 30–5
endoscopic ultrasound (EUS)
acute pancreatitis 185
benign oesophageal strictures 12, 13–14
bile duct stones 124–5
biliary obstruction 148
chronic pancreatitis 199
malignant oesophageal obstruction 27, *29*
miniprobes 201
pancreatic pseudocyst drainage 189
endoscopy (general)
see also specific techniques
complications 4–6
diagnosis of benign colonic obstruction 221
general procedures 3–6
nursing and endoscopy assistants 4
preoperative procedures 2–3
recovery and postoperative care 4
use for feeding tube placement 100, 101, 101–6
enemas
before endoscopy 3
benign colonic obstruction 220
enteral nutrition 95–120
acute pancreatitis 187
advantages and disadvantages 99
choice of tube 106
complications 106
contraindications 99
controversial issues 117–19

oesophageal obstruction, malignant (*cont.*)
    staging 28–30
    type of therapy choices 30
oesophageal perforation
    during dilatation 45
    during endoscopy 21
    during stenting 38–9
oesophageal tear causing GI bleeding 69
oesophageal transection for variceal bleeding 90
oesophageal varices
    causing GI bleeding 69, 70
    and enteral feeding 101
oesophagitis
    causing GI bleeding 69, 70
    ulcerating *13*
oesophagojejunostomy feeding 100
oesophagopharyngeal pathology causing dyphagia 96, 97
oesophagus
    Barrett's 54
    bird's beak *10*
    corkscrew *10*
oestrogen-progesterone therapy of lower gastrointestinal
    bleeding 274
Ogilivie's syndrome 224
omeprazole therapy for GI bleeding 71
opiates before endoscopy 3–4
oral cancer and enteral feeding 101
oropharyngeal cancer causing dysphagia 97
oropharyngeal conversion to nasopharyngeal tube 103,
    104
overtube 84, *85*
oxygen therapy
    acute pancreatitis 186
    prior to bile duct stone endoscopy 129

p53 marker
    biliary obstruction 146, 148, 155
    biliary tree malignant strictures 173–4
pain
    in acute pancreatitis 183
    in benign colonic obstruction 218
    in biliary obstruction 144
    in biliary tree malignant strictures 170
    in chronic pancreatitis 198, 199, 200
    following polypectomy 249
    in upper GI malignancy 42
    relief for malignant oesophageal obstruction 28
painting technique for upper GI malignancy 45–6
palliation of colorectal cancer 251–61

pancreas
    abscess 186, 188
    carcinoma, cytology 148
        differentiation 166, 200
        surgery 170
        survival curve *172*
    drainage tubes 208
    enzyme supplementation 200–1
    function tests 199
    necrosis 187–8
    pseudocysts 186, 188
        deep 205
        management 201–5
        recurrence 201, 205
    sphincterotomy 208, *210*
        small biliary 208
        for sphincter of Oddi dysfunction 214
    ultrasound 168
pancreas divisum 198, 212–13
pancreatic duct
    damage from stents 211, *212*
    leaks and disruptions 205–8
    stones 208, *210–11*
    strictures 209–11, *212*
pancreatitis
    acute 181–95
        aetiology 182–3
        causes 172–82
        classification 182
        controversial issues and decision making 190–3
        diagnosis 183–6
        incidence 182
        management and evidence 186–8
        management techniques 188–90
        predicting severe attacks 185–6
        presentation 183
        prevention of further attacks 193
        role of endoscopic biliary drainage in acute pancreatitis
            190–3
        role of surgical biliary drainage in acute pancreatitis 190
    chronic 157, *158*, 197–215
        aetiology and pathogenesis 198
        biliary obstruction 214
        classification 200
        cytology 148
        diagnosis 199–200
        differentiation from malignancy 200
        endoscopy 201
        grades of severity and prognositic factors 200

T - #0570 - 071024 - C304 - 276/216/14 - PB - 9780367455088 - Gloss Lamination